Spiritual and Mental Health C in Globalizing Senegal

Spiritual and Mental Health Crisis in Globalizing Senegal explores the history of mental health in Senegal, and how psychological difficulties were expressed in the terms of spiritualism, magic, witchcraft, spirit possession, and ancestor worship.

Focused on the effervescent and fruitful early post-colonial years at the Fann Hospital, situated at the famed University of Dakar, Cheikh Anta Diop, this book reveals provocative treatment innovations via case studies of individuals struggling for health and healing, and thus operates as a suspension bridge between scholarship on witchcraft and magic on the one side and the history of psychiatry and psychoanalysis on the other.

Through these case studies, this book creates a new route of exchange for healing knowledge for a broad array of West African spiritual troubles, mental illness, magic, soul cannibalism, witchcraft, spirit possession, and psychosis.

Alice Bullard (Ph.D. & ESQ) is a lawyer specializing in human rights, trafficking, personal status, and mediation. Previously, she was a professor of history at Georgia Institute of Technology, U.S.A.

Routledge Research in Health and Healing in Africa and the African Diaspora

Health and healing have been critical in African and African-descended communities across the globe. As a result, this series will publish monographs and edited volumes on aspects of health and healing on the African continent and in the African Diaspora.

We welcome proposals on a variety of topics in particular, public health, global health security, health care delivery, innovation in health, epidemics, women and children's health, masculinity and health, mental health, traditional healing, and community initiatives. We seek publications from a range of disciplines, or that are interdisciplinary in nature, from the social sciences, public and global health, clinical sciences, and the humanities. In addition, we seek research and analyses from area studies that transcend health issues, including African Studies, African American Studies, Caribbean Studies, and Women and Gender Studies and work that is transnational and that may straddle more than one country or region.

Series Editor:
Donna A. Patterson, Delaware State University, USA

Spiritual and Mental Health Crisis in Globalizing Senegal
A History of Transcultural Psychiatry
Alice Bullard

For more information about this series, please visit: www.routledge.com/Routledge-Research-in-Health-and-Healing-in-Africa-and-the-African-Diaspora/book-series/HHAADA

Spiritual and Mental Health Crisis in Globalizing Senegal

A History of Transcultural Psychiatry

Alice Bullard

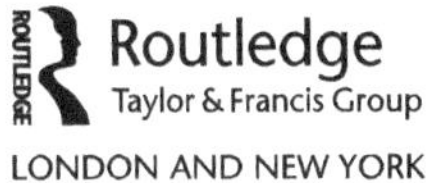

LONDON AND NEW YORK

First published 2022
by Routledge
4 Park Square, Milton Park, Abingdon, Oxon OX14 4RN

and by Routledge
605 Third Avenue, New York, NY 10158

Routledge is an imprint of the Taylor & Francis Group, an informa business

British Library Cataloguing-in-Publication Data
A catalogue record for this book is available from the British Library

Library of Congress Cataloging-in-Publication Data
Names: Bullard, Alice, author.
Title: Spiritual and mental health crisis in globalizing Senegal : a history of transcultural psychiatry / Alice Bullard.
Other titles: Routledge research in health and healing in Africa and the African diaspora
Description: Abingdon, Oxon ; New York : Routledge, 2022. |
Series: Routledge research in health and healing in Africa and the African diaspora | Includes bibliographical references and index.
Identifiers: LCCN 2021057781 | ISBN 9780367631000 (hardback) | ISBN 9780367744267 (paperback) | ISBN 9781003112143 (ebook)
Subjects: LCSH: Psychiatry, Transcultural—Senegal—Case studies. | Mental illness—Treatment—Senegal—Case studies | Mental health—Senegal—History. | Ethnopsychology—Senegal—Case studies. | Traditional medicine—Senegal—Case studies.
Classification: LCC RC455.4.E8 B853 2022 | DDC 362.19689009663—dc23/eng/20220121
LC record available at https://lccn.loc.gov/2021057781

ISBN: 978-0-367-63100-0 (hbk)
ISBN: 978-0-367-74426-7 (pbk)
ISBN: 978-1-003-11214-3 (ebk)

DOI: 10.4324/9781003112143

Typeset in Times New Roman
by Apex CoVantage, LLC

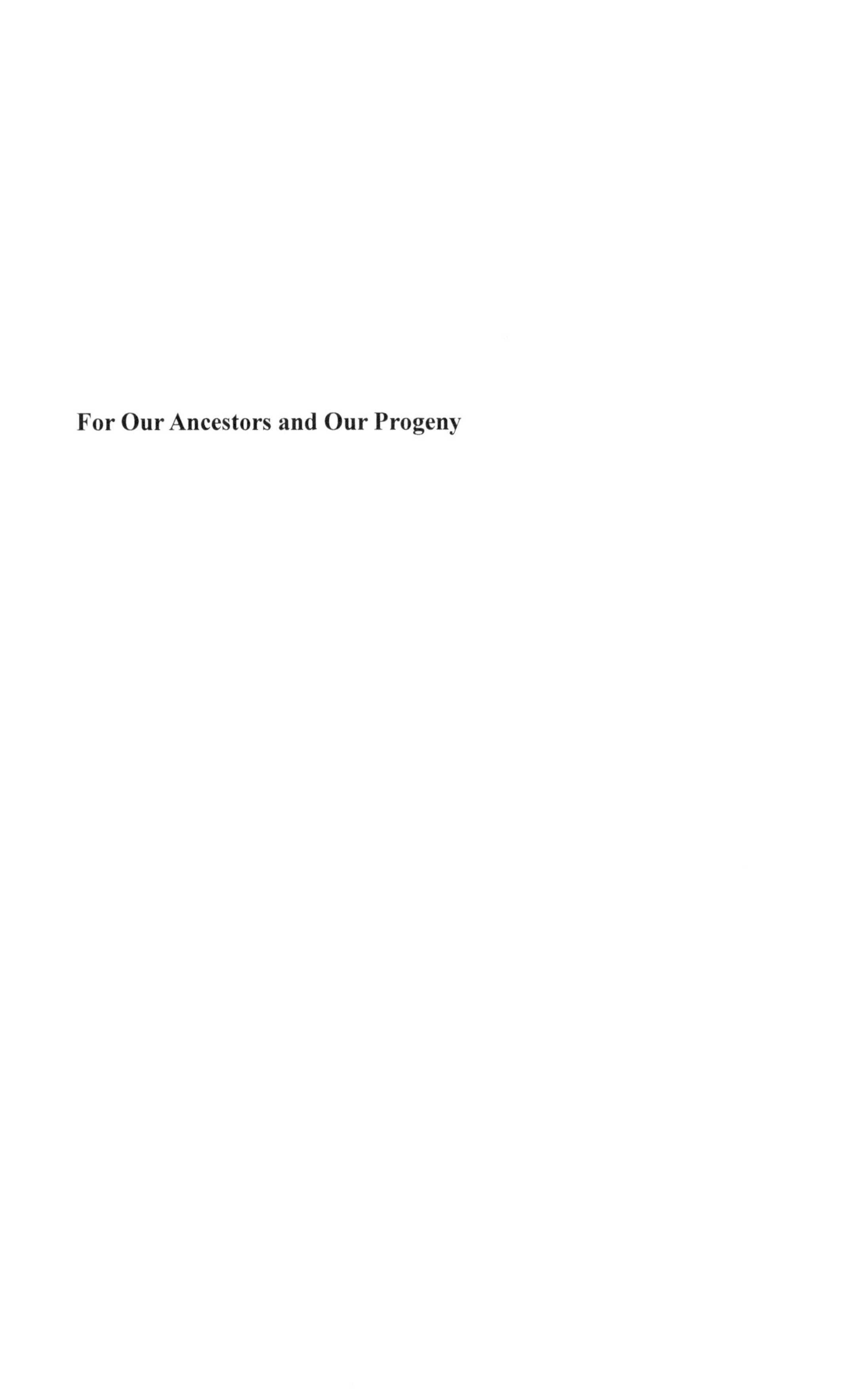

For Our Ancestors and Our Progeny

Contents

Acknowledgments

This book grew throughout many years. Over that time, I have benefited enormously from scholars, clinicians, friends, and colleagues. This is an interdisciplinary and international book; the network in which I have worked is vast and highly differentiated. I am deeply grateful for fellowship support from the National Endowment for the Humanities, the Social Science Research Council, the Camargo Foundation, and the American Council of Learned Societies (ACLS) that enabled the early stages. I owe much to individuals who consented to interviews and who enriched this book, even perhaps unwittingly, through conversations and commentary. Many of these debts are old, but I have not forgotten. Many, many thanks to Marie-Cécile and Edmund Ortigues, Barbara Sobol, Rector of University Cheikh Anta Diop, Ibrahima Thioub, Charles Becker, David Robinson, René Collignon, Mamadou Diouf, Susan Terrio, Matt Matsuda, Panivong Norindr, Frédéric Angleviel, Martin Jay, clinicians at the Fann Hospital, the Director of the national archives of Senegal, Saliou Mbaye, staff at the Institut Fondamental Afrique Noire (IFAN), WARA, Randall Packard and the Johns Hopkins University history of medicine cohort, the editors of *Studies in Gender and Sexuality*, Ellen Corin, Gilles Bibeau, Laurence Kirmayer and the editors of *Transcultural Psychiatry*, Deborah Jenson, Warwick Anderson, Richard Keller, Ranjana Khanna, Hans Pols, Didier Fassin, John D. Cash, Joy Damousi, Christiane Hartnack, Mariano Plotkin, Katie Kilroy-Marac, Mamadou Sikam Sy, Jeanne Koopman, Ellen Foley, Elizabeth Ann McDougall, Carina Johnson, Dan Segal, Peter Redfield, Sybille Nyeck, Katherine Mansfield Cleary, Awa Wade, Joel Bullard, Jonathan Sadowsky, Amber Jacobs, Dagmar Herzog, Omnia El Shakry, Erik Linstrum, Sloan Mahone, Megan Vaughn, Matthew Heaton, Sanjeev Jain, Gary Wilder, Alice Conklin, Ana Antic, Carol Colatrella, Mary Frank Fox, Jonathan Schneer, Kavita Philips, Susan Ross, Leah Rosenberg, Jahnavi Phalkey, Jennifer Cole, Pasquale Pasquino, Molly Vitorte, Martha Willcox, Biram Dah Abeid, Fatimata M'Baye, Abderahmane N'Gaïdé, Mohamed Cheikh Mkhaitir, Nancy Chodorow, Dipesh Chakrabarty, Brahim Bilal Ramdhane, Aminata Moctar, Gregory Nobel, Steve Usselman, the estate of Angelo Hesnard, and Donna Patterson, Chair of History, Political Science, and Philosophy, Director of Africana Studies at Delaware State University, and series editor in the History of Medicine and Africa. This book owes much to these people and more. With good luck, the conversations will continue. My apologies for any weaknesses or omissions.

Introduction

This history knits together knowledge from patients, medical innovators, dedicated clinicians, bureaucrats, philosophers, historians, and anthropologists. In the years of research and learning from which this book is written, I have been repeatedly stunned and thrilled by the dedicated expertise of numerous scholars of diverse specialties. The COVID-19 pandemic forced the cancelation of a final research trip to Senegal, but the sudden flourishing of internet-based seminars brought far-flung scholars into my office. As well, the cancelled trip to Senegal allowed space for more emphasis on contemporary psychotherapeutic literature. Meanwhile, my own previous publications on the history of transcultural psychiatry form a knowledge base for this book (Bullard 2000, 2001, 2002, 2005a, 2005b, 2007, 2008, 2011, 2011–2012, 2015a, 2015b). This earlier work nourishes and enriches the material presented here, but due to lack of space, this book cannot include all the scholarship cited in those essays, nor revisit those historiographical debates. Written for a wide audience, this present book can be approached either as complete in itself, or as a larger project situated with these previous publications.

The Senegalese peoples' beliefs and practices, caught here in the gesture of early post-colonial transcultural psychiatry, form part of a global history and an open civilization (Diagne 2019) of experiences shared across the human species, including magic, denial, dissociation, mythic space, witchcraft, soul theft, possession by ancestral spirits, spiritual healing, plants inhabited by spirits, and more. This history of transcultural psychiatry relates the healing legends, beliefs, and practices reflected largely in the printed case studies, *Psychopathologie Africaine*, in its first ten years of publication, 1965–1975. It carries forward from previous scholarship such as, for example, l'Association des Chercheurs sénégalaise (D'Almeida *et al.* 1997), René Collignon (1978, 2000), Didier Fassin (1992, 2003), Ellen Foley (2010), and Katie Kilroy-Marac (2019). Patients' experiences at Fann Hospital in the 1960s and those who sought to heal them – whether traditional healers, *marabouts*, or biomedical personnel – provide the focus. *Psychopathologie Africaine*, the Fann Hospital's journal, published a vast abundance of rich and compelling documentation, of which only a highly select portion could be included in this volume. The ensuing chapters present cases, diagnoses, and treatments, within the incongruence of the post-colonial transcultural moment.

DOI: 10.4324/9781003112143-1

We grapple with the enigmas of extreme fears and persecutions, magical and mystical moments, and biomedical clinical work within a metaphysical culture.

This book plunges readers into a world of metaphysics and intuition, by which, in some version, all of humanity lives. The great Irish poet and collector of folktales, W.B. Yeats, wrote, "[E]very one is a visionary if you scratch him deep enough. But the Celt is a visionary without scratching" (Yeats 1986 [1892], p. iv). The same might be said of the Senegalese. Largely a culture of peasants, herders, and fisher folk, the diverse peoples of Senegal inhabit a world deeply comparable to the Celts in terms of reliance on spiritual knowledge and metaphysical forces to guide, protect, make fecund, heal, and otherwise succor the people as they made their lives as best they could within frequently harsh and demanding circumstances. The Senegalese, like the Celts, are saints, scholars, poets, and, not infrequently, "touched by the fairies." Although in Senegal, one is touched by *djinn* or *seytané*, or inhabited by *rab*, not fairies. This Celtic comparison is meant as one example of numerous possible comparisons to specific versions of magical and folkloric knowledge. All of humanity, it is clearly documented by careful scholarship, is susceptible to magic and witchcraft (Behringer 2004, and *e.g.* Hoff and Yeates 2000; Vélez 2015).

Mental illness troubles a significant portion of human individuals, along with their families, friends, and broader communities. No matter how resolutely one might wish to ignore mental illness or argue for its essential non-existence (thus shunting the suffering to a problem of politics or religion), individuals continue to suffer and to seek healing. By and large, modern biomedicine has struggled valiantly, but without definitive success, against mental illness. The many excellent critical histories of psychiatry reveal dire situations. Psychiatric and mental health services are frequently difficult to access and plagued with overuse of partially effective drugs, inhumane restraints, and (in the U.S.A. in particular) incarceration rather than treatment (Roth 2018). Struggles with other-worldly spirits, magic, enchantment, and vampirism or devouring by witches, prompt individuals and families to seek relief via divination, trance, potions, fumigation, or similar spiritualist methods, or via biomedical mental health treatments. Thus the case studies presented here are highly individual and also at the same time, through this individuality, both culturally rooted and an embodiment of enduring species-wide phenomena.

Irrational beliefs and fears cause real problems in people's lives and in broader societies. They can lead one astray or kill one's children. Previously, I have discussed how investigating these powerful forces of unreason mandates emotional distancing (Bullard 2011). Getting too close can be dangerous. The lives of Henri Collomb's designated successors at Fann, both of them overtaken by illness as they worked in the hospital, sound a cautionary note against trespass into the spirit realm. Once the gates of unreason are opened, unexpected forces operate more freely. Physiological regulation and dysregulation can be contagious. Countervailing healing rituals balance the dangers posed by malign and terrorizing forces. These battles are intimate and daily; they are connected with life-cycles, family, community, nation, and, indeed, with the species as a whole. Beneficial spiritual force is exemplified, for example, in Cheikh Anta Babou's *The Muridiyya on the Move Islam, Migration, and Place Making* (2021), in which he writes of *baraka*, or God-given grace. Ahmadou Bamba, the founder of the Murid brotherhood, had such strong *baraka* that it continues to stream forth from his grave many decades after his death. Millions of pilgrims seek spiritual healing and power from this legacy of Bamba's *baraka*. In contrast, an American psychotherapist recently wrote how a young man performed the spiritual beliefs his parents taught him in order that they would love him. The young man experienced vivid hallucinations of the devil. The therapist interpreted the evil presence as illicit desire or disowned anger on the part of his patient. Unable to express himself directly, for fear of losing his parents' love, he instead hallucinated an evil spirit. The therapist categorically remarked that this cost the young man his sanity (Frederickson 2021, p. XII).

Affective neuroscience is the lens through which this book takes historical perspective on the case studies from Fann Hospital (Porges 2011, 2017). The case studies reveal a magico-spiritualist consciousness broadly comparable across cultures to folkloric tales of fairies, magic, and witches. The human species shares this propensity to narrativize mysterious, visceral, hopes and fears, and to solidify such narratives into belief systems. Affective neuroscience teaches us to place this narrativizing of the visceral, and consequent metaphysical belief systems, within the perspective of evolved higher consciousness that remains intimately dependent upon ancient reptilian autonomic nerves and lower brain structures. On a planet that is five billion years old, our species is young and seemingly unprecedented, both in its intelligence and its destructive capacities. Despite the power of humanity's cerebral intellect, visceral forces of unreason continually re-emerge in each individual as well as in human collectives. Culture, history, and life experiences can mold physiology, but the powerful autonomic neural system reasserts itself nonetheless time and again.

Deep Time/Deep History and Polyvagal Theory

The neural, physiological, and narrative mechanisms of denial, projection, and magic exist in all humans. Affective neuroscience has advanced our understanding, so that we can appreciate our human species' universals and polyvagal truths that are reflected in the richly detailed Fann Hospital case studies of the 1960s and 1970s. Stephen Porges' *The Polyvagal Theory* (2011) helps us to see with new eyes the perennial physiological truths carried in the magical, spirit-and-witch-populated folkloric worldview. Modernity theory to the contrary, that "unreasonable" dimension of our humanity, will not disappear. Subject to discussion, cultivation, and more or less effective management via folkloric healing, mysticism, and various rites and practices including pharmaceuticals and psychotherapy, the visceral stuff of life endures, reasserts itself, and makes continued claims on each of our lives. How could it be otherwise? We live only in and through our bodies, themselves products of billions of years of evolving terrestrial life.

The enormous expanse of cosmic origins and evolution is called Deep Time or Deep History. As discussed in my first book, *Exile to Paradise*, the discovery of Deep Time ripped the conventional historical fabric that was woven from Biblical narratives of creation (Bullard 2000, pp. 20–23). Human history of a few thousand years suddenly expanded into a past of seemingly unfathomable recesses (Swimme and Berry 1992). Thus, Deep Time featured as a chasm that haunted and terrified nineteenth-century writers. Some of them went so far as to describe the indigenous Kanak of New Caledonia as avatars from that unknowable abyss of Deep Time (Bullard 2000, pp. 50–53). No doubt, there has been a disturbing, frightening dimension to human history conceived outside the comforting frame of divine creation.

This present book, however, makes an entirely different inference from Deep Time. Within the nearly unfathomable expanse of 13 billion years of cosmic evolution, there is a close family relationship of human communities to each other, despite their apparent differences. Scratch the surface of culture or physiognomy, and we are all one species with an overriding amount of shared qualities. Indeed, Deep Time also makes our cousins in evolved life, other animals, seem closer to us and more familiar. Human physiology – which directly conditions consciousness and narrative meanings of life – is shared across our species, even if specific habits, environments, and experiences can condition (idiosyncratically or systematically) physiology. The Deep Time perspective reveals global kinship that is much closer than divisive politics likes us to recognize.

The 1960s case studies postulated an opposition between rational biomedicine and irrational mysticism, and between the modern and the traditional. In light of the neuroaffective polyvagal perspective, such oppositions do not compel our understanding nor our historical narrative (Porges 2011, 2017). Indeed, the narrative informed by affective neuroscience's polyvagal theory (PVT) diminishes the distance between cultures and between supposed human historical epochs. Our present history of globalization is miniscule compared to the vast millennium of evolution that produced our brain stem, our amygdala, our hippocampus, and finally, our cerebellum. The expanse of evolutionary time is completely incommensurable with that of conventional histories of human civilization and globalization. For example, if we take the span of globalizing processes to be 500 years, and consider that 500 years in terms of the six million years during which our species to evolved, that span of 500 years of globalization could happen 12,000 separate times. Moreover, the evolution of life on earth is a product of billions of years. The treasures and complexities of our evolved life, and the unifying power of our species' evolutionary history, are routinely underestimated.

The perennial reappearance of unreason conditioned the context in which this book was finalized: the pandemic of 2020–21 and the bloody insurrection in Washington DC of January 6, 2021. The former president of the United States has made a "vast witch hunt" part of common parlance and widespread belief (Cooney 2017). In those events, driven partly by the QAnon online conspiracy, we are confronted yet again with indisputable proof that broad swathes of humanity can be enthralled by unreason. Contemporary social media, itself dependent on highly refined science, can boost hysteria and delusional thinking, even as science produces the COVID-19 vaccines at record pace. These twin forces of reason and unreason will continue to co-mingle and drive our common history, with no expectation that unreason will relinquish its force. Affective neuroscience provides a framework through which this unreason can be classified as a species-specific legacy of the deep evolutionary history of *homo sapiens*. The PVT demonstrates how neuroception gives rise to a physiological state through which individual consciousness interacts with the world (Porges 2017). Consciousness then narrates to oneself and to others, creating meaning that is more or less idiosyncratic or shared, aleatoric or enduring. The deep evolutionary inheritance that is our autonomic neural system ensures each individual's continued susceptibility to unreason as well as the susceptibility of communities and humanity as a collective.

Destabilized physiology distorts perception as well as disrupting communicative behaviors; it bars reason-based consciousness and thrusts forward emotion-laden and highly reactive and distorting consciousness. The PVT models chain of causation, so that we can follow reactions that travel throughout the body and mind. While the physiological reactions are extremely fast, with adequate training, our brains can recognize what is happening and reason with itself and with the body. This process is not easy and requires significant skill, self-compassion, and trust. Calm, loving co-regulation restores physiological balance, which in turn restores sociable activities. In this way, unreasonable narratives can be turned around, negative and delusional beliefs can lose their relevance and power, and psychopathology can recede.

The legacy of Deep Time evolution in our psychophysiology drives contemporary therapeutic practice, especially that informed by attachment and trauma theory. The clinical psychologist Janina Fisher writes, "[t]here are no stronger evolutionary instincts than the attachment drive and its polar opposite, the animal defense survival responses" (Fisher 2017, p. 106). Disruptions to perceived safety, especially in early life, can blossom into on-going disturbances in attachment patterns and affective behavior that adversely impact mental health, quality of life, and social relationships and social status. Psychotherapy helps the individual achieve interior, physiological safety in order that she or he can better build a life that entails exterior, social safety. Compassionate care for individual interior safety – the twenty-first-century therapeutic agenda – belongs to a minor historical tradition of nonetheless enormous consequence. Deb Dana, for example, in her transposition of polyvagal theory into psychotherapeutic techniques, refers unabashedly to the "sacred space of therapy" (Dana 2018, p. 116). This therapeutic mission routinely seeks to heal the wounds inflicted by forces that underwrite extreme hierarchy, debilitating inequality, and subjugation in personal and economic relationships (*e.g.* Levine 2005; Peyton 2017; Zucchetto *et al.* 2020; Frederickson 2021). However, the mechanisms revealed by PVT can be used for better or worse, to uplift and enable, or to denigrate and denude. Those who understand the power of neuroception and induced physiological state – whether they reach this knowledge via science, mysticism, or intuition – can become expert wielders of these forces. Domestic and institutional practices, norms, laws, and other activities can rely on autonomic mechanisms in order to subjugate, control, or exploit, just as much as to heal, nurture, and restore.

The Global and Globalization

What is intended in this book by this term "global"? In the first instance, global references the characteristics that are shared on our *terra* among all members of the human species. Thus, this book contributes to a species-wide neurohistory (Smail 2007, 2014). Persistent mechanisms of unreason that tenaciously re-emerge and up-end individual wellness and social relationships pose on-going challenges. Humans, first and foremost, are a species that emerged from billions of years of evolution on earth. Evolution has gifted us with amazing bodies that are intricate and finely tuned entities. Each and every individual body shares common traits – chief among these is individual consciousness lived within its own individual – organism level – set of circumstances and modalities. Part of the inescapable individuality of the human organism and consciousness are the evolved neuro-physiological commonalities. History, politics, culture, sex, caste, clan, race, and socio-economic circumstances condition these species-level commonalities, yet can never erase them.

Governing ourselves – in ways small and large – so as to guard and strengthen physiological equilibrium and mental health remains a primary challenge for our species. This challenge is a sub-part of the larger twenty-first-century challenge to us *homo sapiens*, the prospect of the destruction of global conditions that sustain evolved life (Bullard 2015b). These challenges of the age are distinctly "something new under the sun" (McNeill 2000). Within the history of mental health and psychiatry, there are abundant incidences of psychic suffering in response to modernity and globalization. Recently Porges (2017) pointed to dimensions of the urban environment that are manifestly antagonistic to internal safety. For example, trucks, airplanes, escalators, elevators, all machines of the urban environment, emit noise that registers as danger to human physiology. This observation is not entirely new: George Simmel in 1903 wrote of how urban dwellers develop a stimulus shield to inure themselves to the constant barrage of unpleasant stimuli (Simmel 1976). However, the physiologically dysregulating intensification of urban conditions continues apace. These urban stressors are joined by other diverse stressors such as school, mobility, wealth inequality, climate-induced dislocation, and social media contagions. We are facing a species-defining moment in the twenty-first century as *homo sapiens* increase in unprecedented numbers and the earth biosphere chokes, burns, and founders in discarded plastics and floods. Global governance to retain a life-sustaining world is posed as a direct challenge to our fractious, only partially rational, species (Bullard 2015b). Indeed, this reckoning with humanity's devastation of the life-sustaining qualities of earth is the urgent issue of our epoch. If anthropogenic climate change, plastics, nuclear waste, and other devastations did not focus our attention on the global, COVID-19 definitively threw the switch. The enormous challenge of effective global solutions to global issues is met by armies of experts, politicians, and interest groups. Yet unreason, in so many ways, rules the day, rules our history, rules even how our best rational efforts are allocated. Unreason makes its mark in nearly every interaction (Kappor 2020). Rooted in our physiology and evident in our higher pursuits, this unreason requires acknowledgement and accommodation.

The unprecedented mixing of populations in the twenty-first century is another facet of globalization with implications for mental health – both for suffering individuals and for professionals who serve those individuals. International networks and population flows send masses of people, some of whom become patients or doctors, back and forth across borders. Whereas in the nineteenth or early twentieth century, the mixing of cultures and populations was relatively constrained, in the twenty-first century there is an increasingly globalized culture of mixed populations enmeshed in international consumer and employment markets and social media. As of 2018, more than two million immigrants from sub-Saharan Africa lived in the U.S.A., whereas in 1980, only 150,000 sub-Saharan Africans had immigrated to this country (Echeverria-Estrada and Batalova 2019). Thus, twenty-first-century sub-Saharan migration now outnumbers the historic forcible transportation of Africans to the Americas during the trans-Atlantic slave trade. Projections for on-going immigration foresee increasing percentages of sub-Saharan migration to the U.S.A. In comparison, the population of Senegal is just under 16 million. France has an enormous immigrant population, up to 30% of its population as of 2017, but within that mix of people, only a small number hail from West Africa or, more specifically, from Senegal.

Cultural beliefs and practices of immigrants form more or less insular or syncretic presences (for discussion of the Senegalese Mouride Diaspora see Babou 2021). Large communities of West African immigrants, for example in the United States in Philadelphia, New York, and the Ohio River region of Ohio and Kentucky, or in France, in the suburbs of Paris and in Marseille and Lyon, carry with them the culturally specific forms of suffering and healing from their homelands. Since at least the 1970s, West African healers have practiced in Paris, and over these years healers have gained increased prominence (Kuckzynski 2002).

With populations from around the globe increasingly mixing, mental health practitioners are aware that they must offer culturally sensitive care. Indeed, the World Health Organization has promoted culturally sensitive care and complementary and traditional medicine (CAM) since 1976 (Bullard 2007, pp. 209–210). As Adam Ashforth wrote in the context of his South African friend who was beset by witchcraft,

> The intermingling in cities of people from different civilizations, religions, and cultures has also produced a ferment of spiritual life. Innovation and imagination are the key ingredients today in the struggle against the ailments wrought of malice and spoken of as witchcraft, just as they are in the struggle for salvation.
>
> (Ashforth 2000, p. 249)

To the global physiology of the human species and the increasingly mixed populations in the twenty-first century, along with their culturally specific suffering and healing, we must add the shared traits in traditional and alternative medicines. Faith healing, for example, is a human universal. Mystical and metaphysical beliefs, while they take many specific forms, are universal human tendencies. Folklore across human cultures has the broad comparative components of magic, spirits, and witchcraft. When traditional healing is brought into focus, and the local stories are preserved and re-told to new generations (perhaps now in Paris or Philadelphia rather than in Dakar or Richard Toll), that local culture takes its place among other local cultures of mystical or metaphysical causes of health and illness, recovery, or death. Specificity and endless variation are features of humanity, and within this bounty of variation, there is the underlying global sameness of human physiology.

Folklore and the Global

This book presents local knowledge that can be integrated into a broad comparative knowledge of folk-understanding of mental illness and traditional or folk healing practices. The broad cross-cultural comparisons facilitated by this book are compelling; important dimensions of apparently highly local beliefs and practices are also shared globally. Neither can we consign the metaphysical or mystical properties in legends and folk medicine to the realm of allegedly distinctly premodern thinking. Rather, the old prototypical theory of modernity, first developed by Max Weber around the time of the First World War, is no longer tenable. Weber thought that humanity would emerge from a magico-religious worldview to a perspective based in relentless rationality infused by scientific knowledge (Weber 1917 cited in Stuart Hughes 1958, p. 332). If such a change can be documented, it is among only a small fraction of the world's population. Even the decline of adherence to formal religion does not bring with it a release from magical thinking. Indeed, humans seem highly susceptible to magical thinking, which seems to be ineradicably rooted in our psyches and our physiology (Bullard 2011). When one form of magical thinking dies out, another arises. As we discuss in detail in Chapter 7, the universal mental mechanism of denial sustains magical thinking.

This book promotes the circulation of the local knowledge of diseases and healing documented by Fann practitioners among globalized networks of students, scholars, and practitioners. Engagement with this specific set of ailments and healing techniques, which are instances of species-wide tendencies, enriches our global community. As our world knits into closer connections and greater interchanges between distant places, we grow our common humanity through learning about these specific forms of suffering along with the specific struggles to surmount spirit afflictions. As we learn from the *bouffée délirante* diagnosis in the concluding chapter to this book, psychological resilience in the face of psychosis is an exemplary contribution to our global open civilization.

"*Wo es war soll ich werden*"/"Where *id* was, *ego* should become" (Freud 1964, p. 80). This classic Freudian dictum enjoins us to root conscious action within the realm of unconscious drives. If that is a mantra for healing somatic expressions of trauma and anxiety, it comes with no promise that the *id* thereby will fade into the recesses of time. Our common reptilian ancestry endures in all of us, in the unmyelinated vagal nerve, autonomic fear responses, neuroception and interoception. Personal liberation can be recorded and taught, but each individual must undertake personal reckoning with these ancient neural pathways. Each individual seeks attachment and is susceptible to bonds – loving or dangerous. Each individual is susceptible to strong or even violent emotions, called into play within social settings with more or less success. Every individual, every day, interacts with these ancient autonomic neural pathways and the impulse to narrativize their workings and ascribe their power to natural or metaphysical causes.

Unreason and Open Civilization

Souleymane Bachir Diagne, in his *Postcolonial Bergson* (2019), discusses the distinctive Senegalese contribution to open civilization elevated by Léopold Sédar Senghor. Open universe, open civilization, open individual destiny: these all arise from

> pure time . . . which is an organic whole in which the past is not left behind, but is moving along with, and operating in the present. And the future is given to it not as lying before, yet to be traversed; it is given only in the sense that it is present in its nature as an open possibility.
>
> (Diagne 2019, pp. 92–93 citing Muhammad Iqbal)

Senghor, the Francophone Serer poet and first president of independent Senegal, described a particular "Black African" consciousness:

> Here then, the Black-African who sympathizes and identities, who dies to himself to be born in the Other. . . . He lives with the Other in symbiosis, his knowing the Other is an act of giving birth to himself through the Other . . . Subject and object are, here, dialectically confronted in the same act of knowing [*connaissance*], which is an act of love. I think therefore I am, wrote Descartes. . . . The Black African could say, "I sense the Other, I dance the Other, therefore I am."
>
> (Senghor 1964, p. 259)

Senghor's poetic vision was inspired by Serer poets. His philosophical outlook enriched French vitalism with a distinctive Serer and Senegalese way of life. Diagne emphasizes the centrality of vitalist philosopher, Henri Bergson, to Senghor's vision (Diagne 2019, see also Jones 2010). As it happens, the physiological tradition is one of the roots of Bergson's vitalism. The cases from the Fann Hospital reflect the popular vitalist Senegalese beliefs and the cases presented throughout this book reveal insights into the culture Senghor promoted as a distinctive contribution to the globalized humanist culture.

"Je con-naît l'Autre"/"I know/give birth to the Other": this phrase from Senghor is closely similar to the widely celebrated *Ubuntu*, local to South Africa but part of globalized philosophy since the victory of the battle against apartheid. Former U.S.A. president Barack Obama's eulogy for former South African president and leader of the anti-apartheid struggle, Nelson Mandela, evokes *Ubuntu* as "the visible bonds of caring for others." To borrow the words of Ken Harrow,

> The African does not regard himself as self-sufficient but as part of a whole, which is the whole essence of the Ubuntu philosophy, "I am because we are." Back to binaries, this philosophy opposes the characteristic Western belief that, "I think, therefore I am."
>
> (2021)

As Senghor said, "I sense the Other, I dance the Other, therefore I am." In like manner, the physiological tradition opposes the cranium-centered brain (the hyper-localized *cogito*). Physiological emphasis on co-regulation of physiological states has a deep affinity for the process, "I give birth to the Other." Bergson's perception of time as duration, mobility, and spontaneity, points to the open destiny of *homo sapiens*. The futurist orientation of Senghor's vitalism resonates with the freedom essential to "the sacred space" of psychotherapy. Our bodies carry the legacy of deep evolutionary past with a scale of time that dwarfs the scale of human history, but wherever we are taken by our emotion, our choice, our very of aliveness, it is an open, un-predetermined destiny.

The Structure of This Book

Chapters 1 and 2 provide chronological and conceptual bookends to this set of case studies and comparative history of diagnosis and treatment. The book opens with innovations at Fann Hospital in the 1960s and then Chapter 2 presents twenty-first-century affective neuroscience polyvagal theory (PVT). The ensuing chapters present case material and diagnostic and treatment history. The case material contributes in itself to Senegalese history and the global folkloric. These narratives, the healing strategies, and the psychological dynamics of individuals and collectives, enrich the tradition of global open civilization. Innovations in the 1960s in transcultural psychiatry are put into historical context, both retrospectively and prospectively. Many of the cases yield even greater knowledge and understanding when viewed through twenty-first-century PVT.

Chapter 1, "Healing at Fann Hospital": This chapter introduces the innovations at Fann Hospital via the case study of a patient named S.C. which features witchcraft and murder. This introduction to the Fann Hospital technique is contextualized by a comparative presentation of both traditional healing and psychiatry in the colonial era. The chapter concludes with a discussion of the global dimensions to the rise of transcultural psychiatry. Rooted in the suburbs of Dakar and in the treatment rooms of the Fann Hospital, this History reflects globalization as much as it does local cultures. Valorizing local healing techniques featured as part of the global medical movement, just as it demonstrated the vitality of biological and psychological shared dimensions of humanity. Spirit crises came to be understood as universal even as recognized healing techniques proliferated through biomedical, psychoanalytic, social, and psychospiritual practices.

Chapter 2, "Physiology of Trauma, Fear, and Anxiety: Polyvagal Theory": The vagal nerve-physiological paradigm includes a sequence of body-based processes – stimulus, physiological state, behavior, narrative, and belief – and in so doing provides an alternative to the cranio-centric paradigm for investigating and treating mental health. Even the term "mental health" carries within it the cranio-centric bias, because mind and cognition are so intimately associated with the brain. This chapter redirects the discussion to a physiological paradigm expressed as the neuropsychiatrist Stephen Porges' polyvagal theory (PVT). PVT proposes a paradigm shift which remains a minority perspective but is highly influential in contemporary psychotherapy, especially for somatic conditions and trauma narratives. Adopted by trauma-informed practitioners, the roots of PVT stretch back into nineteenth-century French psychiatry, especially to Pierre Janet, the theorist of dissociation. PVT provides a paradigm that draws together physiological state, somatic symptoms, narrativized beliefs, social interactions, and the persistent, ongoing feedback cycle between these. The mammalian need for safety figures as the prominent drive in PVT. Lack of exterior safety triggers autonomic fear reactions, including fight/flight, or play dead (fainting, flagging, dissociation). Lack of interior safety triggers anxiety, a decompensation of sense of self. When the body experiences fear, social engagement is physiologically inhibited. Prolonged fear states promote social isolation, which consciousness narrates in ways that can further promote fear and social disengagement. Porges' PVT emphasizes physiological co-regulation, and puts physiological dysregulation at the root of a wide variety of mental illness.

Chapter 3, "A Case of Impotence/Xala": Impotence focused one of the first cases published by Dr. Henri Collomb and Dr. Moussa Diop in *Psychopathologie Africaine*. The case of Mr. N'D, a 60-year-old Wolof man who had recently married a fourth wife, narrates Mr. N'D's accusations of witchcraft and magic as the cause of his impotence. The doctors, however, diagnosed neurotic phobia. This 1965 clinical case has compelling parallels with Ousmane Sembène's *Xala*, a widely celebrated 1974 novel and 1975 film. This chapter explores these parallels, considers the symptomatic accusations of witchcraft, and the diagnosis of neurotic phobia. PVT is used in the final section to consider physiological dimensions evident in the case yet not present in the neurotic phobia diagnosis. The doctors' diagnosis exhibits curious lack of grounding in empiricism while also overlooking details about the wives of Mr. N'D and how their lives featured in the clinical case. Two wives stood accused of anthropophagic witchcraft. Mr. N'D divorced at least one of those. Meanwhile another wife occupied a preferred status. Polyvagal theory provides an alternative explanation of pair-bonding for Mr. N'D's impotence.

Chapter 4, "The Man Who Makes Trees Cry: A Healer's Art": The case of El Hadji Ba presents this Fulani healer's cosmology, mystical beliefs, and healing techniques. His worldview was informed by Islam as well as by pre-Islamic beliefs. Ba's narrative, published in 1969 in *Psychopathologie Africaine*, presents *djinns* (Islamic spirits), *seytané* (parasitic spirits of the underworld), *sukuñabé* (cannibalistic witches), as well as the healing process for a slave and his wife. Researched and recorded in painstaking detail, the healing beliefs and practices of El Hadji Ba constitute a contribution to global folk medicine. Dr. Henri Collomb recommended psychiatrists collaborate with such magical healers as El Hadji Ba, because such healers have special insight into culturally specific psychological suffering and healing. PVT provides perspective to recognize the social and intersubjective nature of mental health and healing portrayed here in both culturally specific and universal dimensions. The hierarchal healing relationships established by El Hadji are compared to the psychotherapeutic relationship and the ideal of individualistic illness and healing.

Chapter 5, "Witch Narratives: Stolen Souls and Aggression": This chapter plunges into narratives about witches, stolen souls, and interpersonal aggression. The impulse to devour the other and the fear of being devoured are habitually expressed as witchcraft. This chapter discusses the process of Fann Hospital personnel psychologizing their patients' metaphysical beliefs, and weighs the costs of such psychologizing. The Fann Hospital clinical approach to witchcraft is considered in context of diverse scholarship on witchcraft and modernity. PVT promotes understanding how physiological state is adopted into narrative and beliefs. The ancient autonomic neural processes, including autonomic dorsal vagal fear reactions, neuroception, and interoception, reveal the species-wide physiological basis of contagious fear and psychotic aggression. The colonial perspective, including the 1920s witch trials among the Diola of the Casamance region, is contrasted to the post-colonial Fann Hospital perspective. In conclusion the mid-twentieth-century assumption that witchcraft would fade away with increasing technological modernity is challenged by Senegalese futurism that integrates magic, witchcraft, and relational identity.

Chapter 6, "Devoured by Fear in Childbirth and Haunted "No-Good" Children": The terror that frequently directed Senegalese lives is evoked in this chapter via devouring fear in childbirth and the alternating promise and terror of "no-good" children (*l'enfant nit ku bon*). The physiological perspective is emphasized with respect to each. Childbirth and children figure in this chapter as crucial vectors for ancestral spirits or other metaphysical forces to enter and disrupt lives. Childbirth, governed by autonomic physiological processes, figured as a moment of significant peril for many Senegalese women. The supreme social significance of motherhood is achieved via the birthing process that opens women to the spirit world. If her post-partum body did not close properly, women suffered on-going torment and persecution. Social insecurity – difficulties with husband or co-wives – figured prominently in these case studies as did intense physiological dysregulation. The cases exhibit disturbances of interoception (*cenestopathie*), feeling that animals lived under the skin (*zoopathie interne*), and feelings of being eaten, and burned. Ideation included persecution by witchcraft, magic, and (less frequently) spirit possession. The perils of childbirth sometimes nonetheless produced "no-good-children" (*l'enfant nit ku bon*). The "no-good child" is characterized by its ability to choose death at any moment; the child seems to belong more to the spirit world than to the world of humans. A *nit ku bon* might bring unexpected good fortune to the family or might endanger the whole family and community. Spells and rituals forced the child to declare its true identity, encouraged it to stay among the living, or made it return to the spirit world where it belongs. Khady Fall's births contributed to her becoming a priestess of the *rab* (a *ndöepkat*). Binta's case concludes the chapter with reflection on the illness of a teen on the verge of adulthood struck down by spirits in the marketplace.

Chapter 7, "Trauma Defenses: Denial, Dissociation, and Magical Thinking": The physiological autonomic fear reaction ensures that humanity will continue prey to fear of the occult and witches. Trauma via physical injury or emotional betrayal causes sensations that are overwhelming, engulfing, devouring, blood-sucking, and soul stealing. Fear arises as a physiological response to the absence of safety and gives rise to anxiety. Denial is one prominent defense to such rapacious and devouring fear. Denial is explored in this chapter as a psychological mechanism that suppresses vulnerability and anxiety, and enables adult magical thinking. Stephen Porges' PVT renders denial, dissociation, and magical thinking legible in contemporary psychological theory. Denial is a form of dissociation that creates an interior psychological perception of safety within unsafe experience. Contemporary psychotherapy still struggles to accept dissociation into common practice even though in the first half of the twentieth century Dr. Henri Aubin wrote extensively on denial as a universal defensive psychological strategy (Bullard 2011, 2011–2012). Theorized in the late nineteenth century by Pierre Janet, denial arises from a process that starts with a trauma of some sort, whether emotional or physical, proceeds to repression or forgetting of the trauma, and then followed later, sometimes years later, by emergence of somatic symptoms. Denial is intimately tied to stymied, fractured, or disowned desire, as well as to dissociation. The consequent psychological world is one built on symbolic realities that are narrativized from a defensive, segmented, affective state. Betrayal or other trauma that is denied creates a realm of the unknowable, or the unspeakable, composed of obliterated bonds and fractured desire. Aubin termed that the realm of the crypt. That obliterated desire re-emerges as magical thinking, creating contagious affective states discussed in ethnography as taboo and *mana*. Ritual dance and erotic spirituality access the crypt and seek to rework the individual's relation to such occulted energy.

Chapter 8, "Ancestors": Among patients at the Fann Hospital, disrupted relationships with the ancestors could provoke a wide array of illnesses or misfortunes. Doctors Henri Collomb and Henri Ayat observed among migrants that the absence of relationships with the living as well as the dead was a chief source of mental illness. The Serer *lup* and the Lebou *ndöep* celebrate and enshrine the status of the possessed individual as an abode of the ancestors, and of this individual's family as one that hosts the ancestral spirits in their home and worships them at their altar. These rites confer a specific, recognizable status on the possessed, and ensure an on-going beneficial relationship with the spirits. All religions are based in the intervention of a spirit into the world of humans, but so long as the spirit has not revealed its name, this relationship is one-sided. The ancient question, "Who are you?" must be answered so that the relationship between the spirits and the person can be reciprocal. At the Fann Hospital, the temptation to look for enlightenment and inspiration from traditional understanding of spiritual crises stumbled against Senegalese men's increasing obedience to Islamic opposition to these rites. Women continued to disproportionately practice traditional rites, which recognized female ancestral spirits and the maternal lineage. In the twentieth century the rites became "a women's affair" and at the turn of the twenty-first century they were subject to feminist debate. The chapter concludes with a polyvagal theory informed reflection on competing narratives and the indisputable ancestral legacy of our autonomic dorsal vagal neural system.

Chapter 9, "Bouffée Délirante: Living Myth and Madness": The experience that Dr. Henri Collomb called *bouffée délirante* involved loss of home or a milieu of collective sentiments projected or hallucinated onto the terrain (*éspace vécu*), frenetic anxiety, fears of persecution, and other disruptive behaviors. This crisis befell Africans who migrated from their home villages to urban centers, whether within Africa or overseas. Collomb subdivided *bouffée délirante* into four distinct kinetic phases: 1) loss of homeland or ethnic milieu; 2) fear of *sorcellerie, rab, djinn,* or magic; 3) intense anxiety; and 4) delusions. *Bouffée délirante* is not included in the DSM, but is included in the *International Classification of Diseases* (*ICD*). Typically *bouffée délirante* onset is sudden, with felt experience of soul theft. The acute disorder allows full recovery. Disruption of lived space (*éspace vécu*) arises from loss of shared affective projections (hallucinatory space or myth). Diagnostic disputes that attempt to clearly separate *bouffée délirante* from schizophrenia endure. *Bouffée délirante* is also said to border on depression or other affective disorders, including hysteria. These diagnostic disputes grapple with historical dynamics characteristic of globalizing capitalism, including migration, urbanization, racism, and coterminous cultural changes. *Bouffée délirante* contrasts in a revealing manner with the U.S.A.- based diagnosis of protest psychosis among African Americans. Polyvagal theory provides a unifying paradigm for *bouffée délirante* that simultaneously accounts for the universal physiological reactions and allows for culturally specific narratives. The documented resilience in the face of psychosis contributes distinctively to our open civilization and recalls us to the powerful truth so elegantly expressed by Senghor: we live through each other, we dance with each other, we give birth to each other.

Works Cited

Ashforth, A., 2000. *Madumo*. Chicago: Chicago University Press.
Babou, C.A., 2021. *The Muridiyya on the Move Islam, Migration, and Place Making*. Athens: Ohio University Press.
Behringer, W., 2004. *Witches and Witch-Hunts*. Cambridge: Polity.
Bullard, A., 2000. *Exile to Paradise*. Palo Alto, CA: Stanford University Press.
Bullard, A., 2001. The Truth in Madness. *South Atlantic Review*, 66 (2), 114–132.

Bullard, A., 2002. From Vastation to Prozac Nation. *Transcultural Psychiatry*, 39 (3), 267–294.
Bullard, A., 2005a. The Critical Impact of Frantz Fanon and Henri Collomb; Race, Gender and Personality Testing of North and West Africans. *Journal for the History of Behavioral Sciences*, 41 (3), 225–248.
Bullard, A., 2005b. Oedipe Africain, a Retrospective. *Transcultural Psychiatry*, 42 (2), 171–203.
Bullard, A., 2007. Imperial Networks and Postcolonial Independence: The Transition from Colonial to Transcultural Psychiatry. *In*: S. Mahone and M. Vaughan, eds., *Psychiatry and Empire, Cambridge Series in Imperial and Post-Colonial Studies*. London: Palgrave Macmillan, 197–219.
Bullard, A., 2008. Sympathy and Denial; A Postcolonial Re-Reading of Emotions, Race, and Hierarchy. *Historical Reflections/Réflexions Historiques*, 34 (1), 122–142.
Bullard, A., 2011. La Crypte and Other Pseudo-Analytic Concepts in French West African Psychiatry. *In*: W. Anderson, D. Jenson and R. Keller, eds., *Unconscious Dominions: Psychoanalysis, Colonial Trauma, and Global Sovereignties*. Chapel Hill, NC: Duke University Press, 43–74.
Bullard, A., 2011–2012. Le déni, la crypte, et la magie: Contributions à l'inconscient global à partir de la psychiatrie coloniale française en Afrique de l'Ouest. *Psychopathologie Africaine*, XXXVI (1), 59–102.
Bullard, A., 2015a. Neither Melancholic nor Abject: A Lebou (West African) Inspiration for Feminine Empowerment. *Studies in Gender and Sexuality*, 16 (1), 63–81.
Bullard, A., 2015b. Environmental Crisis and Human Rights. *Ekonomska e Ekohistorija (Economic and Eco History) Special Issue on History and Sustainability*, 11 (11), 75–92. Available from: http://repository.usp.ac.fj/8649/2/eko-komplet_copy.pdf [Accessed 13 November 2021].
Collignon, R., 1978. Vingt ans de travaux à la clinique psychiatrique de Fann-Dakar. *Psychopathologie Africaine*, XIV (2–3), 133–356.
Collignon, R., 2000. Santé mentale entre psychiatrie contemporaine et pratique traditionnelle, (Le cas du Sénégal). *Psychopathologie Africaine*, XXX (3), 283–298.
Collomb, H. and Diop, M., 1965. A propos d'un cas d'impuissance. *Psychopathologie Africaine*, 1 (3), 487–511.
Cooney, S., 2017. President Trump Has Now Appropriated Witch Hunts. *Time Magazine*, 18 May. Available from: https://time.com/4784158/donald-trump-witch-hunt-history/ [Accessed 10 September 2021].
D'Almeida, L. *et al.*, 1997. *La Folie au Sénégal*. Dakar: CODESIRA.
Dana, D., 2018. *The Polyvagal Theory in Therapy: Engaging the Rhythm of Regulation*. S.W. Porges, foreword. New York: W.W. Norton.
Deleuze, G., 1966. *Le bergsonisme*. Paris: Presses Universitaire de France (2nd ed., 1998).
Diagne, S.B., 2019. *Postcolonial Bergson*. L. Turner, trans., J.E. Drabinski, foreward. New York: Fordham University Press.
Dols Garcia, A., 2020. Trafficking, Ritual Oaths and Criminal Investigations. *Forced Migration Review*, 64, 50–53. Available from: www.fmreview.org/sites/fmr/files/FMR downloads/en/issue64/dolsgarcia.pdf [Accessed 28 February 2021].
Echeverria-Estrada, C. and Batalova, J., 2019. *Sub-Saharan African Immigrants in the United States*. Migration Information Source, Newsletter of the Migration Policy Institute. Available from: www.migrationpolicy.org/article/sub-saharan-african-immigrants-united-states-2018 [Accessed 20 July 2021].
Fassin, D., 1992. *Pouvoir et maladie en Afrique*. Paris: Presses universitaires de France.

Fassin, D., 2003. *Les Enjeux politiques de la santé: Études sénégalaises, équatoriennes et françaises*. Paris: Karthala.

Fisher, J., 2017. Healing the Fragmented Selves of Trauma Survivors: Overcoming Internal Self-Alienation . London: Routledge.

Foley, E.E., 2010. *Your Pocket Is What Cures You: The Politics of Health in Senegal*. New Brunswick, NJ: Rutgers University Press.

Frederickson, J., 2021. *Co-Creating Safety: Healing the Fragile Patient*. Kensington, MD: Seven Leaves Press.

Freud, S., 1964. *New Introductory Lectures on Psycho-Analysis and Other Works*. London: Hogarth Press and Institute of Psycho-Analysis.

Harrow, K., 2021. *The Toyin Falola Interviews, a Conversation with Professor Kenneth Harrow*. Part 4B. H-Africa. Available from: H-Net.org [Accessed 13 November 2021].

Hoff, J. and Yeates, M., 2000. *The Cooper's Wife Is Missing: The Trials of Bridget Cleary*. New York: Basic Books.

Jones, D.V., 2010. *The Racial Discourses of Life Philosophy: Negritude, Vitalism and Modernity*. New York: Columbia University Press.

Kappor, I., 2020. *Confronting Desire: Psychoanalysis and International Development*. Ithaca: Cornell University Press.

Kilroy-Marac, K., 2019. *Impossible Inheritance: Postcolonial Psychiatry and the Work of Memory in a West African Clinic*. Berkeley, CA: University of California Press.

Kuckzynski, L., 2002. *Les marabouts africains à Paris*. Paris: Éditions du CNRS.

Levine, P.A., 2005. *Healing Trauma*. Boulder, CO: Sounds True.

Maddox, B., 1999. *Yeats's Ghosts: The Secret Life of W.B. Yeats*. New York: HarperCollins.

McNeill, J.R., 2000. *Something New Under The Sun: An Environmental History of the Twentieth-Century World*. New York: W.W. Norton.

Metzl, J., 2003. Mother's Little Helper: The Crisis of Psychoanalysis and the Miltown Resolution. *Gender & History*, 15 (2), 240–267.

Nagle, L.E. and Owasanoye, B., 2016. Fearing the Dark: The Use of Witchcraft to Control Human Trafficking Victims and Sustain Vulnerability. *Southwestern Law Review*, 45, 561–604. Available from: www.stetson.edu/law/studyabroad/netherlands/media/Trk2.Wk3.Day3.Nagle.Fearing-the-Dark.pdf [Accessed 28 February 2021].

Panksepp, J., 2004. *Affective Neuroscience: The Foundations of Human and Animal Emotions*. New York and London: Oxford University Press.

Peyton, S., 2017. *Your Resonant Self*. New York: W.W. Norton.

Porges, S.W., 2011. *The Polyvagal Theory: Neurophysiological Foundations of Emotions, Attachment, Communication, Self-Regulation*. New York: W.W. Norton.

Porges, S.W., 2017. *The Pocket Guide to the Polyvagal Theory: The Transformative Power of Feeling Safe*. New York: W.W. Norton.

Roth, A., 2018. *Insane: America's Criminal Treatment of Mental Illness*. New York: Basic Books.

Senghor, L.S., 1964. *Liberté I*. Paris: Le Seuil.

Simmel, G., 1976. *The Sociology of Georg Simmel*. New York: Free Press.

Smail, D.L., 2007. *On Deep History and the Brain*. Berkeley, CA: University of California Press.

Smail, D.L., 2014. Neurohistory in Action: Hoarding and the Human Past. *Isis*, 105 (1), 110–122.

Solms, M., 2015. *The Feeling Brain*. London: Routledge.

Solms, M., 2020. *The Hidden Spring: A Journey to the Source of Consciousness*. New York: W.W. Norton.

Stuart Hughes, H., 1958. *Consciousness and Society: The Reorientation of European Social Thought, 1890–1930*. New York: Vintage Books.
Swimme, B. and Berry, T., 1992. *The Universe Story: From the Primordial Flaring Forth to the Ecozoic Era, a Celebration of the Unfolding Cosmos*. New York: HarperCollins.
Vélez, K., 2015. By Means of Tigers: Jaguars as Agents of Conversion in Jesuit Mission Records of Paraguay and the Moxos, 1600–1768. *Church History*, 84 (4), 768–806. Available from: www.jstor.org/stable/24537512 [Accessed 27 February 2021].
Wright, Z.V., 2020. *Realizing Islam, Sustainable History Monograph Pilot OA Edition: The Tijaniyya in North Africa and the Eighteenth-Century Muslim World*. Charlotte, NC: University of North Carolina Press. Available from: www.jstor.org/stable/10.5149/9781469660844_wright [Accessed 13 November 2021].
Yeats, W.B. 1986 [1892]. Introduction. *In*: W.B. Yeats, ed., *Irish Fairy and Folk Tales*. New York: Dorset Press, iii–xi.
Zucchetto, J., Jacobs, S. and Johnson, L.V., 2020. *Understanding the Paradox of Surviving Childhood Trauma: Techniques and Tools for Working with Suicidality and Dissociation*. New York: Routledge.

1 Healing at Fann Hospital

The Case of S.C.

In the very first issue of *Psychopathologie Africaine* in 1965, Dr. Henri Collomb, Dr. Paul Martino, and sociologist-ethnographer András Zempléni published the case of S.C., a man consigned to psychiatric care because he had murdered someone he thought was a witch (Martino *et al.* 1965). This case captures some of the most enduring complexities of transcultural psychiatry. Martino and Collomb were psychiatric medical doctors trained in Lacanian psychoanalysis. Zempléni was trained as a sociologist. Zempleni's employment at Fann already demonstrates the atypical practice that included substantial interests in social dimensions of mental health and healing. These men observed that S.C.'s case demonstrates the singular position of Western psychiatry in an African milieu, including diagnostic difficulties and the artificiality of nosographical categories (Martino *et al.* 1965, p. 151). The life-world of S.C. differed so significantly from that of the French hospital personnel that it stymied their psychiatric methods. The signature Fann technique responded with meticulous attention to the specifics of the individual's life, so that the S.C. case history reads almost like a condensed murder-mystery.

We learn immediately that S.C. had never suffered any previous psychological problems. He was employed on the railway and had earned an iron cross during his military service in France. He was clean living and neither smoked nor drank. His daughter F.C., however, was known as a bad character; she was insolent and had frequent altercations with other people (Martino *et al.* 1965, p. 151). One day at the local fountain she quarreled with a young neighbor woman. This woman's father-in-law reproached F.C., "I'll get you and you will never again see your father or your mother" (Martino *et al.* 1965, p. 151).

That night F.C. became very agitated, she thrashed about and cried: "they're going to get me, they're going to kill me." Subsequent headaches and nose bleeds were followed the next day by lethargy. Her whole family was extremely upset and the father (S.C.) rushed to the sorcerer to beg for his forgiveness and for his help. The sorcerer came to F.C.'s bedside and in an attempt at a cure applied a secret ointment and Qu'ranic verses. The next day, however, the girl was worse. She could no longer see and appeared to be almost dead. In a panic the family

DOI: 10.4324/9781003112143-2

took her to the hospital. S.C. (the father) returned to the sorcerer and begged him again to aid his daughter. The sorcerer this time said no, he had already done all that he could.

At this point S.C. was overcome with rage and attacked the sorcerer, killing him. He also wounded the sorcerer's wife who tried to intervene (Martino *et al.* 1965, p. 152). Once the sorcerer was dead, the daughter's health returned to normal. From his jail cell, S.C. regretted the murder, but was happy to have saved his daughter.

While S.C. was in jail, the wife of the sorcerer took up her dead husband's cause and began persecuting S.C. Each night she would leave her body, take on the shape of birds or a lion, and come to attack S.C. She used, according to S.C., magic formulas that could kill without a trace. S.C. professed to know other magical formulas that alone could deter this black magic, and he shared these formulas willingly with his doctors (Martino *et al.* 1965, p. 152).

The doctors' physical exam of S.C. revealed no pathologies. Mentally and emotionally, he was in good form. Only his dreams plagued him, and he believed in all earnestness that they were real. Martino, Zempleni, and Collomb placed S.C.'s convictions within the context of broader African and specifically Wolof belief in witchcraft, reflecting that,

> among the Wolof attacks by witches remain frequent and feared. The sorcerer *döem* is a man whose human appearance is identical to other men. He has the power to take on animal forms or to become immaterial in order to attack. It is generally agreed that only the soul of the sorcerer transforms itself. His fleshy envelop does not participate in these attacks. Attacks are generally carried out at night. The victim is devoured through two essential organs, the liver and the heart, which are reservoirs of *fit* (vital energy).
>
> (Martino *et al.* 1965, p. 153)

This devouring brings on certain, usually sudden, death. In some cases, however, these vital organs are set aside to be shared with a sorcerer's confraternity: this brings on a slower death.

What constitutes mental illness in this scenario? According to S.C.'s community, his mental illness was demonstrated by the fact that he acted on his own impulse and without the support of his community. Martino, Zempleni, and Collomb acknowledged this community standard of mental illness, emphasizing that S.C. did not have the right to kill the sorcerer because he and his family had not obtained a community consensus about the witchcraft. The usual course of events should have involved a consultation with a healer who might have removed the curse or identified the witch. Instead, in this case, S.C. brought the witch to his daughter's bedside, begging him to undo his own magic. When that failed, he killed the sorcerer. It is because he violated the customary practices concerning witchcraft – not because he believed his daughter had been bewitched, nor even because he murdered the man he suspected of witchcraft, but because he did so without having followed the communal procedures – that his peers considered S.C. mentally ill.

From a Western psychiatric point of view, S.C. was suffering from delirium. The murder committed by S.C., according to Dr. Collomb, Zempleni, and Martino, was a first manifestation of an "acute psychosis or systematic complex delusion with themes of persecution" (Martino *et al.* 1965, p. 155). The original French used the term "*bouffée délirante*," which is a specialized French diagnosis discussed in Chapter 9. For the present discussion, "acute psychosis" suffices. The attacks suffered while in prison, including visual and verbal hallucinations and sensory disorientation, in the doctors' estimation, confirmed this diagnosis (Martino *et al.* 1965, p. 156). Zempleni, Martino, and Collomb, however, were troubled that their diagnosis confirmed the social view of S.C. – that he was suffering from mental illness – but that they arrived at this conclusion very differently than did S.C.'s community. The medical team were confounded by the fact that two very different logics upheld the same conclusions about S.C.'s behavior. For the doctors, S.C.'s hallucinations were the chief indicator of mental illness. These doctors were aware, however, that among the Wolof, it was not at all unusual to have perceptions without an objective cause (Martino *et al.* 1965, p. 156). From the Wolof point of view, S.C.'s transgression of the ancestral law is the chief sign of his madness, but such transgression from a psychiatric point of view was of little or no consequence (Martino *et al.* 1965, p. 156).

The judges from the criminal court, meanwhile, focused on yet another topic. They wanted to know if S.C. was a danger to society. Would S.C. murder again? Martino, Zempleni, and Collomb considered this medico-legal concern carefully. They weighed their psychiatric knowledge – which gave S.C. a good prognosis for recovery – against the prospect of him falling victim to witchcraft again. This was very possible, but they happily reported that S.C. had protected himself from further attacks by securing the services of a *bilédio* (a Toucouleur witch chaser and in this case a very renowned one who lived near the Senegal river). The *bilédio* would protect S.C. from further attacks, so Zempleni, Martino, and Collomb decided S.C. posed a minimal threat to the community and most likely would not murder again.

S.C.'s case prompted the team of doctors to reflect that Western psychiatric diagnostic criteria could be employed in such situations only tentatively and with reservations. The people of Dakar and wider Senegal accepted as normal experiences what to Western medical eyes appeared as delirium and hallucinations. On the other hand, such experiences were common and a part of the normal fabric of Senegalese life. In this social milieu, French (or, biomedically trained) doctors lost their chief diagnostic criteria. In Western biomedical psychiatry, delirium and hallucinations composed the hallmarks of mental illness (Martino *et al.* 1965, p. 157). At the Fann Hospital, and working with the diverse West African population of Dakar, the doctors had to learn to define mental illness differently. They adopted a standard that abstracted from the local perspective: the individual dangerously out of step with communal expectations became the chief indication of mental illness. This psychiatric standard for mental illness in Senegal was an abstraction from the Wolof aversion to transgressing ancestral rules. This standard also reflected a perspective on psychiatry informed by Georges Canguilhem and

Michel Foucault, for whom dangerous deviation from the norm is constitutive of mental illness (Canguilhem 1943; Foucault 1961). The physiological perspective, discussed in-depth in the next chapter, integrates the individual who is somehow out of sync, within an understanding of physiological regulation and dysregulation. The rhythm of the heart – which in a sociable state is patterned, and in an excited state beats steadily with unrelenting speed – enables the prosody of voice. Social engagement via micro-facial gestures, the perceptive tilt of the head, or a subtle crease of the eyelids carry an individual in to successful social relationships. Unsuccessful relationships produce physiological dysregulation which in turn impedes other social relationships. The narrativized environment enmeshes with physiological processes, whether those are regulated or dysregulated, and in either case, whether habitual or acute and transient. Acute dysregulation can give rise to sudden mental distress. Habitual dysregulation can express as long-term and entrenched spiritual and psychological difficulties. The narrativizing of physiological states is a powerful force not just for categorizing experience but also for decision-making and on-going participation in further narratives, whether collective, individual, traditional, innovative, or idiosyncratic.

Driven by Western expertise in psychiatry, psychology, sociology, and philosophy, the 1960s and 1970s transcultural project at Fann Hospital aimed to prioritize Senegalese beliefs and practices. This proved a tantalizing enterprise that drew hospital personnel to local rituals related to spirit possession, witchcraft, and magic, and yet which also relied on at least some Western biomedical, philosophical, and psychological assumptions. In effect, the transcultural psychiatrists aimed to integrate widely disparate narrative practices: including medical doctors, psychologists, traditional healers, and sociologists, all within a unified search for healing.

Marabouts and Healing at Fann Hospital Compared to the Colonial Era

The early years of the Fann Hospital journal, *Psychopathologie Africaine*, reflect the enthusiasm and creativity of the efforts of these Western-trained psychiatrists, psychologists, and sociologists to integrate Western psychiatry and psychoanalysis into a therapeutic regime that accepted as well a wide variety of Senegalese healing practices. This creativity, however, never completely shook free of the cultural and racial hierarchies of the colonial period.

Martino and Marie-Cécile Ortigues addressed the disparity between the treatment administered at Fann and the pervasive interest among Fann personnel in Senegalese beliefs and practices regarding troubles of the spirit. For their patients from Dakar – patients who most commonly were Wolof, Lebou, or Serer – the doctors were viewed as men of science to which one could trust one's body, but the doctors were also always, irredeemably, "foreigners" (Martino and Ortigues 1965). Therapeutic relationships that could heal the spiritual troubles of these patients escaped the competence of these foreign disciples of science and fell instead to those referred to generally as *marabouts*. For the patients at Fann

Hospital, according to M-C Ortigues and Martino, Western-trained doctors could calm and strengthen the fragile body, but true healing required a parallel treatment of the soul by a local healer. In effect, then, the personnel at Fann worked within a recognized limit to their competence. As much as they were fascinated by the therapeutic rites of healers, they themselves remained largely tied to biomedical treatment of the body and mind.

Nonetheless, witchcraft and spiritual healing figured prominently at Fann, both within the course of treatment of patients and within the medical the personnel. Moussa Diop – the sole Senegalese doctor at Fann in 1965 – and Henri Collomb evoked the complicated array of healers within the region of Dakar with the remark that in Senegal, a country Islamized already for several centuries but also preserving pre-Islamic practices, the term *marabout* was used broadly and could signify "authentic marabouts as well as charlatans and other 'turbaned healers' (*guerisseurs enturbannés*)" (Diop and Collomb 1965). Marabout is the French version of the Arabic, *mrâbot*, which in turn derived from the Almoravide, *al-Murabit* (Monteil 1980, p. 154; Fassin 1992, p. 73). Used in a strict sense, the term *marabout* refers to Muslim religious leaders imbued with Islamic religious learning and earning, thereby, spiritual and political charisma or *baraka*. Maraboutic healing linked Senegal to this broader Arabic and Islamic tradition of medicine. However, as Diop and Collomb pointed out, in the 1960s the term was used relatively indiscriminately, referring variously to sorcerers, magicians, fetishers, shamans, and medicine men, who all were thought to possess magico-religious powers by virtue of which they could heal – or provoke – illnesses, including spiritual crises or psychiatric disorders. They rely on Mircead Eliade's pioneering scholarship as a guide to distinguishing the mentally ill from the gifted, spiritual healer (Eliade 1951, vol. 1, p. 38). The term *marabout*, for example, was often used in place of the Wolof word, *sérigne*, which refers not only to those learned in the Qu'ran, but also to visionaries, fortune tellers, charlatans, and healers who draw part but not all of their technique from Islamic traditions (Diop and Collomb 1965, p. 306; compare to Lateef 1973 on *zeema* in Niger). Mystical healers enter into relation with various types of spirits – *rab*, *seytanés*, *djinns* – and risk losing their own equilibrium in the process. License to travel into the spirit world without incurring harm was one of the signs of the skilled healer.

Diop and Collomb explained that their patients viewed *djinns* as ambivalent spirits that generally work for the good, offering protection and conferring magico-religious power and mystical knowledge. *Seytanés* were considered bad spirits; they used their powers against people and frequently caused insanity, even among healers (Diop and Collomb 1965, p. 307). *Rab*, meanwhile, are ancestral spirits that can insist on communicating with certain individuals and, in doing so, pose repeated spirit crises until the proper rituals name the spirits and provide a fixed abode for them in the form of a domestic altar. Diop and Collomb themselves found it useful to divide the healers into marabouts (who use methods linked to Islam) and traditional psychiatrists (who use techniques of animist religions) (1965, p. 306). The *bilédio*, for example, was a traditional psychiatrist who specialized in treating those suffering from witchcraft and the Lebou *ndöepkat* healed possessions via trance rituals (1965, pp. 305–306). Despite this effort at clarity, Diop and Collomb caution that Senegalese culture was deeply marked by syncretism, so that any effort to separate out Islamic from animist healers was inevitably frustrated.

These observations did not rest in the world of academic mental health science, but actively operated among patients at Fann and among the Senegalese personnel, in particular in the life and death of Moussa Diop and in the life and death of his successor, Babakar Diop. Moussa Diop took ill and died suddenly in 1967, just two years after the publication of these remarks on how traditional healers protect themselves from the spirit world. The sudden illness deprived the Fann Hospital of the designated successor to Collomb's leadership. The cause of death was liver cancer. Of course, witches are said to eat the livers of their victims, and it is widely recounted and believed that Moussa Diop died because of unprotected transgression in matters of the spirit world. Dr. Babakar Diop also fell ill after he took on the role of hospital director. Katie Kilroy-Marac discusses this haunting of the pioneering Senegalese psychiatrists: "Moussa Diop's death marked the field of psychiatry in Senegal with fear, self-doubt, and a suspicion that would never quite be allayed" (2019, p. 151). In Senegal, fear of medical engagement with spirit troubles persists even despite on-going engagement in the field.

In the case of the marabout Sékou C. presented by Diop and Collomb, a mystical rite of communion with *seytané* and *djinns* led to persistent mental illness marked chiefly by compulsive and disruptive animal noises, compulsive arm movements, and rocking and rotating of his head (Diop and Collomb 1965, p. 311). These somatic symptoms appeared after a failed *khalva* meditation during which Sékou C. fell asleep and dreamed of a white woman, dressed in European clothing, who was bigger and stronger than him. In his dream, this woman came and sat next to him, inviting him to make love. Sékou C. refused and the woman mastered him by seizing both his arms. At that point Sékou woke up (1965, p. 311). After the dream and onset of symptoms, Sékou tried during several months to heal himself through prayers and exercises, but finally his symptoms became so persistent and debilitating that he was forced to try the white man's hospital. Sékou claimed adamantly that his illness was caused by a *djinn*, but the expense of seeking a maraboutic treatment was too much for him and his family. At the hospital – and in their subsequent article – the doctors were greatly interested by Sékou's dream, his life story, and the symbolic dimensions to his symptoms. Reflecting on Sékou's treatment, Collomb and Diop regret the missed opportunity to observe a purely psychological and maraboutic cure. Under their medical care, Sékou's treatment at Fann Hospital centered on the anti-psychotic tranquilizer chlorpromazine hydrochloride. Developed in a French pharmaceutical laboratory, Largactil (also called Thorazine) was the first anti-psychotic on the market (Rosenbloom 2002). In addition to the Largactil, Sékou received six electro-shock treatments (Diop and Collomb 1965, p. 311).

The Fann Hospital clinicians inhabited a dilemma. They valued the symptoms of their patients as vital cultural and symbolic dimensions of their patients' illness. Indeed, many among the personnel were influenced by Freudian, Jungian, and

Lacanian psychoanalysis. However, they habitually resorted to strong biomedical treatments that suppressed these symptoms. The biomedical interventions calmed the body even if they did not produce a cure. Respect for the authority of local healers, whose narratives provided the meaning of symptoms, allowed the Fann personnel a window onto maraboutic treatment. In the case of Sékou, for example, a healer who befriended Sékou announced that the white woman in Sékou's vision was a *djinn* with whom Sékou should have joined forces. Refusing the *djinn* was what had provoked his madness. Ceding the interpretative ground to the healers, moreover, limits our own post-colonial interpretation as much as it did for the Fann personnel. It is tempting to make much of a huge white woman forcing Sékou to have sex, but on what grounds can we make any interpretive claims that go beyond those made by the healer or the patient? The historian of Nigerian psychiatry, Jonathan Sadowsky, reflected that "the content of madness *demands attention*; it should not be treated as a distraction" (1999, p. 96). Investing the symptoms with meaning, however, is an act of appropriation – licensed appropriation in the case of the healers described here, and unlicensed appropriation when performed by foreigners, whether medical clinicians or historians. It is doubtful that we can claim to be more acutely aware of the dynamics of race, gender, and power in this early post-colonial context, or that we have a special understanding of the power Sékou might gain via an alliance with *une grande femme blanche*. What we do know is that Sékou lamented his missed opportunity, and sought in vain to revisit his dream and consummate his union with the white woman *djinn* (Diop and Collomb 1965, p. 321).

Rather than interpreting the symptoms as individualized expressions, Fann personnel tried to think the mental illness through the cultural idioms of their patients. Sékou, for example, fell into a disoriented crisis – that is, he was overwhelmed by an internal sense of chaos – because in his *khalva* dream his spirit had voyaged into the invisible universe and had not successfully returned to the physical world. His soul had left his body, in a type of anticipation of death, and this had created engulfing anxiety and mental illness. The successful union with the *djinn* (the huge white woman) would have allowed Sékou to return to the world in an adaptive, integrated manner. Because the *khalva* had succeeded in opening the spirit world, but his voyage had reached a bad end, he was abandoned in chaos and mental illness (Diop and Collomb 1965, p. 321).

The Fann personnel also adopted a tactic of interpreting the broader social context and processes surrounding the patient and their cure. The patient, as Collomb and his team recognized, might be symtomatic, but he was not responsible or guilty because of his symptoms. The other – whether person or spirit – made him sick. The other – a healer of some sort – cured him. Collomb and Diop commented that this turn to the other was not a renunciation of individual power, but rather a correlative of the tight, unifying dependences between people (Collomb and Diop 1965, p. 231). Redolent of psychoanalytic and philosophical freight, *l'autre* as used by Collomb and Diop resonates with Maurice Leenhardt's description of Kanak personage in *Do Kamo*. Leenhardt described the Kanak psyche as essentially disaggregated. The Kanak "gained identity through a complex system of relationships" between people and between people and animals, plants, or even features of the landscape (Leenhardt 1947 cited in Bullard 2000, pp. 180–181). That the European personnel at Fann see themselves, and presumably other whites, as outside the realm of "others" – capable of provoking illness or promoting healing – seems to be a blind spot. Collomb and Diop emphasized that the Dakaroise society permitted delirium and integrated the impacted individual into social relationships. To this "African" formulation, they contrasted the dominant Western view: "the crazy person does not have a place in human society, delirium is not permitted, the sick is alone with his sickness for which he alone is responsible" (Collomb and Diop 1965, p. 231).

The relative openness to marabouts and traditional psychiatrists was one of the significant innovations at the Fann Hospital. The role of healers within the hospital, however, was only a small part of the transcultural project. Persecution complexes and hallucinatory experiences featured much more prominently among the patients at the Fann Hospital than would be the case in Europe. As described by Martino and Marie-Cécile Ortigues, the professionals at Fann had difficulty determining the line between a healthy mind and a delirious one, because persecution and hallucination formed such a widely accepted part of the culture (Martino and Ortigues 1965, p. 248). For example, allegations of witchcraft among the Senegalese did not signal a persecution complex, but rather conveyed an accepted and usual social event. A patient who complained of being devoured by a witch expressed an accepted social reality. The family of the patient participated with the patient in the truth of such complaints. Indeed, the family accepted the allegations, and often enriched them by making them more specific. In such a context, is everyone delirious? Or is no one delirious? Ortigues and Martino remarked that the mental health professional gained as much as was lost in this situation. If the distinction between delusion and sanity was blurred, nonetheless the hospital personnel found themselves working in a situation in which the mentally ill were not isolated from society, but rather deeply enmeshed in it. The mentally ill treated at Fann were not "alienated" but rather remained a part of his or her social group. Ortigues and Martino contrasted this socially rooted sufferer to the *aliéné* of French psychiatry, marked distinctly by singularity, removed from social bonds, and isolated from reciprocal understanding (Martino and Ortigues 1965, p. 248).

According to Martino and Ortigues, the fluid boundaries between the delirious were replicated in cases of hallucination as well as psychosis. Visions, dreams, and hallucinations, remarked Martino and Ortigues, were common currency in the Dakar milieu, distinguished only for how ordinary they were. In all these fluid states, whether persecution, delusion, or hallucination, the evil (or trouble) was not located within the individual but was exterior, and the group agreed that this was the case. This was a fundamental truth in the psychology of those who came for treatment at Fann: "guilt is not interiorized" (Martino and Ortigues 1965, p. 249). Paired with this, according to Martino and Ortigues, there was little or no emphasis on linear temporality in the consciousness of their patients or their patients' relatives (Martino and Ortigues 1965, p. 250). Establishing the relative dates of major events – the death of a mother or father, previous major illnesses and how long they lasted – ordinarily produced confusion.

Marabouts *in the Colonial Era*

Missing in Diop and Collomb's case of Sékou is a sense of the post-colonial as a legacy, an outgrowth, and an escape from the colonial. During the colonial era, the African healers were subject to prosecution for practicing, while Western psychiatric treatment for Africans was largely unavailable, and if available, consisted of frequently lethal incarceration. The post-colonial era of Fann marked a dramatic shift, with the sudden valorization of traditional healers by the director of the major psychiatric hospital in Dakar.

Throughout the colonial era, the marabouts' power was a force the French struggled to mitigate and contain. The medical role of these powerful individuals, however, is less often discussed, in part because the medical power of such men was not clearly separate from their power as holy men and political leaders, and in part because spiritual healing did not much interest nineteenth- and early twentieth-century medical professionals. The historian Jan Goldstein recounted the battle in France between the emerging science of psychiatry and the authorities of the state and the Catholic Church (Goldstein 1987). This field of medicine gained professional status in fits and starts over the course of the nineteenth century. The emergence of psychiatry parallels the emergence of French Republicanism, itself a famously tumultuous history that began in the Revolution of 1789, through the Napoleonic era, the Restoration, the July Monarchy, the Revolution of 1848, and the Second Empire, on through to the 1871 establishment of the Third Republic in the wake of the twin devastations of the Franco-Prussian War and the Paris Commune. Throughout this long century of political turmoil, the revolutionary Republican agenda included a pro-science and anti-clerical dimension. Psychiatry thrived with the revolutions, and suffered with the revival of the monarchy and religion. During the Restoration, the government closed down the medical faculty in Paris for two years, 1822–23, and forbade all private medical courses except those granted special authorization (Goldstein 1987, pp. 255, 261). Physiology, to which the nascent field of psychiatry adhered, grounded the science of mental illness in biology. This materialism subverted religion as well as the socio-political order enshrined in monarchy (Goldstein 1987, p. 255). The pioneers of the early nineteenth century studied autopsies closely, seeking lesions in the gut or brain, in order to find the organic cause of insanity (Goldstein 1987, pp. 250–257).

French medical men of nineteenth-century psychiatry, thus, struggled to break from metaphysics and religion, and like the political revolutions that colored their time, this break was violent, with categorical rejection of the former order. This violent break characterizes the sometimes rigid mindset of scientific materialists. Only through unequivocal rejection of superstition and metaphysics could psychiatrists pursue their quest to reach a truer understanding of illness. Neutrality toward religion was not an option (Goldstein 1987, p. 230). Thus, in the nineteenth century a whole series of books, the *Bibliothèque diabolique*, reinterpreted famous episodes of spirit possession as hysteria (Goldstein 1987, p. 236). Nonetheless, through the mid-nineteenth century, relatively frequent spiritual visions and possession experiences arose in such places as Morzine, La Salette, Marpingen, and Lourdes (Harris 1997, p. 461). Even into the mid-twentieth century, according to Julia Kristeva, illiterate Breton women exhibited classic possession crises, although the medical establishment had long since adopted the secular language of hysteria (Clémont and Kristeva 2001, p. 9). Moreover, psychiatrists reported a collective bewitchment delirium that embroiled a small Normandy village from 1947–53, which delirium had roots in a vicious property dispute (Letailleur *et al.* 1955).

The doctors working abroad in the French colonial administration came out of the French medical schools that had fought religious authorities and faced down religious truths throughout France. To these doctors, superstition was superstition, no matter where and no matter the language of the villagers or peasants. Dismissive and combative toward spiritual healing in France, doctors generally were not appreciative of such practices in Senegal either. The tight trio of healing powers, religious charisma, and political leadership appears in General Louis Faidherbe's description of the Tidjani marabout, Ahmadou Cheikhou. The 1868 famine and cholera outbreak, reported Faidherbe, "produced great religious euphoria among the natives of Cayor and Walo, in the river-region of Southern Senegal" (Faidherbe 1889, p. 288). Cheikhou offered protection of health and welfare, a point of political loyalty, and the opportunity to achieve martyrdom through holy war. Cheikhou professed that those who pledged loyalty to him would be spared the ravages of hunger and disease. He attracted so many people that he had soon raised an army for a holy war against the French. Faidherbe's portrait of Ahmadou Cheikhou, as well as of El Hadj Omar and other marabouts, brings home the intertwining of religious, spiritual, and military power that posed such a formidable threat to French rule as well as to the establishment of medical ideas and standards that were independent of religion (Faidherbe 1889, pp. 158–161).

As the French colonial presence gained strength, the administration used doctors in an effort to win people's confidence and loyalty. A medical career in the colonies provided French men an opportunity for heroism, according to the colonial administration, as well as an opportunity to occupy the frontlines of the civilizing mission. French policy required doctors who accompanied military troops or administrative personnel to operate clinics and pharmacies, and to grant medical consultations for anyone who asked for care. These medical consultations were free, and according to the 1896 report on health in colonies, "are greatly appreciated by the locals whose confidence in our doctors grows stronger every day since the opening of medical posts six months past in Thioro, Sedbiou, Carabane, Kaedi, and Thiès" (Anon. 1896).

In 1906 the French sought to measure the success of their medical missions by gathering statistics. While certain doctors resisted this modern innovation and the figures gathered were none too exact, nonetheless a comparison can be made between the figures of 1905 and 1906. In 1905, doctors in Senegal reported treating 54,300 patients, and doctors from across French West Africa (the A.O.F.)

reported treating 165,261 patients. These figures rose significantly in 1906, when doctors in Senegal reported treating 187,146 patients and doctors across the A.O.F. reported treating 634,547 patients (Anon. 1906, p. 94). In 1906 there were 61 centres médicaux d'Assistance; 15 of these were in Senegal. Two of those were in St. Louis, and one each were in Dakar, Rufisque, Bakel, Podor, Louga, Kaolack, Tivaouane, Zinguinchor, Gorée, Thiès, Sédhiou, Bignona, and Dagana (Anon. 1906, p. 44).

Marabouts, traditional healers, and local chiefs posed on-going resistance to the French doctors. Notable sites of resistance included Casamance, Timbuktu, Niamey, and Gao. In particular Niamey and Gao were cities of active warfare. Meanwhile, the local doctor in Casamance, Doctor Boudriot, reported that "the population is completely dominated by the marabouts and native healers" (Anon. 1906, p. 52). "Frequently," reported Boudriot,

> I learn of a man or a woman in some location who is really very sick, but whom we have never treated. We go to visit this person, and always find that he or she is in the hands of an "empiric."

According to Boudriot, the French practice of medicine in Casamance was limited to treating syphilitics or those suffering ulcers but "the truly ill never come to us for care" (Anon. 1906, p. 94). He opined that this resistance to European medicine would continue

> as long as the sorcerers and healers of all sorts can continue to live off of public credulity with impunity. Against this we can do nothing except to arm ourselves with patience and to continue our efforts to dissipate bit by bit the reserve that the natives hold toward us.
>
> (Anon. 1906, p. 52)

Marabouts reportedly saw European doctors as an affront to their own prestige and as a threat to their lucrative commerce in protective cords, pouches, and amulets known as *gris-gris*. The efforts to extend biomedical care, however, did prompt West Africans to seek medical treatment, even while they maintained their preference for local healing practices. The healers, moreover, were excluded from colonial medical circles and subject to prosecution for pursuing their trade. The colonial administration also tried to dislodge healers by training West Africans as medical aides, auxiliary doctors, and midwives (Grimaud 1978).

Documents on the plague portray the struggles between the colonial authorities and healers in asserting dominance over stricken villages. For example, in the plague year of 1924, three marabouts from Baol were sentenced to three to four years' imprisonment (Anon. 1924). These marabouts had infringed on the public health laws by traveling in infected areas (including N'Doutte Diasane and Meché M'Bar) in order to treat patients. The administrative report reflects disdain for the marabouts' medical practice as well as outrage at their flaunting of the travel prohibition, stating baldly, "they traveled in the infected regions . . .

in order to exploit the population by selling them *gris-gris* and medications" (Anon. 1924).

The disdain for the marabouts juxtaposes curiously with the admitted failure of the French medical practices. In this episode of plague, out of 1,650 known infections, 1,085 individuals died. Administrators explained this chillingly high death rate by recalling "the impossibility of extending medical care to individuals in their isolated huts with little in the way of comforts and where the prescribed hygienic practices cannot be applied" (Anon. 1924).

This inability of the French to provide adequate medical treatment surely worked to the advantage of the marabouts. The maraboutic power, in turn, further fed the French fear of the political-spiritual-medical power of the *marabouts*. Put simply, the marabouts offered a compelling alternative to allegiance to the French (Robinson 2000; Babou 2007). Even colonial officials acknowledged that the marabouts emanated an "occult power" capable of attracting allegiance from diverse ethnic groups, even including the allegiance of the mixed-race Catholics. Their converts willingly donated large sums of money, which were used in part to build mosques, themselves a symbol of the marabouts' power and a rallying point for their followers. "There is a danger in this occult power that I must point out," reported one local official. "This is a peril for our administration" (Rapport Politique 1926).

Psychiatry at Fann and Before

Throughout the nineteenth century, psychiatric care had very little presence in colonial French West Africa – as was the case throughout most of the French colonies. The French law of 1838 that mandated asylum treatment of *aliénés* was not adopted into Senegalese or French West African law. That law of 1838 occasioned a massive confinement throughout metropolitan France. Very few people were confined in French West Africa. Indeed, across the entire French empire in 1885 only 338 people were in psychiatric custody. Statistics from 1885 reveal only 13 people (most likely Europeans) were interned in Senegal (Anon. 1885). L'hopital de Saint Louis held one woman suffering paralytic insanity. Doctors had diagnosed seven men and four women in the same hospital with "idiocy." The military hospital held one epileptic man. No other cases from Senegal were reported (Anon. 1885). Various healers filled the demand for spiritual counsel or mental health care in the colonial era, and they continue to provide the majority of such care to this day. Nonetheless, there was a certain amount of French psychiatric activity in French West Africa, including the occasional psychiatric confinement and transportation.

The treatment of aliénés in Senegal emerged as a politic issue in 1896, when the Félix Faure presented an exposé on the conditions of the mentally ill to the Conseil Général of Sénégal (Reboul and Régis 1912, p. 82). This 1896 debate followed close upon the formation of the AOF and the mounting concern for the health of the workforce in West Africa. Faure's report is animated by a humanitarian desire to alleviate the suffering of the ill, and to provide modern medical attention to the extent possible. The report documents shocking conditions. In general, those confined for mental health difficulties received treatment no better than prisoners. The Director of the Interior described the deplorable situation at l'hopital civil in Saint Louis:

> they are confined in isolated, narrow cells that can be compared to privies without ventilation. I saw a gasping native, clutching at the grill on the window, climbing like a monkey in order to breath some fresh air through the narrow bars of his prison.
>
> (Reboul and Régis 1912, p. 82)

Reboul and Régis reflected on this debate of the Grand Conseil:

> it is easy to see how precarious the situation is for the insane in these various establishments, and how little their situation differs from that of prisoners. All the same, we can rightly say that often observations have been made on this state of affairs and that the good intentions repeated many times have not been realized.
>
> (Reboul and Régis 1912, p. 88)

Indeed, the tight colonial budget constrained the good intentions of the doctors. Certainly as well, the negligent mental health services reflected a narrow understanding of the needs of West African patients. These constraints added to a general reluctance to take mental illness among Africans seriously. Indeed, mental illness among Africans was nearly invisible to the colonial authorities. Traditional healers and marabouts had highly developed techniques for caring for the mentally ill, who usually were reintegrated back into their families and villages. Only the most severely stricken, or those without wealth or family, would have become errant vagabonds and drawn the attention of the authorities. Yet the colonial doctors took a dim view of the healers and marabouts, who were viewed as enmired in hopeless superstition and unreason and given to violent treatment of the mentally ill.

Dr. Gustave Martin and Dr. Huot exemplify a colonial medical perspective on marabouts and healers. They reported from Gabon to provide more material for the comprehensive Reboul and Régis report of 1912 (Reboul and Régis 1912, p. 101). They expressed exasperation at the reluctance of the Gabonese to fault the guilty, and recriminated against their attribution of mental illness to evil spirits:

> For them, every *aliéné* is a victim of an evil genie (*N'Kinda*), or of the spirit of an enemy dead for any length of time (*Iguambé*), who out of vengeance haunts his brain, troubles his reason, blinds his understanding, annihilates his personality and makes him commit the most disorderly acts.

They characterized the treatment for madness as reminiscent of former French beliefs in spirit possession and described the violent methods used to encourage the evil spirit to leave the person's body. The patient was "tied up, denied food, and ridden with blows in a direct attempt to drive the spirit to abandon its victim" (Reboul and Régis, p. 101). Dr. Huot contended, and Reboul and Régis concurred, that this view of mental illness was nothing other than "the doctrine of demonic possession, as old as the world" (Reboul and Régis, p. 101). The professional psychiatrist's disdain for belief in demon possession prevented any more nuanced interpretation of the Gabonese beliefs or practices. This dismissive perspective was first corrected in professional writing by Roger Bastide's discussion of possession in 1958. The reported brutality of the healers' methods contrasts sharply with post-colonial Fann reports.

During the 1896 debate, M. Aumont championed the idea of transporting severe and chronically ill individuals to asylums in the south of France. This plan promised improved care for the ill without entailing the expense of building an asylum in Senegal. This ambitious plan of transportation, however, failed to consider how French doctors would offer therapeutic care for the transported West Africans. The chief source on this internment in France is Dr. Borreil's 1908 medical thesis. As with other reports on West Africans and psychiatry from this period, this report by Borreil was adopted into the Reboul and Régis report of 1912. The language barrier frequently posed difficulties in West Africa, where nonetheless translators might be found for minor dialects. Such translators were unavailable in the south of France. This was just one of many incongruities to the humanitarian transportation plan. The Conseil General adopted Aumont's proposal in 1897 and made plans to ship the severe or chronically ill to the Saint-Pierre asylum in Marseille. For the price of two francs per day, the Marseille asylum provided all necessary medical care, food, clothing, and general up-keep. In choosing to send their *aliénés* to the Saint-Pierre asylum, the civil authorities of Senegal copied a tactic from the French military. As early as 1886, Senegalese who served in the French military were sent to Saint-Pierre. The government of Senegal first approved a nine-year contract with Saint-Pierre, and then in 1905 renewed this contract for another term. However, a cholera epidemic at Saint-Pierre forced a change. Beginning in 1911, Senegalese soldiers in the navy shipped instead to the Pierrefeu asylum in Aix-en-Provence. Shortly after, Algerian soldiers also went to Pierrefeu. In 1905 Guinee signed a transportation agreement with the Marseille asylum (Reboul and Régis 1912, p. 95).

Of the four shipping companies doing business between France and Senegal in 1912, only one accepted African mental patients for transportation to Marseilles. A relatively well-equipped ship from Ligne de l'Atlantique occasionally transported European mental patients. However, their specially outfitted room, a spacious and airy 16 cubic meters, was off-limits for the Africans. The company Transports Maritimes booked African patients onto cargo ships, where they were lodged pell-mell, as the captain saw fit. The authorities condensed their shipments, sending prisoners along with the *aliénés*. The *transportés* were accompanied, depending on the size of the group, by one or two nurses, as well as by a police officer and a gendarme (Reboul and Régis 1912, pp. 90–91).

According to Dr. Alombert-Goget, the head doctor at Marseille, from 1897 to the end of 1911, the hospital received 126 transported *aliénés* (Reboul and Régis

1912, p. 93). In the same report, Alombert-Goget provided precise diagnoses for 119 of the 126 transported: 32 cases of mania, 31 cases of degeneration, 20 cases of melancholy, 11 cases of alcoholism, ten cases of dementia, eight cases of systematic delirium, five cases of epilepsy with psychological complications, one *folie circulaire*, and one general paralysis. Out of these, 94 died. That is a mortality rate of 74%. Of 35 West African women admitted in Marseille, no one was ever discharged and 29 had died by 1911. Of 91 West African men admitted, 65 died. The death rate from tuberculosis alone was 55%. Harshly critical of the transportation program, Alombert-Goget commented: "look at what has been produced by the treatment of native *aliénés* in metropolitan asylums. One would not dare to imagine anything more regrettable" (Reboul and Régis 1912, p. 93). In the 14 years from 1897 to 1912 only 13 Senegalese were discharged from the asylum. Eight of these – six alcoholics, one maniac, one melancholic – were judged to be cured, and five – diagnosed with mental debility – had their health significantly improved (Reboul and Régis 1912, p. 93).

Dr. Paul Borreil's 1908 "Case-Study Three" concerned a Diola woman admitted for dementia to the hospital in Saint Louis in November 1906. The impersonal moniker "Diola woman" is oddly fitting, since neither the personality nor individual life story of this woman is present in the documents. Named like an abstract ethnic prototype, she appears for us as she appeared to the personnel in the Marseilles asylum: bereft of identity, unable to communicate, a stranger. Even in Saint Louis she was unable to speak with anyone, not in French, nor in Wolof, Lebou, or Serer. In Marseille her isolation was all the more complete. Borreil described her as speaking non-stop, performing bizarre dances, and making incoherent gestures. Borreil reflected the French inability to read the body language of the Senegalese. He painted a portrait of "a Black dancing an erratic 'bambo dance' in the middle of the courtyard, making bizarre gestures and noises" (Borreil 1908, p. 25). He confessed openly that French doctors have no idea how to understand this woman. The bizarre aspect of this Diola dancing in French eyes is reflected in the contemporary French slang, "*il a le coup de bambou*," meaning "he's mad, crackers, nuts." Borreil portrayed the French doctors' consternation in the face of this physical display. For patients such as this, the doctors simply did not know: "Is the man agitated? Is he suffering? Or is he addressing a perfectly legitimate prayer to his God?" (Borreil 1908, p. 25).

The inability to read body language extended as well to the ignorance of sacred ornamentation. Diola woman is described as covered with various trinkets, bracelets, necklaces, and so forth. Certainly some, if not all, of these "trinkets" were *gris-gris* designed to ward off witches' spells and evil spirits. Yet the medical personnel in France did not recognize these as protective amulets. This woman's profound isolation might have lessened if the doctor or nurses recognized these trinkets as protective amulets. If they recognized these items as a Diolan version of, for example, a Saint Christopher's medal, or a medallion of the Holy Virgin, the basic dimensions for doctor-patient rapport might have blossomed. Meaningless to the attending physician, the *gris-gris* nonetheless testify eloquently to that woman's search for protection from the spirits that plagued her (Borreil 1906, p. 41).

Diola woman, Case Number Three, died 14 months after her arrival in Marseille. By that time, she was emaciated and prematurely aged. In death, her body finally spoke a language the doctors understood. Their autopsy revealed advanced tuberculosis and an enormous kidney stone. Tuberculosis was the common cause of death of the interned Senegalese. The kidney stone, however, illuminated the Diola woman's psychiatric profile. Normally quite agitated and maniacal, after some months in Marseille she had also suffered spells of subdued, seemingly depressive behavior. The kidney stone revealed that in fact she had not suffered depression, but from intense convulsions of pain (Borreil 1906, p. 25).

Meanwhile, the early twentieth-century mental health services in Senegal, and across West Africa remained rudimentary. In 1910 Dr. Morin wrote a comprehensive report on the *aliénés* in Senegal. Large sections of Morin's report are reproduced verbatim in Henri Reboul and Emmanuel Régis' comprehensive report of 1912, "L'assistance des aliénés aux colonies." Morin, Reboul, and Régis record that in the early twentieth century the few Senegalese in custody for mental illness were usually confined in the Hôpital civil of Saint Louis. In the first decade of the twentieth century, that hospital held less than 200 mental health patients. The routine diagnosis for all of these patients, 188 to be precise, was *aliéné*. Nothing more was recorded by way of diagnosis. We can take perfunctory diagnosis as an indication of the rudimentary medical attention delivered. L'hopital de Gorée, exclusively for Africans, during those same years reported treating 43 individuals for mental illness (Reboul and Régis 1912, p. 88). African military personnel with severe mental problems were confined in the l'hopital colonial de Dakar; between 1903–09 this hospital reported receiving 158 European mental patients and only 22 African mental patients (Reboul and Régis 1912, p. 88).

The conditions of hospital confinement were harsh. Doctors working at l'hopital civil in Saint Louis protested the conditions of the mentally ill under their care. They described confinement there as unpleasant and un-therapeutic. The rooms reserved for the mentally ill consisted of five small cells that measured two by two meters. These cells had barred doors and windows. They sat at the back of the hospital, next to the latrines. By way of furniture, one cell had a wooden bed-frame, and another cell had a mattress. The remaining cells had no furnishings at all (Reboul and Régis 1912, p. 87). Conditions at the other Senegalese hospitals for the mentally ill were similarly miserable. L'hopital colonial de Dakar, that served military personnel, had three rooms for African aliénés. These had doors and windows secured with heavy bars and locks. L'hopital de Gorée treated indigent Europeans (very rare in the colony) and civil or indigent Africans. With only one small (three by two and half meters, two meters high) cell available for the insane, confinement at l'hopital de Gorée was strictly short term. Chronic cases were sent on to l'hopital Civil in Saint Louis (Reboul and Régis 1912, p. 86).

Even after 1911 and the end of transportation of patients to France, Western psychiatric services in Senegal underwent only slight development until the end of colonialism. Plans to build a psychiatric hospital languished, apparently due to lack of funds. In 1938, however, the Governor General of French West Africa formally instituted a psychiatric service (d'Almeida *et al.* 1997 gives the text of this law, pp. 244–249). This new law expressed the intent that psychiatric doctors, rather than regular medical doctors, provide mental health care. The 1938 law also adopted a somewhat decentralized approach to mental health care. It stipulated that individuals released from care should return to their normal residence. The village leader had an obligation to look after individuals who might relapse or pose a danger to the others. The onset of the Second World War, however, delayed further reform.

Wartime, on the other hand, provided individual psychiatrists with significant experience treating West African soldiers. The First World War and the aftermath saw the earliest, most serious, efforts of French psychiatrists to treat mentally ill Black Africans. The *tirailleurs senegalaise* who fought for the French suffered psychological wounds from the war, just as soldiers from the other countries. Shell shock emerged in the Great War as a much-debated grievous injury. Angelo Hesnard collaborated with Antoine Porot to write two books in which they described Black Africans' responses to the war (Porot and Hesnard 1918, 1919). Hesnard figures large in the history of psychoanalysis in France; his 1914 book co-authored with his mentor Emmanuel Régis, *Psychoanalyse des névroses et des psychoses*, is credited with bringing Freudian analysis into the French psychiatric community. Hesnard contributed substantially to developing a distinctive French school of Freudianism (1927 and 1946). Porot, the leader of the Algiers School of colonial psychiatry, has a reputation for biological racism that in retrospect makes him an unlikely collaborator with Hesnard (Keller 2007a, 2007b). However, Hesnard's work in colonial psychiatry was less prominent than his position in the psychoanalytic community. He founded the *société psychanalytique* of Paris, and the *société de l'évolution psychiatrique*. Eventually he rose to the rank of Colonel in the Navy. He was a student and follower of Emmanuel Régis, who with Henri Reboul compiled the comprehensive report of French colonial psychiatry published in 1912. At the time of his collaboration with Porot, Hesnard was a *médecin de premier classe de la Marine*, and specialist in neuropsychiatry. Hesnard later on became Henri Collomb's training analyst. Porot had already served as the head of the medical center at Lyon. During the First World War Porot directed a military neuro-psychiatric clinic (Keller 2007a).

The collaboration between Porot and Hesnard linked the psychiatry of Black Africans with that of North Africans. According to Hesnard and Porot, violent outbursts, mania, deliriums of persecution, and anxious melancholia characterized the pathological reactions of Black soldiers to warfare. These reactions were "noisy and ephemeral and often susceptible to cure in the hospital." Above all, remarked Porot and Hesnard, the continued mental health of the Black troops depended on their milieu, "it is important not to let them feel uprooted and so to group them according to their home regions and dialects" (Porot and Hesnard 1918, p. 46). Subsequently, the two doctors described "Blacks and Senegalese" as comparable to North Africans (described in highly racist fashion) and yet, because they lacked the North African "resigned passivity," they appeared even more "openly childish and lively."

Post-Colonial Fann

Psychiatric precursors to Fann-style transcultural innovations in French West Africa include Dr. Cazanove and Dr. Henri Aubin. Like Hesnard, Aubin worked for a time with Antoine Porot. His interest in ethnopsychiatry can be traced to his years working in Algeria (Keller 2007a; Bullard 2011). Proving an exception to the dominant trend of biological racial stereo-typing in colonial psychiatry, Cazanove in the 1920s and 1930s and Aubin in the 1930s to 1950s called for detailed attention to the role of culture in psychopathology (Cazanove 1933; Aubin 1938, 1939, 1956). Cazanove and Aubin recommended that all psychiatrists study ethnography. By the 1950s some psychological testing tried to integrate ethnographic dimensions (Bullard 2005a). Aubin went a step further, to advocate for psychiatric villages in French West Africa (Aubin 1938, p. 164). Psychiatric villages became a favorite project for Collomb, who much preferred them to asylums, and used them as a chance to bring patients into closer contact with their own culture and healing traditions. The resonance of Cazanove and Aubin with the Fann Hospital group suggests that the cultivation of local knowledges at Fann was not just an overcoming of the colonial antipathy for African healing, but that it was also continuous with a certain counter-current in the colonial era.

As the AOF sought independence from France, one of the French tactics for maintaining ties in the region was to create the University of Dakar. This university developed quickly into an important center of learning. Modeled precisely on French universities, the University of Dakar was also endowed by the French in 1957. The French financed the university and furnished and paid for the original faculty. From 1916 through 1953, l'École Africaine de Médecine et de Pharmacie de Dakar produced 581 African doctors and 56 pharmacists. From 1950, West Africans could transfer to France to complete a French medical degree. The University of Dakar's medical school became a full-fledged department in 1962. The Fann psychiatric hospital was housed on the University grounds, adjacent to the main hospital. Fann Hospital replaced the Ambulance du Cap Manuel – a colonial asylum used indiscriminately for such "dangers to society" as lepers, tuberculosis patients, others with contagious diseases, and those suffering mental illness – that was constantly guarded by armed soldiers and cannons (Rainaut 1981). Another late colonial asylum, at Dantec Hospital, consisted of a cage which confined half-nude men and women, who were prevented from any contact with the outside world (Aubin 1938, p. 154). In contrast to these institutions of confinement – and in tune with the broad criticisms of asylum-based psychiatry in the 1960s – Collomb developed Fann as an open facility, which welcomed those seeking aid, their families, and traditional healers in an open-air setting (Collomb 1973). Innovations under Collomb's leadership testify to his efforts to integrate Senegalese cultures into a reformed psychiatric practice. Motivated by an African acceptance of the "mad" as especially meaningful members of society, Collomb opposed the isolation and alienation of individuals in asylums and fashioned Fann as an open-door therapeutic center. Collomb had traditional houses constructed in the courtyard of the psychiatric unit. The doctors instituted a type of "village council" known by the Wolof name of *penc* for the patients and personnel. To integrate the hospital experience into the patient's social world, each patient needed to be accompanied during his or her stay by a family member. The desire to emphasize social context and sense of belonging led Collomb to advocate psychiatric villages (rather than asylums) as the model for care. In addition to creating a sociable and African atmosphere at Fann, the doctors sometimes collaborated directly with traditional healers, and generally worked with an on-going assumption that any patient was likely working with healers alongside their treatment at the hospital.

In apparent contradiction of these innovations, Collomb's appointment as the Director of Fann in many ways mirrored colonial medical careers. A military appointment was the norm for doctors in the French colonies, including, for example, Porot, Cazanove, Aubin, Planques, and others. Indeed, Collomb was a product of a network of colonial, military, psychiatrists. He studied medicine at a military school (l'École du Service de santé de la Marine et des Troupes Coloniales in Bordeaux) and later taught at l'École d'Application du Service de Santé de la France d'Outre-Mer. Angelo Hesnard, a co-author with the colonial psychiatrist Antoine Porot, was Collomb's training analyst. Collomb began his appointment at Fann as a Lieutenant Colonel. In 1962 he was promoted to Doctor Colonel; then in 1966 to Doctor General. Collomb's salary at Fann, along with the salaries of his research team and of the more than 150 other faculty members at the university, was paid by the French state (Crowder 1967, p. 118). Funding for the researchers at Fann – René Collignon communicated privately in 2003 – came largely from the CNRS or from university salaries. After the mid-1970s the Senegalese state took over more of the budget, which drew in more diverse funders such as the World Health Organization (WHO), the United Nations UNESCO, European countries other than France, and some humanitarian organizations (whether religious or of the NGO variety). That opening to global funding hit the financial roadblock that was neo-liberal structural readjustment, drastically curtailing funding for staff, faculty, pharmaceuticals, and the building itself (Kilroy-Marac 2019, pp. 155–184). That globalization of the hospital, however, was still in the future, when Collomb took on the role of director.

Collomb was a military man, and an employee of the French state running a psychiatric hospital at a university built, funded, and staffed by the French. All of this makes it appear unlikely that he would be a champion of traditional healing and a persistent advocate for psychiatric renewal and reform in Senegal. Yet his years at Fann were marked by innovations that continue to provoke interest and admiration, if not uncritical praise. The first president of independent Senegal, Léopold Sédar Senghor, extolled Collomb's work for embodying what he called *l'ésprit de Dakar* or the desire to create an Afro-centered post-colonial nation (Senghor 1979, p. 4). Senghor wrote:

> Professor Collomb questioned the traditional [Western] methods of psychiatric medicine . . . following the example of Black African healers he saw patients as ill, not abnormal. And he used the healing methods of Black

> Africa, that is, healing patients by peaceful methods, using culture and art rather than violence and constraints.
>
> (Senghor 1979, p. 4)

The work accomplished at Fann, and published from 1965 through 1975 in *Psychopathologie Africaine*, earned an international reputation for the personnel at Fann. The scholarship of this large group of clinicians and scholars produced a flood of important publications. The group at Fann was largely French or European-derived Francophone (i.e., Belgian or Swiss). Moussa Diop, a Senegalese doctor, and András Zempléni, a Hungarian who researched *ndöep* and *samps*, are notable exceptions. Marie-Cécile Ortigues was a French student completing her doctorate in psychology when she joined the clinical team at Fann. Her husband, Edmond Ortigues, directed the philosophy department at the University. Together the Ortigues wrote a psychoanalytic study of patients at Fann, *Oedipe Africain* (1984; see also Bullard 2005b). Simone Valantin and Jacqueline Rabain pursued studies of mothers and childhood development (1979). This sampling of the Fann researchers includes just a fraction of the skilled sociologists, psychologists, and psychiatrists who spent years of their lives at the hospital. At least one of this group, René Collignon, a Belgian psychologist who came to Fann in the 1970s, continued until well into the twenty-first century to work part of each year at the hospital and edited *Psychopathologie Africaine* until it ceased publication. Collignon has emerged as a major historian of Fann and published a comprehensive bibliography in 1978.

Collomb tempered the European dominance at Fann by training students drawn from across French-speaking Africa in psychiatry, so that their work became increasingly prominent in the journal by the 1970s. Moussa Diop was an early collaborator with Collomb and was designated to be Collomb's successor, but as discussed earlier, he died in 1967. Babakar Diop, a Senegalese Lebou, emerged as the eventual successor to Collomb. Eric Gbodossou, who had some of his medical training with Collomb, hailed from Benin and went on to become a champion of traditional healing (Gbodossou 2004).

In Nigeria, Dr. Thomas A. Lambo's efforts to accommodate African culture within Western biomedical psychiatry slightly pre-dated Collomb's efforts, and would likely have influenced his trajectory (Lambo 1963; Heaton 2013). Further inspiration for the turn toward African traditional healers is found in the work of French anthropologists such as Jean Rouch and Roger Bastide (Rouch 1963; Bastide 1958). In Accra in 1954, Rouch filmed the annual festival of the Hauka religious sect, which became the basis for his 1955 film, *Les maîtres fous*. Rouch's film documented the possession crises of the Hauka, and explored their cathartic and functional dimensions. Subsequently, Rouch continued on to publish a study in 1963 of the prophet Albert Atcho in Brégbo. Similarly, in 1958, Bastide argued persuasively for the psychotherapeutic value of *candomblé*. Prefiguring the Fann group's respect for Serer and Lebou's divination and trance rituals, Bastide argued that, "contrary to what doctors who first happened upon *candomblé* thought, these rites have a useful role in the mental life their adherents" (1958, p. 227).

If Collomb and the Fann group followed a current that originated in the colonial era and grew more resonant in the early post-colonial, their cultivation of traditional African healing was also part of a counter-trend to the post-colonial centralizing regimes exemplified by the *Diagnostic and Statistical Manual III* (*DSM-III*) and the *ICD*. In the twilight years of colonialism, international organizations, such as the World Health Organization, the World Federation for Mental Health, and the Scientific Council for Africa South of the Sahara, called for integrating local healing into Western medical protocols. At a 1958 conference in Bakuva the final report took note of a widespread interest among psychiatrists in learning from local healing techniques, and recommended further investigation of traditional healing, along with a study of the possibility of the progressive development from one system to the next (Anon. 1958, p. 9).

Yet starting in the 1960s, research led by Norman Sartorious at the World Health Organization (WHO) undertook the creation of a systematized, universal language for mental health diagnosis and treatment. This campaign for international psychiatry has enjoyed many successes, and has positioned a newly universalized language of psychiatric care as the accredited, scientific medium (De Girolamo Girolamo *et al.* 1989, but see criticism by Kleinman 1987; Watters 2010). A new orthodoxy, this time geared toward the needs of "universal scientific research and a universal language of psychiatry" (and, within the global marketplace, of the pharmaceutical industries and insurance companies) replaced the imperial orthodoxy of French supremacy. The *DSM-III* was first published in 1980 (Kirk and Kutchin 1992). The international classification of mental and behavioural disorders: clinical descriptions and diagnostic guidelines, known more commonly as the *ICD 10*, appeared in 1992 (Jablensky 1999). Efforts at the Fann Hospital and the resurgence of traditional healing challenged this post-colonial, globalized, techno-scientific hegemony.

In an effort to explain his own career path and transformation from colonial military doctor to advocate of "traditional healers," Collomb reflected:

> I've been in Africa for many, many years and I've let myself be contaminated. Certain among my colleagues would say that I've lost all scientific judgement and adopted superstitions. Well, I think also that I've reflected long on what goes on around me, and the approach of the healers invited me to think that perhaps something else other than science exists, that explains some types of healing.
>
> (1979a, p. 26)

Collomb recommended parapsychology as a domain even the most materialist scientists should exploit. In yet another article, he criticized Western psychiatry for "banishing the spirits," which, in effect, doomed the mad person to become a "nothing" among his family and friends. "When they look at the 'crazy,' moderns see only illness, nothing else," wrote Collomb, "whereas traditional healers saw the mad as messengers from the spirit world" (1979a, p. 460).

In one of his most widely read articles, Collomb described what he viewed as the optimal relation of a Western psychiatrist to African cultures (Collomb 1973). Every year, recounted Collomb, young Europeans leave for Africa as if they are going on a pilgrimage. Eager for new ways of living, eager to discover values beyond those offered by consumer society, they seek to immerse themselves in Africa, "what they find is a measure of their own sensibility, their openness (*disponibilité*), their own authenticity." Very few, according to Collomb, are actually capable of immersing in African culture, most "play with deculturation, more or less fascinated by the desires they project in a society where they are not subject to the constraints of their own culture" (1973, p. 347).

The psychiatrist who follows this route, according to Collomb, would be able to become a follower of a local healer, and learn his techniques. Once liberated from prejudices that discredit the mentally ill and from Western biological and psychological models, immersion in local healing traditions could allow such a psychiatrist to discover a "new" psychiatry (Collomb 1973, p. 347). However Collomb cautioned that such deep immersion is no less difficult for a psychiatrist than for any other Westerner; despite the best intentions one always remains a foreigner. Moreover, he emphasized that translating the African psychiatry into French forces the recognition that the African beliefs are relatively inaccessible and that they cannot be used by the Western psychiatrist (Collomb 1973, p. 348).

Despite these obstacles, Collomb saw real merit in this type of immersion. Beyond the willingness to question one's own culture and Western science, the positive attitude toward healers and toward traditional psychiatry would inevitably influence his psychiatric practice. This influence could foster better relationships with Africans, whether or not they were patients, and could help inform the general organization and goals of his psychiatric practice.

Collomb's desire to bring traditional healing into the psychiatric arena was susceptible to criticism. Edmond Ortigues, Collomb's contemporary and fellow faculty member in Dakar (he was the director of the Department of Philosophy), criticized Collomb for viewing traditional healers as doctors. This was criticism from close quarters. Edmond Ortigues was married to Marie-Cécile Ortigues, who was completing her doctoral residency in psychology under Collomb's supervision at the Fann Hospital (Ortigues 1984; see also Bullard 2005b). To the Ortigues' way of thinking, traditional healers practice religion, and confusing this with medicine does no one any good (Ortigues 1984). The historic link between medicine, magic, and the divine is undeniable and in cultures where these are indissolubly bound up with each other no easy distinction between them can be made. Such is the contradiction described by Edmond Doutté's book on religion and magic in North Africa (1908). But the Ortigues' point remains worth considering. As the elderly couple explained in a personal interview in Paris, June 2003, once the distinction between medicine and religion has been made – as it was in European psychiatry in the nineteenth century – for a Western-trained psychiatrist to behave as though it had not, risks abandoning science and creating a sentimental medicine.

If dangerous deviation from the norm is the chief marker of mental illness, practicing psychiatry in post-colonial Dakar, in other words in a milieu in which norms were rapidly changing, increased the difficulty of choosing standards by which to recognize mental health or illness. Individuals suffering mental crises, as portrayed in the following chapters, faced similar difficulties. Those navigating a mental or spiritual crisis might call upon fragile or fading beliefs of past generations, Western imports, or Dakaroise local innovations. We might now call such practice neo-traditional medicine, or "invented traditions," or, if the practitioner proved inept and insincere, charlatanism (on invented traditions see Ranger and Hobsbawm 1983).

Among the complications of appropriating "traditional healing" into a Western medical practice is the likelihood of hijacking"tradition" from its own meanings and agendas to those of Western biomedicine. Medical collaboration with traditional healers deliberately appropriates their practices to effect healing. But such collaboration does not participate fully in the rituals and beliefs of the healers. In effect, in collaboration with biomedicine, the healers' art is instrumentalized and shorn of much of its deeper meanings and broader repercussions. The role of the healer as a mediator of social tensions is especially attenuated in Western medical practice that locates disease within an individual body (Collignon 2000).

Cultivating a knowledge of "traditional healing" also involved a problematic project of determining (perhaps unwittingly) what constitutes tradition and who can claim to speak for it. Taking seriously the thrust of historical change makes it difficult to invest the term "traditional healer" with a clear meaning. While Collomb was not unaware of historical forces, he did not turn his accomplished intellect to sociologically profile "traditional healers," nor even to give a clear definition of what he considered a traditional healer, versus for example a "charlatan." Indeed mental health researchers in the 1960s and 1970s were not especially interested in the politics involved in "inventing tradition." The small treatise published in 1974 by Danielle Storper-Perez, *La folie colonisé*, is the notable exception. Only in 1983 did scholars gain a much-needed critical edge on the complexity of inventing traditions (Ranger and Hobsbawm 1983).

In 1974 Collomb joined the efforts of traditional healers to organize a demand for state certification or testament to their status and skill as healers. Collomb envisioned such accreditation leading to their increasing integration into psychiatric services (Collomb 1973, p. 356). Collomb's advocacy reflected a broad current in post-colonial medicine concerning the difficult position of traditional healers in the 1970s, since they had no official status or recognition (for a sense of this era see Ademuwagun *et al.* 1979).

In July of 1975 Senegalese law 75–80, prompted in part by the research of the Fann group, recognized the role of traditional healers in treating mental illness (Collignon 2000). Notably, restrictions on healers practicing in areas of general medicine have not been relaxed in Senegal as they have, for example, in 2004 for *sangomas* in South Africa. The Senegalese legislation was re-enforced by the

WHO policy of promoting the use of traditional healers to provide primary health care around the globe. First articulated in 1976, this policy was reiterated during the 1978 WHO conference on primary health care in Alma-Ata that recommended that states should rely overtly on traditional healers to bring more health care to rural areas (Collignon 2000, pp. 291–292). At the same time, in an effort to minimize costs and maximize availability of care, the WHO aimed to integrate mental health care with primary health care. This policy has been cramped by the strains suffered by healers in working with WHO and by the difficulties some medical professional have accepting healers (Bibeau 1983; Koumare *et al.* 1992). The WHO also commissioned a Beninian doctor who had made his career in Senegal to compile an *Encyclopedia of Traditional Medicine*, thereby encouraging the development of a written, text-based practice out of an oral culture (Fassin 2003, pp. 90–91). It is unclear if this project came to fruition, but significant contributions in this area have been made by Erick Gbodossou, the leader of Prometra (which stands for Promotion de la Medecine Traditionnelle) in Dakar, and Alexis Amoussou, who was the first Beninois psychiatrist and who worked in Senegal in the 1950s.

The WHO policies gave rise to *tradipraticiens* who "invented a tradition" that combined African pharmacopia with some elements of biomedical science. Collomb commented on this development:

> the new interest of international organizations in African traditional medicine (the WHO, OUA/Organisation de l'unité Africaine, CAMES/Conférence Africaine et Malgache pour l'Enseignement Supérieur) is pushed by the desire of the people to rediscover a cultural identity in the process of decay. The current situation is very ambiguous.
>
> (Collomb 1979a, p. 459)

This ambiguity signaled by Collomb endures.

Works Cited

N.b.: citations to works in the National Archives in Senegal are denoted by "ANS." *N.b.*

Ademuwagun, Z.A. *et al.*, 1979. *African Therapeutic Systems*. Waltham, MA: Crossroads Press.

Anon., 1885. French Archives Nationales at Aix-en-Provence, Fonds Ministeriels. *Affair Politiques*, carton 1206, dossier 1.

Anon., 1896. *Rapport Santé*. ANS 2 G 1-7.

Anon., 1906. *Service Sanitaire Rapport*. ANS 2 G 6-21. Available from: https://www.santepubliquefrance.fr/a-propos/services/service-sanitaire.

Anon., 1924. *ANS Sous-serie 6M, Dossier 323*. Available from: https://archives.haute-garonne.fr/n/rechercher-un-dossier-de-naturalisation/n:376.

Anon., 1958. *Report and Recommendations from the 1958 Bakuva Conference*. Sponsored by the CSA/CCTA [Scientific Council for Africa South of the Sahara/Commission for

Technical Co-operation in Africa South of the Sahara], WFMH & WHO issued in London, 14 April.

Aubin, H., 1938. L'Assistance psychiatrique indigène aux colonies. *Congrès des Médecins Aliénistes et Neurologistes de France et des Pays de Langue Française*, XLII, 147–176, 6–11 April.

Aubin, H., 1939. Introduction a l'étude de la psychiatrie chez les noirs *Annales MédicoPsychologiques*, I, 1–29, 1 January.

Aubin, H., 1956. Discussion du Rapport de Psychiatrie. *Congres des Médecins Alienistes et Neurologistes de France*, LIV session, 162.

Babou, C.A., 2007. *Fighting the Greater Jihad: Amadu Bamba and the Founding of the Muridiyya of Senegal, 1853–1913*. Athens, OH: Ohio University Swallow Press.

Bastide, R., 1958. Psychiatrie, Ethnographie et Sociologie; Les maladies mentales et le Noir brésilien. *In*: *Desordres mentaux et santé mentale en Afrique au Sud du Sahara*. London: Reunion CCTA/CSA, FMSM, OMS de Specialistes sur la Santé Mentale, CSA, 223–232.

Bibeau, G., 1983. Regards Anthropologiques sur une Encyclique Sanitaire peu Orthodoxe de l'OMS. *Psychopathologie Africaine*, XIX (2), 231–238.

Borreil, P., 1908. *Considerations sur l'internement des Aliénés Sénégalais*. Montpellier: G. Firmin, Montane et Sicardi.

Bullard, A., 2000. *Exile to Paradise: Savagery and Civilization in Paris and the South Pacific, 1790–1900*. Palo Alto, CA: Stanford University Press.

Bullard, A., 2005a. The Critical Impact of Frantz Fanon and Henri Collomb; Race, Gender and Personality Testing of North and West Africans. *The Journal for the History of Behavioral Sciences*, 41 (3), 225–248, Summer.

Bullard, A., 2005b. Oedipe Africain, a Retrospective. *Transcultural Psychiatry*, 42 (2), 171–203, June.

Bullard, A., 2011. La Crypte and Other Pseudo-Analytic Concepts in French West African Psychiatry. *In*: W. Anderson, D. Jenson and R. Keller, eds., *Unconscious Dominions*. Chapel Hil, NC: Duke University Press, 43–74.

Canguilhem, G., 1943 [1991]. *The Normal and the Pathological*. C.R. Fawcett and R.S. Cohen, trans. New York: Zone Books.

Cazanove, C., 1933. Les Conceptions Magico-Religieuses des Indigènes de l'Afrique Occidentale Française. *Les Grandes Endémies Tropicales*, 5, 38–48.

Clémont, C. and Kristeva, J., 2001 [1998]. *The Feminine and The Sacred*. J.M. Todd, trans. New York: Columbia University Press.

Collignon, R., 1978. Vingt ans de travaux à la clinique psychiatrique de Fann-Dakar. *Psychopathologie Africaine*, XIV (2–3), 133–356.

Collignon, R., 2000. Santé mentale entre psychiatrie contemporaine et pratique traditionnelle, (Le cas du Sénégal). *Psychopathologie Africaine*, XXX (3), 283–298.

Collomb, H., 1973. L'avenir de la psychiatrie en Afrique. *Psychopathologie Africaine*, IX (3), 343–370.

Collomb, H., 1979a. De l'ethnopsychiatrie à la psychiatrie sociale. *Canadian Journal of Psychiatry*, 24 (5), 459–470, August.

Collomb, H., 1979b. *Henri Collomb, 1913–1979; Son Oeuvre, Son Humanité*. Préface par Paul Bournay, Private publication in Valbonnais, not available for public sale. Published on the occasion of Dr. Collomb's death. Available from: https://www.academia.edu/3161787/Imperial_Networks_and_PostcolonialIndependence_The_Transition_fromColonial_to_TransculturalPsychiatry_in_Psychiatry_and_Empire.

Collomb, H. and Diop, M., 1965. Bouffées délíriantes en psychiatrie Africaine. *Psychopathologies Africaine*, 1 (2), 167–239.

Crowder, M., 1967 [1962]. *Senegal; A Study of French Assimilation Policy*, rev. ed. London: Methuen.

D'Almeida, L. *et al*., 1997. *La Folie au Sénégal*. Dakar: CODESIRA.

De Girolamo, G. *et al*., eds., 1999. *Promoting Mental Health Internationally in Honour of Professor Norman Sartorius*. London: Gaskell.

Diop, M. and Collomb, H., 1965. Pratiques mystiques et psychopathologie: A propos d'un cas. *Psychopathologie Africaine*, 1 (1), 304–322.

Doutté, E., 1908. *Magie et Religion dans l'Afrique du Nord*. Algiers: Adolphe Jourdan.

Eliade, M., 1951. *Le chamanisme et les techniques archaiques de l'extase*, vol. 2. Paris: Payot.

Faidherbe, L., 1889. *Le Senegal, La France dans L'Afrique Occidentale*. Paris: Hachette.

Fassin, D., 1992. *Pouvoir et maladie en Afrique*. Paris: Presses universitaires de France.

Fassin, D., 2003. *Les Enjeux politiques de la santé: Études sénégalaises, équatoriennes et françaises*. Paris: Karthala.

Foucault, M., 1961 [2006]. *History of Madness*. J. Khalf, ed., J. Murphy and J. Khalfa, trans. New York: Routledge.

Gbodossou, E., 2004. *The African Concept: From God to Man; An Introduction to African Spiritualism*. Dakar, Senegal: Prometra.

Goldstein, J., 1987. *Console and Classify: The French Psychiatric Profession in the Nineteenth Century*. Chicago: University of Chicago Press.

Grimaud, A.H., 1978. *Les Médecins Africains en AOF: Etude Socio-historique sur la formation d'une elite coloniale*. Memoire de matrise, sous la direction de M. Abdoulaye Bathily. Dakar, Senegal: IFAN.

Harris, R., 1997. Possession on the Borders: The 'Mal de Morzine' in Nineteenth-Century France. *The Journal of Modern History*, 69 (3), 451–478.

Heaton, M.M., 2013. *Black Skin, White Coats: Nigerian Psychiatrists, Decolonization, and the Globalization of Psychiatry*. Athens, OH: Ohio University Press.

Hesnard, A., 1927. *Les syndromes névropathiques*. Paris: G. Doin.

Hesnard, A., 1946. *Freud dans la société d'après guerre*. Geneva: Editions du Mont-Blanc.

Jablensky, A., 1999. Beyond ICD-10 and DSM-IV: Issues in Contemporary Psychiatry. *In*: G. de Girolamo *et al*., eds., *Promoting Mental Health Internationally in Honour of Professor Norman Sartorius*. London: Gaskell, 47–56.

Keller, R., 2007a. *Colonial Madness: Psychiatry in French North Africa*. Chicago: University of Chicago Press.

Keller, R., 2007b. Taking Science to the Colonies: Psychiatric Innovation in France and North Africa. *In*: S. Mahone and M. Vaughan, eds., *Psychiatry and Empire, Cambridge Imperial and Post-Colonial Studies*. New York: Palgrave Macmillan, 17–40.

Kilroy-Marac, K., 2019. *An Impossible Inheritance: Potcolonial Psychiatry and the Work of Memory in a West African Clinic*. Berkeley, CA: University of California Press.

Kirk, S.A. and Kutchin, H., 1992. *The Selling of DSM: The Rhetoric of Science in Psychiatry*. London: Routledge.

Kleinman, A., 1987. Anthropology and Psychiatry: The Role of Culture in Cross-Cultural Research on Illness. *British Journal of Psychiatry*, 151, 447–454.

Koumare, B., Coudray, J.-P. and Miquel-Garcia, E., 1992. L'Assistance psychiatrique au Mali; B propos du placement des patients psychiatriques chroniques auprès de tradipraticiens. *Psychopathologie Africaine*, XXIV (2), 135–148.

Lambo, T., 1963. *African Traditional Beliefs: Concepts of Health and Medical Practice*. Ibadan: Ibadan University Press.

Lateef, N., 1973. Diverse Capacities of the Marabout. *Psychopathologie Africaine*, IX (1), 111–130.

Leenhardt, M., 1971 [1947]. *Do Kamo: La personne et le mythe dans le monde mélanésien*. Paris: Gallimard.

Letailleur, M., Demay, J. and Morin, J., 1955. Délire collectif de sorcellerie. *Congrès des Medecins aliénistes et neurologistes de France et des pays de langue française*, LIII, 254–258.

Martino, P. and Ortigues, M.C., 1965. Psychologie Clinique et psychiatrie en milieu Africain. *Psychopathologie Africaine*, 1 (2), 240–253.

Martino, P., Zempleni, A. and Collomb, H., 1965. Délire et représentations culturelles (à propos du meutre d'un sorcier). *Psychopathologie Africaine*, 1 (1), 151–157.

Monteil, V., 1980. *L'Islam noir; Une religion à la conquête de l'Afrique*. Paris: Seuil.

Morin, D., 1910. *Rapport*. ANS versement 163, 1 H 74. Available from: https://core.ac.uk/download/pdf/14520157.pdf.

Ortigues, M.C. and Ortigues, E., 1984. *Oedipe Africain*, 3rd ed. Paris: L'Harmattan.

Porot, A. and Hesnard, A., 1918. *L'Expertise mentale militaire*. Paris: Masson & Cie.

Porot, A. and Hesnard, A., 1919. *Psychiatrie de Guerre; étude clinique*. de M. le médecin-inspecteur Simonin, Préface. Paris: Felix Alcan.

Rabain, J., 1979 [1994]. *L'enfant du lignage; du sevrage B la classe d'âge*. Paris: Payot.

Rainaut, J., 1981. Historique de la creation du service de neuropsychiatrie de Fann. *Psychopathologie Africaine*, XVII, 431–435.

Ranger, T. and Hobsbawm, E., 1983. *The Invention of Tradition*. New York: Cambridge University Press.

Rapport Politique, 1926, *Sous Serie 6M 323*. Available from: https://fr.wikipedia.org/wiki/Raymond_Poincar%C3%A9.

Reboul, H. and Régis, E., 1912. *L'assistance des aliénés aux colonies*. Rapport au Congrès des médecins aliénistes et neurologistes de France et des pays de langue française, XXII session, Tunis. Paris: l'Académie de Médecine, 1–7 avril.

Régis, E. and Hesnard, A., 1914. *Psychoanalyse des névroses et des psychoses, ses applications médicales et extra-médicales*. Paris: F. Alcan.

Robinson, D., 2000. *Paths of Accommodation; Muslim Societies and French Colonial Authorities in Senegal and Mauriania, 1880–1920*. Athens, OH: Ohio University Press.

Rosenbloom, M., 2002. Chlorpromazine and the Psychopharmacologic Revolution. *Journal of the American Medical Association*, 287 (14), 1860–1861.

Rouch, J., 1954. *Les maîtres fous* (film). Available from: https://en.wikipedia.org/wiki/Les_ma%C3%AEtres_fous.

Rouch, J., 1963. Introduction à l'étude de la communauté de Brégbo. *Journal de la société des Africanistes*, XXXIII (i), 129–202.

Sadowsky, J., 1999. *Imperial Bedlam: Institutions of Madness in Colonial Southwest Nigeria*. Berkeley, CA: University of California Press.

Seck, B., Stephany, J., Koumare, B., Stach, H., Dia, S. et Gbikpi, P., 1981.Un modèle de désinstitutionnalisation au Sénégal; Le dispositif itinérant d'Assistance aux Malades Mentaux (D.I.A.M.M.). *Psychopathologie Africaine*, XVII (1–3), 271–278.

Senghor, L.S., 1979. Lettre. Reproduced *In*: H. Collomb, ed., *Professeur agrégé de médecine, 1913–1979; Son Oeuvre, Son Humanité*. Préface par Paul Bournay, Private publication in Valbonnais, not available for public sale. Published on the Occasion of Dr. Collomb's Death, 4. Available from: https://www.persee.fr/authority/38870.

Storper-Perez, D., 1974. *La folie colonisé*. Paris: Karthala.
Watters, E., 2010. *Crazy Like Us: The Globalization of the American Psyche*. New York: Free Press.

****

****

2 Physiology of Trauma, Fear, and Anxiety

Polyvagal Theory

Introduction

Psychiatry and psychotherapy seek to heal those afflicted with cognitive and emotional disorder, yet sure advances in this field remain difficult and controversial. This chapter provides a twenty-first-century book-end, to clarify our perspective on 1960s and 1970s Fann clinical practice. Advanced theory in affective neuroscience and psychophysiology boasts of roots in the work of the nineteenth-century French physiologist Claude Bernard (1872). To Bernard and to Charles Darwin, who followed Bernard's work, the vagal nerve – that connects the heart, lungs and viscera directly to the brain stem – provides biological proof of the direct link between mind, body, and emotion. Darwin wrote,

> When the mind is strongly excited, we might expect that it would instantly affect in a direct manner the heart; and this is universally acknowledged and felt to be the case. Claude Bernard also repeatedly insists, and this deserves special attention, that when the heart is affected it reacts on the brain; and the state of the brain again reacts through the pneumo-gastric nerve [now known as "the vagal nerve"] on the heart; so that under any excitement there will be much mutual action and reaction between these, the two most important organs of the body.
>
> (1872, p. 69, as cited in Park and Thayer 2014)

This chapter presents an emergent paradigm in physiological mental health research and treatments. This physiological perspective remains a minority outlook and the most popular statement of it (Stephen Porges 2011, 2017a, 2017b) has met some criticism. Nonetheless, this physiological paradigm is a deeply useful corrective to the standard cranio-centric perspective on sciences and medicine concerning disorders treated by psychiatrists and psychologists. Notice in the directly preceding sentence, the complicated dance to avoid the term *mental* health. Indeed, in the very term "mental illness" we encounter the bias for a cranio-centric focus. The physiological perspective might more easily be said to focus on malfunctions of the autonomic nervous system that give rise to chronic physiological dysregulation and broken social relationships that are narrativized

DOI: 10.4324/9781003112143-3

and fed back into an on-going lived cycle. "Mental health" and "mental illness," from the perspective of PVT, are inept if pithy summary expressions of such complex cycles of dysfunction. This chapter presents the physiological paradigm, and concludes with reflections on how this paradigm helps us to achieve a new historical perspective on the mid-twentieth-century innovations at Fann hospital.

Physiology and Mind

French psychiatry originated in the materialist science of physiology (Goldstein 1987). Pioneers in the field – including Philippe Pinel, Jean-Etienne-Dominique Esquirol, François-Joseph-Victor Broussais, and Franz Josef Gall – assiduously studied autopsies in order to discover the organic lesions that they insisted had provoked symptoms among their patients (Goldstein 1987, p. 251). This emphasis on physiological origins of mental illness opposed the dominant metaphysical and religious perspectives on the human soul or spirit. For example, in 1818 Esquirol claimed that "the traverse colon was often displaced into a perpendicular or oblique position" in melancholics and others who had died while mentally ill (Goldstein 1987, p. 251). The physiologist's interest in displaced viscera as the organic disorder at the root of mental symptoms finds a distant echo in the PVT currently advanced by Stephen Porges. Moreover, these early physicians of the psyche acknowledged the reciprocal conditioning of the individuals' physical and moral state (Goldstein 1987, p. 264). Disequilibrium of the body provoked disequilibrium of the mind, and once in a fearful and anxious state, the mind itself could drive further physical symptoms.

The nineteenth-century physiological point of view is represented in the writings of the immensely influential Auguste Comte. To escape metaphysical thinking that postulated an indissoluble soul, Comte physicalized the self. He joined with Francis Gall and Johann Spurzheim, and studied as well the cerebral neurology of Joseph Broussais (Bullard 2000, p. 111). Human nature, he explained, is not primarily locatable in the intellect. Rather, Comte argued for recognition of "the relations which unify the affective life and the active life to the heart and to the character" (Comte 1851, as cited in Bullard 2000, p. 111). Abstracting the mind from the body, or abstracting the intellect from emotions, vitiated that which it meant to study. Comte did not even believe that thoughts arose first in the mind. Rather he squarely centered the instigation of thoughts in the physicality of desire and instinct. Comte insisted that "man only thinks and knows in order to act or to love, that is, to love oneself or to love another" (Comte 1851, as cited in Bullard 2000, p. 112). Comte expressed the same thought more pithily when he wrote that humans "act out of affection and think in order to act" (Comte 1851 as cited in Bullard 2000, p. 111). The key to human liberty, for Comte, was the freedom to express one's desires, to choose one's allegiances and loyalties.

The physiological self, in Comte's mid-nineteenth-century portrait, consisted of numerous sensations and drives, unified and given direction by emotion. Without the coherence of a driving emotion, the self wafted into diverse tendencies. "Distinct, fully independent powers pull [the self] in many different directions, and it is only with great effort than any equilibrium is maintained. At most, *le moi* could be said to consist of a cerebral synergy, always relative and incomplete" (Comte 1851 as cited in Bullard 2000, p. 111). That cerebral energy arises from blood, muscles, heart, and breath rate. It is in the bodily organs that emotions take hold. Scientists such as Comte battled the nineteenth-century religious received wisdom. As French science increased its domain at the expense of religious doctrines and metaphysics, a dense web of scientific studies replaced the formerly unitary doctrine of the soul. The very density of these scientific communities, however, contributed to the unreconciled polarities of treatment at Fann Hospital in the mid-twentieth century. Thus, for example, the ultimate success of Paul Broca in localizing in a specific lesion a specific impairment (aphasia) has prompted on-going efforts to localize mental illness in specific brain regions. The entities scientists research, however, differ markedly. Pharmaceuticals work on the molecular level, and neural networks are measured in centimeters (Boes *et al.* 2015). The best clinicians might combine advanced science of the smallest dimensions all the way through neural networks, physiological state, emotions, and narrativized/expressed beliefs. These so-called top-down and bottom-up explanations are mutually enriching. No comprehensive understanding of mental illness can be achieved from one distinct approach, but the fields of expertise are dense, specialists are jealous of their turf, and knowledge remains incomplete.

At the Fann Hospital in the 1960s and 1970s the clinical practice ranged across a very wide spectrum. At one end: the clinicians eagerly recorded symptoms and the detailed narratives of the patients about the origins and supposed meaning of their symptoms. This top-down narrative focus reflected the vogue for psychosomatic talking treatments in the grand tradition created by Pierre Janet, Sigmund Freud, and Jacques Lacan. On the other end of the spectrum, the clinicians did not hesitate to treat with electro-shock and Western biomedical pharmaceuticals. These "bottom-up" interventions into biochemistry and the body's energy-state proved powerful even when inexplicable. In the Fann scholarship, these disparate clinical dimensions co-existed without reconciliation. The long narrative case studies full of detailed descriptions end with a simple notation of dosage of injections and number of electro-shock treatments. The unreconciled rift between narrativized somatic symptoms and direct biomedical intervention is not a shortcoming peculiar to the personnel at Fann. Precise biochemical or physiological causation of mental illness, despite concerted scientific research agendas, continues to elude scientists. Clinicians continue to prescribe drugs that work on the molecular level and whose impacts are not fully understood. Individuals continue to struggle with physical symptoms and involuntary ideation that they narrate to themselves and to therapists, in more or less helpful or harmful fashion.

Within this trammeled clinical terrain, we must admit that the bi-directional connection between body and mind – already remarked by the earliest French psychiatrists – has been largely overlooked in Western biomedicine (van der Kolk 2014, p. 76). The narratives of the Fann Hospital cases reflect this schism. Elaborate efforts to understand Senegalese cultures and collective beliefs were paired with pharmaceutical injections and electro-shock, but no mediating explanation bridged these domains.

In 1994, however, this type of rift was at least partially bridged by the neuropsychiatrist Stephen Porges in his theory of the role of the vagal nerve in emotional regulation, social interaction, and a variety of behaviors associated with mental impairment (Porges 1995, 2011, 2017a). The multiple functions of the vagal nerve system illuminate previously murky connections of physical symptoms, physiological states, social behavior that gives rise to narrative, and psychological (dis) equilibrium. The vagal nerve system, already recognized by Bernard and Darwin as a crucial conduit between mind, emotion, and physiology, comprises major nerve pathways that connect the brain stem to all the major life-sustaining organs, including the heart and lungs, as well as to sub-diaphragm organs including the stomach, liver, gall bladder, small intestine and bowels, and the genitals. These autonomic neural systems are shared throughout the species, so that this contemporary physiological understanding is global, although, as we discuss later, intra-species inflections can be integrated into the physiological fundamentals.

Porges' polyvagal theory (PVT) has been criticized for lack of scientific precision and general over-reach (Grossman 2019). A more recent integrated model of neurovisceral integration in emotion regulation and dysregulation is less expansive (Thayer and Lane 2000). Indeed, some in the psychophysiology research community have declared PVT dead, despite the fact that PVT is widely influential and the vagal nerve is the compelling focus of on-going research. Thus for example, recent research has demonstrated that the vagal nerve indeed does facilitate human ability to recognize emotion (Colzato *et al.* 2017; Sellaro *et al.* 2018). As well, the vagal nerve stimulates release of epinephrine that boosts memory consolidation in the amygdala (Hassert *et al.* 2004).

Clinical therapists, especially those in trauma-informed practice, have integrated PVT into treatments. J.M. Karemaker, who largely agrees with Grossman's criticism of PVT, pointed to why PVT nonetheless continues to be powerful:

> [W]e know that the vagus nerve is involved not only in heart rate control, but also in efferent and afferent control of the gastro-intestinal tract and other organs (liver, lungs, etc). On top of that it is probably the link between the brain and the immune system. . . . In particular the electroceutical use of vagus nerve stimulation is finding more and more applications, not only for its peripheral effect on the heart but also for central effects, where it had already been in use for suppression of epileptic seizures. . . . [L]et us now look at the broader picture of what the vagus nerve might be capable to do, the functions that have escaped us while we were looking in the other direction.
>
> (Grossman 2019)

That "other direction" to which scientists have been looking is the cranium-centered brain. This return to physiology is, as well as a return to a body-centered self, a self not reducible to what is in the brain.

Porges' PVT re-focuses mental health discussions from the cranium-centered brain to the physiological interaction of the body and brain via the vagal nerve network. Clinical psychotherapists who focus on mind-body connections seek pathways to healing through strategies of physiological regulation – including co-regulation and self-regulation. Notably, van der Kolk's book, *The Body Keeps the Score*, follows Porges' and the nineteenth-century investigations of Claude Bernard and Charles Darwin that documented the intimate connection, via the vagal nerve, between the brain, the heart, the lungs, and the gut (2014, p. 76). These are bi-directional neural connections: sensory input from the major organs travel via the vagal nerve directly to the brain and messages from the brain travel back through the vagal nerve to the organs.

In this chapter we consider the PVT not as definitive theory – even in 2021 empirical research is still a long way from demonstrating all the precise mechanisms – but rather as an attempted paradigm shift in the science of mental health away from the cranio-brain to the vagal neural system and physiological states that interact with higher brain processes. Indeed, Porges, in 2007, described PVT primarily as a perspective that creates a paradigm within which questions can be posed and research pursued. A scientific theory contrasts to a paradigm in that a theory proposes an explanation which can be proven or disproven, whereas a paradigm provides a broad framework for asking questions and seeking understanding. Only within the broader perspective of a paradigm do specific facts become more or less salient (Kuhn 1962). More important than what scientists do not yet understand about the vagal nerve network is the simple fact that the vagal nerve, and physiology more generally, has been overlooked and discounted by the cranio-centric brain science of the late twentieth and early twenty-first centuries. The shift of paradigm from the cranium to the vagal neural network, to exterior stimulation and interior bodily sensations, and in general to physiological regulation or dysregulation, opens up different research questions and different therapeutic processes than does a focus on neurochemistry and the cranium-seated brain. The PVT paradigm encourages research and therapy focused on the vagal nerve's role in feeding body-based sensations to the brain, and on how physiological states condition cognition, beliefs, and behavior.

Porges' PVT is one example of the broad impact of the affective turn in neuroscience on the therapeutic community. Porges developed his theory over a 30-year career of focused empirical double blind and placebo-controlled research. In the wake of such prolonged focus on minute data points he turned, beginning in 1994, to address broader audiences about his insights into trauma and physiological and behavioral state regulation and co-regulation. Through collaboration with leaders in the field of trauma and somatization, including Peter Levine, Bessel van der Kolk, and Pat Ogden, Porges developed a physiological explanation for a two-tiered reaction to lack of safety. The imperative of safety is part of the long-term conditioning force on the evolution of the human brain. As a physiological state, safety is achieved via bonding and proximity to other caring humans. For all mammals, safety is a key facet of survival, necessary to birth, raising the young, and endurance of social groups. When an individual is in a state of safety the ventral vagal nerve slows and patterns the heart rate, and facilitates social engagement via striated facial muscles, head movements, and prosodic vocalization.

The specific neural network that composes the social engagement system (known as SES) ceases normal operation in situations of physiological stress. Danger provokes a first-tier fight or flight response from the sympathetic nervous system. A second-tier response from the dorsal vagal complex (DVC) relies on an ancient reptilian evolutionary legacy of the ability to feign death. Fear responses – whether via the sympathetic nervous system fight or flight response, or via the dorsal vagal feigned death and immobility response – disrupt our physiological ability to engage socially. That is, there is a disruption of the neural mechanisms that allow socially engaging expressions via the head, the face, and the voice. For example, stress causes affect and tone of voice to go flat. When the SES is disengaged, relationships are impaired. Lack of safety, hence, impairs relationships and those impaired relationships can contribute to on-going lack of safety. We shall see how this feedback can escalate to produce chronic instability and dysfunction.

Double Departure

Porges came of age as a researcher during the years when artificial intelligence, computer science, and engineering fostered cognitive science expansion into brain imaging and electrophysiological techniques. His own early scientific research, even before those advances, constituted a double departure. In the first instance, he broke with the "top-down" cortico-centric orientation toward mental processes which overlooks or even intentionally stifles bodily feelings and impulses (Porges 2017a, p. 33). This turn away from the cranium-encapsulated brain to the lower brain and radiating neural systems features among traumatologists such as the previously mentioned van der Kolk, Levine, and Ogden. Those convinced that "the body remembers" and "the body speaks" go so far as to speak of battling against a predominant cranium-brain bias. Such cranium-brain bias is the dominant paradigm; it is broadly shared by major research initiatives and focuses pharmaceutical companies.

Porges departed as well from B.F. Skinner's behaviorism, in which emotions could only be studied as a factor of motivation and were demonstrated through experiments with laboratory rats (Porges 2017a, p. 35). Early in his career, Porges instigated an innovation in the standard psychological stimulus – physiological response experimental model. The stimulus–response equation, for example, featured in Porges' demonstration of heart rate variability and respiration. Inspired in part by a very early twentieth-century German physiologist, H.E. Hering, Porges demonstrated that the heart's pacemaker, which causes the heart to beat at a steady rate, is habitually slowed and patterned by the ventral vagal nerve. When that brake by the ventral vagal nerve is released, the heart races and the sympathetic nervous system engages to produce a physiological state of fight or flight.

Porges advanced his field by recognizing that autonomic physiological states must be recognized in stimulus–response research models. The physiological state of the organism (O) henceforth figured as a crucial dimension of S–R, such that the S–O–R became Porges' new interpretative paradigm. Within this new S–O–R model, he focused on the autonomic neural state as the platform from which behavior and psychology arise (Porges 2017a, p. 41). The emphasis on physiological state as deeply conditioning of behavior and consciousness has more recently prompted the reworking of psychoanalytic theory to prioritize the physiological state (Solms 2021).

Physiological state is easily apparent if we consider roller-coaster rides or thrilling films. These activities induce physiological state changes. Tension, fear, and the rush of adrenaline: this type of thrill is sought out frequently enough to make amusement parks and horror films lucrative businesses. After the roller-coaster ride, the euphoria gradually dies down. Perhaps there is an impulse to go on another ride. When fear happens in more realistic and demanding settings, the impact of the changed physiological state can save a life. However, if a person is in an aroused and fearful physiological state and is required to engage in sociable activities, that poses difficulties. The physiological state will hamper even the best intentions at sociable behavior. The only reliable way to regain a sociable demeanor is to calm down, to regulate one's physiological state, and regain sociable, physiological equilibrium.

Porges' controlled research studies sought to advance understanding of specific neural pathways that connect neural stimuli to specific physiological responses that in turn directly impact social and emotional behavior and beliefs or narratives about the ensuing behavior. For thousands of years, traditions of religion, literature, and folklore have carried intuitive knowledge of these visceral dimensions of humanity. Deep breathing, cultivated by religious chanting and meditation, for example, works to engage the vagal nerve that slows heart rate and reduces anti-social physiological arousal (Porges 2017b). Porges and other scientists in affective neurophysiology hold out the prospect that we will eventually have even more specific knowledge of neural pathways and mechanisms for what previous generations have experienced as instinct, gut reaction, visceral response, mystical experiences, and seemingly inexplicable emotional behavior.

Even without consideration of social and historical factors, far-ranging implications follow from Porges' focus on physiological state. Fear reactions impede social engagement, and lack of social engagement encourages fear. Fear generated by social isolation feeds further maladaptive fear states, and that fear in turn generates more extreme social isolation. In this way fear compounds fear and physiological dysregulation and narrativized explanations grow more entrenched and more complicated. Porges explains that the physiological fear reaction shuts down the social engagement system. Once socially disengaged, any person can be subject to various strategies of ostracizing, stigmatizing, scapegoating, teasing, bullying, violent attacks, and the like. If such anti-social behavior continues or escalates, further fear and isolation push the physiological reaction into further extremes, and consciousness invents more narratives to support such extremes. Fear generates anti-social behavior and that anti-social behavior meets with further rejection of that individual via other peoples' visceral responses and disengagement of social mechanisms. In this process we see the interpersonal, social genesis of illness. The dysfunction is interpersonal, not strictly located in an individual. Words might be exchanged or not, but that interaction will be translated, in each person involved, into narrative understanding. Idiosyncratic narrative typically bears the label "ill." Whereas collective or dominant narratives govern as normative. Only exceptionally are collective beliefs recognized as pathological. All experience in life is susceptible to narrative, however obscure or banal those narratives might be. With a disruptive trauma, the narrative of that trauma becomes a focal point, a type of inflected origin, so that a stream of meaning and action flows from there. The escalation of broken relationships, endangerment, isolation, and then further or magnified endangerment, might continue in geometric growth and complexity. Tangled in the bowels in unsolvable knots, fear reactions engender numerous diagnostically recognized states. Indeed, linking such belief and behavior to diagnosis is central to the existing mental health professions, however cranium-centered medical models wrongly isolate out cognition and behavior from the bi-directional physiological networks.

Neuroception and the Safety Imperative

Porges explains how an individual's physiological state controls and directs consciousness. In his early research Porges explored the "ventral vagal brake" on the heart's pacemaker and how this brake is disengaged via sympathetic neural fight of flight reactions. The sympathetic nervous system reacts with a flight or fight response within 100 milliseconds (Dana 2018, p. 19). This activation brings a burst of adrenaline. If danger continues then the hypothalamic-pituitary-adrenal response will release cortisol within about two minutes. The physical indications include dilated pupils, sweating, and increase of breath and heart rate. These are the characteristic features of the fight or flight physiological state (Dana 2018, p. 20). If this sympathetic neural response is unsuccessful, say, because the individual is trapped or tied down, then the physiological response shifts to the gut, where the dorsal vagal nerve rules. A gift from our ancient, long extinct, reptilian ancestors, the dorsal vagal system can freeze the organism in a feigned pose of death or immobility. The dorsal vagal fear mechanism can release fecal matter and frequently entails dissociation and/or depersonalization (Porges 2017a, p. 58).

Neuroception, in Porges' PVT, is "the neural process that evaluates risk in the environment without awareness" (Porges 2017a, p. 43, citing Porges 2003). The mechanisms of this newly named "neuroception" is incompletely explained by Porges, and has generated criticism, but the immediate sensation of the environment and physiological response is well documented. However, in individuals with chronic physiological dysregulation, neuroception can be distorted. This distorted neuroception and consequent distorted interoception drive an individual's social isolation. Porges explains how bodily response is contingent on mind as much as on stimulus. He maintains that "[t]he debilitating effects of challenges to our mental and physical health, which are often defined as stressing and calibrated via changes in cognitive performance, are frequently less dependent on the physical features of the event than they are on our bodily responses" (2017a, p. 44). In other words,

Porges emphasizes that an individual's physiological state controls and directs consciousness.

Porges distinguished neuroception from perception: instantaneous neuroception instigates physiological state change. Only in the wake of state change does consciousness take note. It bears emphasis, again, that Porges defines neuroception as a neural process that does not involve cognition (2017a, p. 68). Rather, Porges explains that the autonomic nerves evolved to perceive cues and instantly produce the individual organism's physiological response. Routing this mechanism through cerebral regions would slow response and expose the individual to further danger.

In addition to putting the body into specific physiological states that prompt defensive behaviors, neuroception underwrites our "exquisitely tuned capacity" to read other people's state and intention which we derive "from the tone and rhythms of their voice, their facial expressions, their gestures, and their posture" (Porges 2017a, p. 44). Such reading of another's state and intention is normally automatic and unconscious. Porges remarks to clinical therapists, "[w]e may not have the words for this information, but if we listen to the way they make us feel, it will inform our practice" (Porges 2017a, p. 44). Note that the physiological state of the first person here implicates and evokes a physiological state in her interlocutor, so that the two states exist in relationship with each other. This interpersonal physiological acclimation, one to the other, is co-regulation. Ideally co-regulation promotes calm and safe conditions, but individuals can also co-regulate in high nervousness, anger, or other states. Chronic inability to co-regulate in order to reach a physiological state of safety with others is constitutive of a malaise that can be diagnosed as mental illness. Co-regulation can be difficult to achieve: "[t]he process of obtaining the state of shared inter-subjective experience is metaphorically like entering the code into a combination lock; suddenly the tumblers fall into place and the lock opens" (Porges 2017a, p. 49). The communication of safety and trust are vital to produce co-regulation of physiological state. Or, as Porges phrases it, to be "safe in each other's arms" (Porges 2017a, p. 49). Merely looking at another person is a complicated act of engagement and of "projection of the bodily state of the observer" (Porges 2017a, p. 48). Like inter-subjective co-regulation, the system dynamics on the neural level, that is, the information traveling along the vagal nerve, he notes, is bi-directional. As much as 80% of that neural traffic is from neuroception to the cranium, while the remaining 20% is from the brain to the various organs.

Even without conscious recognition of physiological state change, that state change will nonetheless impact the social engagement system and color the individual's experiences and perceptions of on-going events. The individual's physiological state will, as well, register with and condition, the physiological states with those with whom he interacts. Porges reflects on the contemporary American dismal of bodily sensations: "Our culture really doesn't have a place for that, so it tries to deal with this [pain or feeling] by suggesting, 'If you feel pain, take medication so you don't feel the pain'" (2017a, p. 143). Gut or gastric problems, in Porges' view, are indicative of the unmyelinated vagus activation in immobilization defense (Porges 2017a, p. 111). Any number of disorders can arise from acute or chronic activation of the unmyelinated vagal defense mechanisms (Porges 2017a, p. 143).

Interoception and Consciousness

Neuroception happens via autonomic nerves without the intercession of consciousness. In contrast, consciousness – implicating cerebral functions – is constitutive of perception. Interoception adds yet another dimension to the interaction of nerves, physiology, and mind. Interoception expresses the perception of bodily processes, interior sensations, and states. That is, interoception is the visceral communication to the brain (Porges 2017a, p. 142). Solms argues that interoception is inherently affective and, in Freudian terms, represents the id (2012, minute 16:28 & 23:20). Consciousness takes form as narrative, which encodes beliefs and in turn those beliefs condition our perception of experience. In this way, for the chronically dysregulated individual, truth can become highly idiosyncratic.

Interoception that is paired with scientific knowledge and narrative can yield highly accurate renditions of physiological processes. However, interoception that is narrated with metaphysical beliefs can link bodily processes into complicated and far-ranging collective or idiosyncratic belief systems. Once narrative and belief are intimately linked to interoception, the individual's body and mind are twined into a mind-body formation that can be extremely powerful. Such a mind-body formation might be of short duration or might be enduring. Thus, a lunge or tug-in-the-gut might not enter into consciousness if a person is not attuned to interoception. If that pull in the gut enters consciousness via interoception, it could be narrativized in any number of ways, including science-based understandings of nervous reactions, fear, or skittishness. By another person, that tug-in-the-gut might be considered common gastritis to be treated with antacids. Yet again, a gut disturbance might be integrated into metaphysical explanations of attacks by evil winds, spirits, or witchcraft. Interoception of a chronically dysregulated individual can give rise to fabulous narratives and beliefs that constitute what we call mental illness.

Looking back at the French physiological tradition, in the very early twentieth century, the emergent medical term *coenesthésie* (also spelled *cenesthésie*) compares to Porges' interoception. *Cenesthésie* at the dawn of the twentieth century expressed

> the sentiment that we have of our own existence via our vegetative and splenetic consciousness along with our sympathetic consciousness. Indeed, all the organs of our body are tied to the brain by this [vagal] nerve which serves the centers of . . . all the diverse biological interactions.
>
> (Lévy 1906, p. 101)

In a clear anticipation of PVT, *cenesthésie* held that the vagal nerve "continually transmits to the brain real organic sensations without our consciousness of them, but from these continual organic sensations we receive a sense of the whole, of our existence, of our individuality" (Lévy 1906, pp. 101–102). *Cenesthésie* could also include sensory perceptions but these remained secondary to "the interior organic sensations which dominated perception of the exterior world and of our own bodies" (Lévy 1906, p. 102).

Cenesthésie in disordered individuals caused deliriums in which the afflicted felt their body invaded by a foreign presence, either a demon or perhaps an animal. Such convictions could arise from ill-informed interpretations of symptoms caused by specific biological causes – such as tumors, ulcers, or tuberculosis. However, absent such organic disturbance, disrupted or disturbed *cenesthésie* could directly cause *possession démoniaque* and *zoopathie* (Lévy 1906). Dr. Lévy recounted how Parisian surgeons in 1906 operated on one young woman who was convinced she had lizards in her stomach. This passed for "psychotherapy" at that time. The aim of the surgery was to play along with the delusion and to convince the patient the animal had been removed (Lévy 1906, p. 119). After that particular sham-surgery, the nurse gave the mother of the patient a small lizard. The nurse assured the mother the lizard came from her daughter's stomach. The affair was only exposed after some 2,000 Parisians flocked to see the liberated animal (Lévy 1906, pp. 135–137). Lévy cautioned that it is impossible to keep such a duplicitous secret and that, at any rate, the surgery itself entails danger (Lévy 1906, p. 138). The dangers of *zoopathie*, however, loomed large and incurable. Progression of the disease included persecution of ineffective doctors as well as supposed *sorciers*, self-mutilation in an attempt to remove animals such as snakes and ferrets, and suicide (Lévy 1906, pp. 127–130). Lévy documented as well that delirious pregnancy and *zoopathie* frequently appeared co-terminously (Lévy 1906, pp. 114–115).

A decade prior to his directorship at the Fann Hospital, Dr. Henri Collomb co-published a case of *zoopathie* combined with a phantom pregnancy experienced by a Wolof man by the name of Antoine Sy (Alliez *et al.* 1956, p. 846). Sy was a Catholic, aged 26, spoke fluent French, and had served in the French army for six years. His illness began with a physical trauma, a car accident in February of 1955, to which he had a psychotic reaction. His initial clinical exam, in the field in French Indo-China, revealed delirious and persecutory ideas, fear of being killed by his fellow soldiers, and auditory hallucinations of insults and threats (Alliez *et al.* 1956, p. 846). Sy was shipped back to l'hopital Michel-Lévy in Marseille where further exams revealed no lesion nor biological abnormalities. However Sy's persecutory symptoms re-emerged with a "sensation that someone was sucking his blood" (Alliez *et al.* 1956, p. 846). He frequently punched at his invisible persecutor. An auditory hallucination told him when the blow had landed. Some days later he strangled another patient, with intent to kill the person whom he "designated the author of the vampirism" (Alliez *et al.* 1956, p. 847). A few days later he became convinced he was pregnant: "I have two little ones in my stomach, I can feel them, a boy and a girl. God gave them to me. I'm so happy. I'll keep them" (Alliez *et al.* 1956, p. 847). Each night Sy "gave birth by his flank, not only to babies, but also to fragments of babies, and to animals" (Alliez *et al.*

1956, p. 847). His hallucinations and delusions increased, vampires plagued him, preying on parts of his body, but he wanted to stay whole so that he could continue his engagement in the army. He saw himself as an angel with wings. He read his prayer book incessantly. He had two boys in his stomach even though, following the will of God, he had already given birth. After several weeks, these symptoms gradually decreased, and Sy was sent back to Senegal (Alliez *et al.* 1956, p. 847).

Alliez, Collomb, and Vidal described Sy's case as a *bouffée délirante* characteristically caused by trauma that is "lived in terror" which prompts a fight or flight response. In Sy's case, first he fought his phantoms, and then he tried to kill another patient. Once "the storm passes," generally a state of denial sets in, followed by spontaneous remission (Alliez *et al.* 1956, p. 847). The delirious pregnancy and *zoopathie* contrasts to European cases, the doctors pointed out, because of the extremely important role of magical beliefs among Africans. Whereas such illness among Europeans entails general mental debility and is incurable (Lévy 1906, p. 131), for a Wolof like Sy, the strong belief in magic allowed him enough mental resilience to recover his health. Some areas in Western France, the doctors allowed, have similarly strong magical beliefs (Alliez *et al.* 1956, p. 848).

Cénesthésie, the body's sensation of itself, Alliez, Collomb and Vidal emphasized, played a large role in Sy's illness. The generalized anxiety, lived as terror, felt to Sy like someone was trying to suck his blood. In Sy's case, that specific interoception, to use the PVT terminology, was strong enough to instigate attempted murder (Alliez *et al.* 1956, p. 849). Interoception also underwrote the delusional pregnancy and the delusional *zoopathie*. For Sy, these delusions profited from his ready belief in magic. His religiosity and "mystical preoccupations" facilitated the inflation of his ego, the erasure of its limits, and his "participation in the ambient *mana*" (Alliez *et al.* 1956, p. 850). Thus elevated into a mystical and magical state, Sy was able to believe that even though he was a man he could be pregnant. Sustained by a mystical and magical worldview, Sy could emerge from his delusions with his intellect intact.

***

Safety

In the persecution complexes of numerous case studies published by the Fann Hospital, the lack of safety is paramount. Patients routinely expressed severe anxiety, with palpable fear they would be killed, drained of their blood, that their liver would be eaten, or their soul stolen. Safety is an evolutionary imperative for all mammalian species. Porges connects the mammalian neural need for safety – social bonds are required to raise infants into adulthood and for the survival of the bonded groups – directly into a prescription for "responsible humans" to "respect the responses of others as we help ourselves and others navigate in an inherently dangerous world to find safe environments and trusting relationships" (2017a, p. 44). That imperative, to respect the physiological need for safety, reflects Porges' commitment to a particular form of psychotherapy that by any measure is not a clinical universal. Porges' emphasis on instilling and maintaining physiological safety is, indeed, an innovation.

As Porges explains, our species' neuroception provides "an exquisitely tuned capacity to derive [other people's] state and intention" from any combination of tone of voice, minute variation of eyelid crinkle, eye brow furrow, head tilt, gesture, and/or posture. Porges addresses himself to the community of mental health practitioners, but many others make concerted efforts to become proficient in interpreting such physiological expressions. Porges wisely keeps himself within the boundaries of his scientific research and his own theory. It is rather for a history book such as this one to connect his theory to some of the numerous ways in which humans have sought to understand and control this neuro-physiological-social matrix – what might, in outmoded terminology, be called the subtle humors of the body.

Human history is commonly written as the history of about 5,000 years, in which cities, trade, and writing are active. When considered in the time-frame of three billion years of terrestrial life-form evolutionary processes, the 5,000-year time-frame of human civilization is a mere flick of one eye-lash during one blink of an eye. Porges oriented his own research to the very long perspective afforded by the Deep Time of evolution in order to understand the vagus nerve regulation of the heart (Porges 2017a, p. 107). On this topic what he lacks in specificity, he claims in paradigmatic power. "Our ancient common ancestor probably had an autonomic nervous system similar to a turtle. What is the primary defense system of a turtle? Shutting down and even retracting the head!" (2017a, p. 107). This turtle metaphor ignites our understanding of our own bodies as carriers of ancient life history. Porges puts humanity into the context of the eons of terrestrial life-form evolution. The Deep Time frame diminishes the conventional span of human civilization to a very short episode within the approximately 150,000 years in which the human species evolved, and then into an even smaller blip within hundreds of millions of years of evolutionary processes. The civilizations of modernity are of paltry, nearly inconsiderable, duration in relation to the five billion years of earth's existent and the three billion years of terrestrial life-form evolution. When we consider the parochial boundary on contemporary humanity, we can recognize more easily the huge amount of commonalities between current cultures and nations. We can also perceive that the recent two or three centuries of technological modernity are a great anomaly in human and earth history, and pose entirely new physiological challenges.

The vagus nerve is the tenth cranial nerve. It connects the brain stem directly to the heart, lungs, and sub-diaphragmatic organs, as well as to neck, facial expression muscles, and the ears. Charles Darwin, as we noted above, called the vagus the "pneumogastric nerve" (Porges 2017a, p. 167, citing Darwin 1872). Bi-directional information flows in the vagus provide direct mind-body connection, with 80% of the information flowing from the body to the brain (Porges 2017a, p. 170). Porges' PVT focuses on distinguishing different pathways and processes within the vagal circuits. Rather than a uniform vagal nerve, he proposes polyvagal processes marked by a distinction between upper organs and sub-diaphragmatic organs. The myelinated upper vagal nerve tissue is distinguished from the unmyelinated sub-diaphragmatic nerve tissue. That unmyelinated vagal complex is the neural center for all the digestive organs and the origin of gut feelings, instincts, and visceral emotions (Porges 2011, p. 48). The unmyelinated vagal nerve evolved earlier. Porges suggests is it a legacy of our ancient reptilian evolutionary ancestors (see also discussion by Steele *et al.* 2017, pp. 11–14, on evolution and dissociation).

The myelinated and unmyelinated vagal nerves link into the brain stem in several places. The nucleus ambiguus (NA) in the ventrolateral reticular formation of the brain stem links with the facial muscles – these are muscles of ingestion, listening, and engaging others – as well as the lungs and the heart (Porges 2011, pp. 27, 29, 2017a, p. 170). The sub-diaphragmatic unmyelinated vagal nerve (the dorsal vagal, also sometimes called the vegetative vagal) that evolved in our now-extinct reptilian ancestor is tied to the dorsal motor nucleus (DMNX) in the dorsomedial medulla section of the brain stem (Porges 2011, pp. 27–28). Yet a third location, the nucleus tractus solitarius (NTS), is the site of reception of afferent pathways that travel from peripheral organs through the vagus into the brain stem (Porges 2011, p. 28). The DMNX and the NA receive input from the NTS and from the amygdala and hypothalamus.

It is worth commenting here that the amygdala and hypothalamus receive a great deal of attention in scientific studies of trauma (van der Kolk 2014). The amygdala is thought to hold implicit body memories that are not conscious and not located in a time-sequenced narrative. The hypothalmus, in contrast, holds narrativized, time-sequenced memories. Porges does not focus on those brain regions, as his focus is on the lower brain stem and the major bodily organs. This befits Porges' overall interest in recuperating bodily feelings and states from general scientific neglect and reorienting inquiry away from nearly exclusive focus on brain-centered cognition to include the body-based neuroception, interoception, and physiological state.

Humans share the unmyelinated vagus with reptiles and fish (Porges 2017a, p. 170): "Phylogenetically earlier vertebrates had only an unmyelinated vagus, . . . which provided ancient vertebrates with an ability to defend by immobilizing, which meant reducing metabolic demands, reducing oxygen demands, and reducing food demands" (2017a, p. 108). For example, "reptiles freeze and immobilize to reduce metabolic activity; they go under water for several hours without breathing" (Porges 2017a, p. 172).

Thus the unmyelinated vagal nerve gifts to us the ancient animal defense mechanism of feigning death. Colloquially, we might speak of playing opossum. The neural mechanisms that control such an extreme physiological reaction can also induce more mild aversion-inducing defenses. Affective behavior that is hesitant, uncertain, too reserved, cold-blooded, or emotionally shut-down, all of these can arise from triggering the unmyelinated vagal response system. The fundamental trigger of a dorsal vagal (vegetative vagal) response is a neuroception of unsafety combined with an inhibition on the fight or flight response.

The myelinated ventral vagal nerve links to the mammalian social-bond-seeking expressions. When this social engagement system is disengaged, the sympathetic neural reaction seeks safety through fight or flight, not freezing or playing dead. The return to vagal regulation of the heart signals deceleration of fight or flight and return to sociable facial expressions, inner ear attunement to human voices, prosodic voice, and lower, patterned heart rate. This type of physiological state change might happen many times each day. While the social engagement system is working, the person's face is expressive and their voice is prosodic, not harsh and flat. Porges emphasizes that the SES also involves "contracting middle ear muscles that facilitate the extraction of human voice from background sounds" (Porges 2017a, p. 76). The inner ear muscle contracts to allow the extraction of human voices from the panoply of ambient sounds, "[w]hen people are smiling and looking at the person speaking, their middle ear muscles are contracting. In this state, they are better able to extract human voice from background sounds, but they are doing this at a price" (Porges 2017a, p. 76). This price is that when engaged for human voice, the ears cannot easily hear predatory sounds. On the other hand, once a physiological state change disengages the SES, then the person can more easily distinguish threatening noises: "[i]n this biobehavioral state, they can hear low-frequency background sounds but now have difficulties in extracting meaning from the higher frequencies associated with human voices" (Porges 2017a, p. 76). The fear reaction is designed to preserve life, but when we shift physiological state, "there is an expense; we now have difficulties hearing and understanding human voice" (Porges 2017a, p. 77). Physiological state that arises from stress, confrontation, or vigilance impedes the body's inherent social abilities.

This physiological shift, as we have discussed, operates via pre-conscious neuroception at an incredibly quick pace. However, a key component of PVT is that the dorsal vagal physiological shift, reliant on the ancient, reptilian, unmyelinated vagus, does not cooperate easily with a return to the mammalian social engagement system. The individual can get stuck in the dorsal vagal, reptilian state. In that physiological state the individual cannot accurately read the social expressions of other individuals. Indeed, their reading of other's cues for safety and unsafety are frequently inverted. Pain threshold is heightened, so that situations that would prompt others to "fight or flight" are perceived not only as within the norm of toleration, but perhaps even as desirable. This provides a renewed perspective on the classic Freudian repetition compulsion. Van der Kolk vividly described such behavior among traumatized Vietnam war veterans, reporting how "they seek out experiences that would repel most of us" (2014, p. 31). Van der Kolk compared this directly to a patient who had been raped and then took up life with a violent pimp (2014, p. 31). The compulsion to re-enact and re-victimize, in the paradigm of Porges' PVT, is at least partially explained by being stuck in the dorsal vagal reptilian reaction and thus being physiologically incapable of distinguishing safety from danger, and incapable of activating the mammalian social engagement system.

If an individual cannot fight or flee danger, the dorsal vagal response is to shut down, to lose muscle tone, to dissociate, and at the limit, to lose consciousness (Porges 2017a, p. 103). Porges aims to instill a sense of wonder and gratitude for this dorsal vagal reaction because it "enables individuals to experience horrendous exposure to abuse and not consciously feel it and, thus, to survive" (Porges 2017a, p. 105). In this manner, he attempts to upend self-critical narratives of survivors who question their own passivity or dissociation in the face of danger. Porges emphasizes that "when our body goes into certain states related to being traumatized, it is acting heroically. The body is helping us, it is saving us, and our body is not failing us – it's attempting to survive" (2017a, p. 151).

Individuals who habitually re-trigger, who dissociate and seem to live within their own world of terror, are trapped in the dorsal vagal fear response. "There is a problem," writes Porges, "when we use the immobilization circuit for defense, since our nervous system doesn't have an efficient pathway to get out of it. Many people are in therapy because they can't get out the immobilization circuit" (2017a, p. 106).

One Time Conditioning

One traumatic experience can suffice to establish a lifetime pattern of easily reactivated trauma. In terms of Porges' PVT this means that once an individual has experienced immobilizing terror, the unmyelinated vagal autonomic reaction is easily and habitually re-triggered. That is, once a person is initially forced into dissociation in response to threat, that physiological response recurs more easily and can become habitual. Thus, a personal history of trauma can create a lifetime pattern of dissociation, vacant stare, trance-like somnolence, and other more or less severe reactions, up to and including death.

Porges likens this habituation to single-trial taste aversion (2017a, p. 162) and thus objects to most models for trauma treatment, which are behavioral models, including "desensitization, visualization, and cognitive behavioral therapy" (Porges 2017a, p. 162). Porges proposes the "one-trial conditioning model in which, with a single exposure, something gets associated and triggers us and puts us into a specific physiological state" (2017a, p. 162). Porges notes that "taste aversion produces a regurgitative response" reliant on the unmyelinated, reptilian vagus. Like immobilization or dissociation, taste aversion aims to preserve life, in this case by ridding the body of vile, potentially lethal, substances. For example, chemotherapy or radiation treatment can produce a nausea response that instills long-lasting aversion to whatever food was regurgitated (2017a, p. 167). "Once the unmyelinated vagus is recruited in defense," Porges emphasizes, "the individual's neural regulation is different and reorganized in a way that is resistant to modification and natural return to former homeostatic state" (2017a, p. 167). Porges analogizes this single-trial taste aversion to the original trauma and trauma sequelae.

The neuroceptive basis for seemingly immediate or unconscious affective behavior, combined with the understanding of how a life history that includes trauma makes this dorsal vagal neural network over-active, stakes out a physiological proposition for the origins of numerous somatic expressions.

Refusal to make eye contact, absence of facial expressions and of socially engaging eye and head movements, discordant voice, and general social avoidance are some root behaviors that stymie individual well-being. These behaviors indicate social unease and, because these behaviors are off-putting to others, they enforce social isolation. Complicated consequences of over-active freeze neuroception include fits of ungovernable anger or rage, violence, depression, dissociation, borderline personality disorder, and psychosis.

The Perennial Physicality of Life

For this present study, what is essential in reference to the polyvagal theory is the reassertion at each and every moment of the irreducible bodily dimension to behavior, communication, and consciousness. Too frequently the bodily dimensions of soul sickness and/or mental illness are submerged, dismissed, or even relegated to the shameful or allegedly lower type of life. Yet only in and through our bodies can we live at all.

Human bodies are truly marvelous. An adept of any time or culture can grasp their body's intelligence via intuition. The one in all of us makes us all one, as Sybille Nyeck expressed the adage inherited from her Cameroonian snail-women ancestors (Nyeck 2017, personal communication). This wisdom tends to greater accessibility when we have fewer distractions from the intuitive.

Porges' polyvagal theory undergirds the intuitive with scientific explanation while simultaneously removing the overlay of religion or metaphysics that often accompanies intuitive grasp of these processes. Porges writes:

> We can detect and interpret how another person feels, because the nerves that control the striated muscles of the face and head are linked in the brain stem to the myelinated smart vagus. We functionally wear our heart on our face. Our brains automatically interpret this information and our body responds.
> (2017a, p. 133)

Porges acknowledges that "smart clinicians" and individuals who are well socialized could already know this, and that his PVT aims to explain the process. Sages, poets, philosophers, prophets, shamans, marabouts, folk lore, and fairy tales: the wealth of traditions on "human nature" is illuminated by this knowledge of fundamental neuro-physiological mechanisms. As we shall see in further discussions in this book, PVT can help us to understand intuitive and culturally enmeshed narratives regarding autonomic physiological states, whether these are narratives of social bonding and unsociable behavior are collective or idiosyncratic. Moreover, we will more deeply understand the minority status of the therapeutic imperative for compassionate inter-subjectivity and fortifying neuroceptive safety. Indeed, such compassionate concern for safety is only rarely the objective in societies or even in families, which tend rather to hierarchy marked by privileged positions, casted status, and social exclusion.

We all of us, across all variations of humanity, have bodies whose physiological state is controlled via the autonomic neural system. Neuroception produces physiognomic state, in and through which interoception generates consciousness.

Notably consciousness only engages via a body already enmeshed in physiological state and already attuned to social engagement or asocial withdrawal. History and culture twine around the physiological fundamentals in a never ceasing, mostly unacknowledged, on-going dance.

Polyvagal Nosology

Many of the chapters of this book are organized around Senegalese reported symptoms and syndromes. Given the incisive criticism of nosological categories implemented via commercialized psychiatry (Porges 2017a, pp. 74–75), there is no great reason to prioritize Western psychiatric terms. The goal of this book, after all, is to foster greater understanding, not to use insurance approved categories to bill for clinical treatment, much less to prescribe medications.

In *Black Skin, White Coats*, Matthew Heaton endorses the criticism of psychiatric diagnostic categories voiced by Nigerian medical experts, Peter O. Ebigbo and U.H. Ihezue from the Department of Psychological Medicine at the University of Nigeria in Enugu. Heaton relates how Ebigbo and Ihezue "found that overall, 'similar symptom clusters attract widely different diagnostic labels even in a single institution'" (2013, pp. 185–186). Heaton continues: "They were unable to determine if this diversity in diagnosis reflected 'uncertainty on the part of the users of the labels' or 'the inadequacy of these labels'" (2013, p. 186). In both cases this inadequacy cuts to the heart of psychiatry. Diagnosis links symptoms to treatment regimes recognized by international biomedicine. Fundamentally, a diagnosis serves to link symptoms to recommended drugs.

This questioning of psychiatric diagnoses and recommended biomedical interventions is echoed by Porges. Indeed, he disregards psychiatric labels in favor of a focus on fundamental symptoms:

> I think there is a common core of features among several psychiatric diagnostic categories. Not a common cause, but more like a shared effect. . . . There has long been an assumption that if you can give the disorder a name, it will lead to improved treatment and will provide a better understanding of the disorder. However, it appears that diagnoses, especially within the area of mental health, have had a greater impact on the finances of clinicians than on understanding the mechanisms underlying the disorder that would lead to improved treatment. In general, diagnostic labels provide the clinician with the ability to use certain billing codes required by insurance, although labeling psychiatric disorders have had little impact on understanding underlying neurophysiological mechanisms.
>
> (2017a, p. 74)

Porges continues his rigorous criticism:

> [t]here are several underlying processes that cross several clinical disorders. These common processes frequently are not of interest to federal funding

> agencies and disease-specific foundations. Research focusing on these common processes is limited and frequently goes unfunded, since funding sources are directed toward identifying "biomarkers" assumed to be specific to clinical diagnosis. Unfortunately, although virtually every mental health disorder is assumed to be biological and is often considered to involve genetics or brain structures, decades of research searching for an elusive biomarker or biological signature has been far from impressive.
>
> (Porges 2017a, pp. 74–75)

Across the broad swath of suffering that arises from conditions as diverse as trauma, depression, schizophrenia, and autism, Porges sees similar interrelated physiological conditions:

> Not only do individuals with these disorders have auditory hypersensitivities, but they have behavioral state regulation difficulties, a flatness of affective tone expressed on their faces, a lack of prosody in their voices, and an autonomic state characterized by higher heart rates and less vagal regulation of their heart that would support defensive behaviors.
>
> (Porges 2017a, pp. 75–76)

Implications of PVT that Porges Recognized and Other Implications

The implications of PVT have inspired many psychotherapists. Porges himself has participated in an initiative to train the inner ear muscles. Called the Safe and Sound Listening Protocol, this inner ear training offers guided practice paired with specially designed music. Porges came to this inner ear training because of the auditory hypersensitivities that are present in many mental health conditions. The protocol strengthens the ear muscles in order to stimulate the SES, a method he developed because of his insights regarding the integrated "neural circuit that relates auditory hypersensitivities to flat facial affect, poor vocal prosody, and dampened vagal control of the heart" (Porges 2017a, p. 75). Porges has also contributed to a hospital design project, with specific recommendations to control undesirable machine noises. If humans truly understood the PVT views on neuroception, safety and social engagement, Porges suggests that we would design our environments to promote visceral safety and invest more broadly throughout society in reducing sound pollution. As with PVT more generally, the component of safety within this paradigm is itself historical and subject to nuance. Controversies over school and work environments that are hostile, abusive, arenas of cancel culture and micro-aggressions give clear historical twist to how we think about safety. Porges, a neuroscientist with deep connections in the medical community, turned his own attention to the architecture of hospitals and the design of therapists' offices. In particular, he focused on mitigating deep, repetitive sounds, such as from elevators or escalators, because these mimic the sounds of ancient predators and thus provoke a physiological fear response.

The more general contribution of PVT to clinical practice, however, arises from the emphasis on physiology rather than the cranio-brain. Porges' theory has a neurobiological focus on safety and risk, as subject to neuroception, which in turn directly impacts physiological state, social behavior, psychological experience [including social and individual meaning], and health" (Porges 2017a, p. 45). PVT thus re-designates disorders recognized in clinical situations as mind-based disorders as in fact problems produced by "difficulties in neural regulation of specific circuits" that turn off "defensive strategies and enabl[e] social engagement to spontaneously occur" (2017a, p. 45). Porges emphasizes the autonomic, involuntary dimension of neuroception. Thus, he does not agree with the dominant view that atypical behaviors are learned and can be "unlearned" via conscious strategies of "association, extinction, and habituation" (2017a, p. 45). While Porges does not reject pharmacological interventions, neither do such interventions target what he views as the primary mechanisms of the neuroception of unsafety and disengagement of the SES.

In contrast, Porges sees promise in the potential for "neural exercises" that promote regulation and co-regulation, so that physiological safety can be obtained (2017a, p. 45). Such safety, he emphasizes, is not just a highly valuable component of growth, learning, and creativity, but a necessary prerequisite (2017a, p. 47). For Porges the physiological state is a type of platform, or basic condition, from which the individual experiences and through which such experience is understood and narrativized.

Compounding the difficulties of physiological dysregulation and coterminous disengagement of the SES, Porges notes that these inevitably give rise to narratives and beliefs that justify the social dislocation. He writes: "[w]hen stuck in [physiological and psychological] states that do not promote social interaction and a sense of safety, individuals develop complex narratives of why they don't want to socially interact and why they don't trust others" (2017a, p. 112). This inevitable integration of disequilibrated states and experiences into a story about the events, or the day, or the week, or one's character, or the course of one's life, is the primary point of reference for discussing mental illness. What starts as a physiological state can quickly transform into a life-narrative, often with metaphysical or even eschatological dimensions. Through these narratives, individuals "provide an interpretation of their visceral physiological feelings" (Porges 2017a, p. 112), but they do so by drawing on generally received ideas. In the case of habitual re-triggering of a dorsal vagal response, an individual detects risk even though there is no objective risk. From that point, Porges explains: "their narrative provides their justification for not being loving, trusting, and spontaneously engaged" (2017a, p. 112).

The root issue, according to Porges, is an autonomic neural response to perceived danger. That "perceived danger," however, sometimes is not real danger. This happens because our individual experiences teach our bodies how to respond and sometimes there is a memory of perceived danger that even years and years later can still trigger the "danger" alert when there is no objective danger. Porges asks:

> [w]hen this occurs, how do you get a person out of that loop of defense and justification? How do you recruit the social engagement system and inhibit both the sympathetic mobilization fight/flight state and enable the person to come out of the dangerous immobilization shutdown state?
>
> (2017a, p. 112)

The first focal point is for the individual to be in a state of safety, both externally (socially) and internally (physiologically). Overcoming visceral distrust and fear, however, is not an easy attainment, especially if an individual has already developed a narrative which re-enforces suspicion and distrust. The individual who is wrapped up in pain and cut off from social engagement is not easily persuaded to trust others. Moreover, that lack of trust will induce a physiological reaction in other individuals, which interpersonal dysregulation will set off another spiral of escalating fear and ostracism. Professional therapists and councilors are trained to resist such physiological reaction, but negative counter-transference nonetheless produces difficulties in clinical sessions. Such professionals received two recommendations from Porges: first, "empower the client to negotiate safety" and, second, "understand the principles of neuroception that enable us to understand that the nervous system, in safe environments, will respond to certain features differently than it will in dangerous situations" (2017a, p. 113).

The twin types of security – exterior and interior – can pose recurrent challenges throughout life. Mental health professionals are trained, however, only to work to help secure the latter, that is, to help secure interior safety. Either the individual seeking consultation has already secured exterior safety, that is, physical safety, or therapy might help them to be more capable of securing such exterior safety. But the exterior world falls largely outside the reach of mental health sciences. This is, of course, a serious limitation and mandates that any truly successful practice open the individual to other avenues to secure social security. Any honest perspective on mental health practices must also admit that clinicians do not always prioritize interior safety. The history of psychiatry is over-burdened with treatments – often brutal invasions of the individual's body via purgatives, restraints, extremes of temperature, electricity, or surgery – that clearly did have a primary goal of establishing a sense of interior safety.

Indeed, working to ensure the patient's interior sense of safety is novel enough that Jon Frederickson in 2021 devoted an entire book to the topic, with the apt title, *Co-Creating Safety*. Frederickson identifies lack of interior safety as a major impediment to successful clinical practice, in particular with individuals who are fragile. A "fragile" individual is one who frequently experiences overwhelming feelings that defeat their normal coping strategies. Fredrickson writes: "The term 'fragility' is both a metaphor patients employ and a theory therapists need. Theoretically, fragility refers to a weakened ability to bear overwhelming feelings when clients' customary coping strategies collapse" (Frederickson 2021, p. XII). The fragile individual whose defenses are defeated feels as though she will dissolve in anxiety. Fredrickson recounts that

> They may become confused, dizzy, faint, or even run out of the office. They feel as if they are falling apart. And, in a way, they are. Their anxiety regulation fails. Their ability to put feelings into words disappears. And their capacity to differentiate fantasy from reality vanishes.
>
> (2021, p. XII)

The fragile patient, trapped by such automatic and unconscious reactions, cannot respond to reality because he is reacting to his own projections. Anxiety and projections color his experiences and control his life. In this way the unconscious learned habits of the nervous system replace conscious will. Without the ability to engage the will and to act freely, the self languishes, bound in a perpetual re-enactment of earlier trauma(s). These projections that imprison the fragile patient are invisible to him but stymie his longing for love and a meaningful life.

Individuals create psychological defenses to secure themselves against anxiety or other emotional pain, but these defenses are a form of inaccurate narrativized belief that amount to lies that "we tell ourselves to avoid the pain in our lives" (Frederickson 2021, p. XV, citing Meltzer 2009). Feelings that generate anxiety induce efforts at avoidance through "maladaptive thoughts, behaviors, relational patterns, or inattention" (Frederickson 2021, p. XV). The goal of therapy, as expressed by Fredrickson, is to help "us see what we avoid and how we avoid and then face what we avoided. Once we face what we avoided, we can live into life again, walking into the unknown" (2021, p. XVI, citing Weinberger 1995).

The drama of the fragile patient – so deeply susceptible to engulfing anxiety – is captured by Fredrickson when he writes:

> He cries out for help yet slaps away the outstretched hand he fears will smack him. Dreading rejection, he conceals his need. The pain is so great, he cannot bear to feel. He dares not think. And, yet, inside his heart, he yearns to be known.
>
> (2021, p. XIII)

Rather than hold a painful emotion inside, fragile people split the painful emotion from their sense of self and experience that "split emotion" as coming from outside their self,

> Splitting and projection remove their painful inner life and relocate it into the cosmos. The client sees feelings outside in others and forgets they reside in himself. But when he exports his feelings or impulses onto another person, he no longer relates to her as she is. Instead, he interacts with the picture he has projected upon her: a supposedly angry person. As a result, the fragile patient

> feels paralyzed in a world populated by his projections. He longs for love but perceives only the images he has placed upon people. As a result, he lives in perpetual fear or anger.
>
> (2021, p. XIII)

The individual who is caught up in his own projections (narratives and beliefs) can lose touch "with the loving person he knew, and thus, with reality" (2021, p. XIII).

The troubled dynamic sketched by Fredrickson centers on the lack of interior safety. Fear is a response to an objective, external threat, whereas "[a]nxiety refers to our response to a subjective, internal threat: a feeling frightens us" (2021, p. 5). This absence of interior safety is the essential feature of anxiety, and it germinates most powerfully in the individual's childhood relationship with their caregivers. Human interdependence requires that infants and children rely on the adults in their lives, but such reliance brings with it exposure to the difficulties those adults endure and pass along. Frederickson sketches the dynamic in which

> the child becomes afraid of the frightened or frightening parent, fearing the loss of a relationship they require for their survival. As a result, they try to hide their feelings to decrease the caretaker's anxiety and to bring security back into their insecure connection. Through repeated experiences, this link between feelings and danger becomes conditioned, contaminating every invitation to love.
>
> (2021, p. 5)

In such an individual, their anxiety signals that "feelings and impulses rising now could endanger the relationship" (2021, p. 5). Anxiety wreaks havoc on the interior sense of self as well as disrupting perception and cognition. A host of physical and mental symptoms of anxiety can arise, including drifting, dissociation, confusion, losing track of thoughts, poor memory, visual blurring, tunnel vision, blindness, sudden loss of feeling in areas of the body, fainting, freezing, fugue states, dizziness, ringing in the ears, hallucinations, and projection.

The Somatic: Physiology Within Culture and History

In 1955 Frantz Fanon wrote of the "haze of an almost organic confusion" through which "the colonized perceives the doctor, the engineer, the schoolteacher, the policeman, the rural constable" (Fanon 1955, p. 121). This insistence on the physiological dimension of malaise that can blossom into mental illness is now expressed in biomedical idiom via Porges' polyvagal theory and affective neuroscience more generally.

Working with Porges' theory, we can perceive a unification of the biomedical with psychodynamic somatic expression. Previously the biomedical perspective has been cast as a method opposed to the psychodynamic, as in the anthropologist Katie Kilroy-Marac's characterization of the Nigerian psychiatrist, A. Lambo

(2019, p. 82). Moreover, the neural network and physiological state within the body exists in dynamic interaction with other people and their physiological states, so that interaction and relationships take on a powerful role in PVT. This contrasts with a widely operative biomedical perspective that locates mental illness in the mind of an individual (Kilroy-Marac 2019, p. 205).

Interpretation and treatment of the somatic and behavioral expression of mental anguish or disequilibrium belongs not only to the varieties of psychoanalysis and psychotherapy, but also to the wisdom carried in literature, folklore, and religious practices. Indeed, the emotional matrices governed by the vagal nerve network form the center of our felt personhood; it is where body and soul mix, mingle, and live out our humanity. Traditions of meditative deep breathing, choreographed group breathing with practiced intonation (singing), chanting, rhythmic movement: all of these are designed to stimulate vagal neural sense of intra-species bonds and security. Porges himself explored some of this terrain (Porges 2017b).

Our species-specific polyvagal system is a global reality. It is a unifier of the biomedical, the narrative, and the somatic and physiological state, in dynamic interaction with other people and the environment. The PVT offers a type of master-key to a profusion of behavior and provides for the underlying physical dimensions that give rise narrativization. Neither can this paradigm succumb to deterministic reduction and objectification of the human individual, because the vagal neural system implicates complicated communication and inter-subjectivity via the twitch of lips, the crease of a brow or crinkle of the corner of the eyes, as well as via the beating pulse, smooth or disrupted digestion, strong breath and voice, or spasmodic gasps and a wavering tone. Human lives are composed via this social engagement system, and are disrupted when social engagement is impeded by dorsal vagal dominance. All of humanity speaks this language via our physiology.

Nonetheless, these processes are impregnated with historical and cultural dimensions that intersect with and condition the physiological processes as well as the consequent narrativizing. Hewing for this present discussion to just a general outline, we can point, for example, to an environment that is built by humans that can deeply influence physiological state. Social expectations and established narratives – especially narratives regarding metaphysics, the divine, evil, and the spirit world – can govern the narrativizing of autonomic behavior. Beliefs about society, status, and human hierarchies can deeply condition what type of behavior is allowed or disallowed to certain individuals, thus underwriting narratives of conformity or of socially disruptive lack of compliance. Technological innovations can give rise to new possibilities for human behavior and thus new narratives arise within which autonomic physiological states take on new roles. As well, resistance to established social expectations and status mechanisms can underwrite behaviors and narratives that are intentionally oppositional and asocial, thus turning the physiology of fear to an intentional purpose of resistance or revolution.

Porges' polyvagal paradigm changes age-old topics of dogmatism and debate. The PVT does not end such discussions, but rather it reorients them. The species' need for neuroceptive safety, while seemingly a straightforward dimension of individual and social life, in fact is anything but simple. Efforts to secure safety, for oneself or one's children and other family, implicates the ancient struggle for survival shared by all evolved life. As a species, we humans have arrived at an age of super-abundance, but inequity and steep hierarchy ensures that the vast majority of humanity endures dire and often insurmountable difficulties. Conversely, femicide and other forms of violence against women and girls is extremely well documented (UNGA Report 75/144). Just as traditions for generating safety are cultivated, so are traditions that generate hierarchy, privilege, subjugation, and outcaste status. Gender hierarchy and various other bases for caste status and discrimination – whether via occupation, religion, tribe, or race – are pervasive inhibitions on securing safety. We can see that our mammalian need for safety, on which Porges places such emphasis, is pursued within complicated human cultures in which safety is, at best, precarious and secured unevenly.

Our species is, indeed, much, much more than its vagal neural network and physiological states. As Steven Pinker remarks in *How the Brain Works*, "the human cerebral cortex does not ride piggyback on an ancient limbic system, or serve as the terminus of a processing stream beginning there. The systems work in tandem, integrated by many two-way connections" (1997, p. 371). Pinker's popular account overlooks the vagal neural network, but even with respect to the amygdala he insists on the interchange between it and "the brain's highest centers" (Pinker 1997, pp. 371–372). There is, indeed, complex interaction between cognition and emotion. This interaction is an on-going dynamic process. As Pinker writes: "The emotions are mechanisms that set the brain's highest-level goals" (1997, p. 373). There is no simple relation between emotions and higher-level reason, but rather they continually interact and condition each other. The highest goal set by a strong emotion in turn sets off a cascade of decisions, actions, interactions, further emotions, and smaller goals within the larger goal. Pinker writes: "an emotion triggers the cascade of subgoals and sub-subgoals that we call thinking and acting" (1997, p. 373). These are woven and nested together, so that "no sharp line divides thinking from feeling, nor does thinking inevitably precede feeling or vice versa" (1997, p. 373).

Within that dynamic process, physiology never simply disengages or disappears; such could be the case only in death. Physiology, even when it is ignored or actively discounted, is nonetheless always in play. Regardless of conditioning forces, physiological state continues to assert itself as a dynamic factor in either well-adapted behavior or in behavior that is somehow dysfunctional and out of step or out of tune with others.

Daniel Smail wrote that "culture is coded in[to] human physiology" (2007, p. 159), but in fact the process is not a one-way encoding, but a never-ending dynamic interaction. The physiological response to specific stimuli might largely pass unperceived, but state change seizes our attention whenever a visceral disconnect occurs between individuals or groups. Autonomic neural conditioning of our physiological state directly impacts social engagement, which behavior and social feedback in turn give rise to conscious interpretations and narratives used to explain the changed sociability and physiological reactivity. This complex system is also subject to individual and cultural specificities. Loyalty, taste, preference, habit, habitat (environment), trauma bond or healthy bond: these are just some manners through which neuroception interacts within culture.

Humans do not make their lives inside a therapy-approved safe-space. Life does not allow perpetual ventral vagal-induced sociable affect to manifest in patterned breathing, variegated heart-beat, crinkled eye lids, friendly and inquisitive brows, and prosodic speech. The mammalian drive for sociability and safety is everywhere subject to desires, constraints, and conditions, that can mandate more or less extreme sacrifices to obtain social bonds. Mental illness, one might say, is one type of response to the organism's habituation of the vagal nerve to lack of safety, or to safety that is conditioned upon unbearable stress. The term unbearable here refers precisely to the dorsal vagal complex (unmyelinated, subdiaphragmatic) kicking into panic mode, so that anti-social behavior repels would-be predators. The panicked dorsal vagal nerve conditions physiognomic responses that include feigning death, fainting, dissociating, freezing, going numb, selective mutism, unresponsive and rigid affect, shunning behavior, and generally off-putting affect. When this spectrum of behavior becomes the default physiognomic response even in objectively non-threatening situations, the ensuing behavior patterns are narrativized as mental illness.

Works Cited

Alliez, J., Collomb, H. and Vidal, G., 1956. Idées délirantes de grossesse chez un Africain de race Ouolof. *Annales Médico-Psychologiques*, 114 (5), 845–851.

Bernard, C., 1872. *De la physiologie générale*. Paris: Hachette.

Boes, A.D. *et al*., 2015. Network Localization of Neurological Symptoms from Focal Brain Lesions. *Brain*, 138 (10), 3061–3075. Available from: https://doi.org/10.1093/brain/awv228.

Bullard, A., 2000. *Exile to Paradise: Savagery and Civilization in Paris and the South Pacific, 1790–1900*. Palo Alto, CA: Stanford University Press.

Colzato, L.S., Sellaro, R. and Beste, C., 2017. Darwin Revisited: The Vagus Nerve Is a Causal Element in Controlling Recognition of Other's Emotions. *Cortex*, 92, 95–102, July. Available from: https://doi.org/10.1016/j.cortex.2017.03.017. PMID: 28460255 [Accessed 7 April 2017].

Dana, D., 2018. *The Polyvagal Theory in Therapy: Engaging the Rhythm of Regulation. S.W. Porges, foreword*. New York: W.W. Norton.

Fanon, F., 1955 [1965]. *A Dying Colonialism*. London: Bloomsbury.

Frederickson, J., 2021. *Co-Creating Safety: Healing the Fragile Patient*. Kensington, MD: Seven Leaves Press.

Goldstein, J., 1987. Console and Classify: The French Psychiatric Profession in the Nineteenth Century. Chicago: University of Chicago Press.

Grossman, P. 2019. *Re: After 20 Years of "Polyvagal" Hypotheses, Is There Any Direct Evidence for the First 3 Premises That Form the Foundation of the Polyvagal Conjectures?*. Available from: www.researchgate.net/post/After-20-years-of-polyvagal-hypotheses-is-there-any-direct-evidence-for-the-first-3-premises-that-form-the-foundation-of-the-polyvagal-conjectures/5cbea925f8ea527d7746d7ec.

Hassert, D.L., Miyashita, T. and Williams, C.L., 2004. The Effects of Peripheral Vagal Nerve Stimulation at a Memory-Modulating Intensity on Norepinephrine Output in the Basolateral Amygdala. *Behavioral Neuroscience*, 118 (1), 79–88. Available from: https://doi.org/10.1037/0735-7044.118.1.79.

Kilroy-Marac, K., 2019. An Impossible Inheritance: Potcolonial Psychiatry and the Work of Memory in a West African Clinic . Berkeley, CA: University of California Press.

Kuhn, T., 1962. *The Structure of Scientific Revolutions*. Chicago: University of Chicago Press.

Lévy, H., 1906. *Les délires de zoopathie interne*. Le Mans: Monnoyer.

Park, G. and Thayer, J.F., 2014. From the Heart to the Mind: Cardiac Vagal Tone Modulates Top-Down and Bottom-Up Visual Perception and Attention to Emotional Stimuli. *Frontiers in Psychology*, 5, 278. Available from: https://doi.org/10.3389/fpsyg.2014.00278.

Pinker, S., 1997. *How the Brain Works*. New York: Norton.

Porges, S.W., 1995. Orienting in a Defensive World: Mammalian Modifications of Our Evolutionary Heritage: A Polyvagal Theory. *Psychophysiology*, 32, 301–318.

Porges, S.W., 2007. The Polyvagal Perspective. *Biological Psychology*, 74 (2), 116–143, February. Author manuscript available in PMC 1 February 2008. Published in final edited form. Available from: https://doi.org/10.1016/j.biopsycho.2006.06.009.

Porges, S.W., 2011. *The Polyvagal Theory: Neurophysiological Foundations of Emotions, Attachment, Communication, Self-Regulation*. New York: W.W. Norton.

Porges, S.W., 2017a. *The Pocket Guide to the Polyvagal Theory: The Transformative Power of Feeling Safe*. New York: W.W. Norton.

Porges, S.W., 2017b. Vagal Pathways: Portals to Compassion. *In*: E.M. Seppälä, E. Simon-Thomas, S.L. Brown, M.C. Worline, C. Daryl Cameron and J.R. Doty, eds., *Oxford Handbook of Compassion*. New York: Oxford University Press, 187–202.

Sellaro, R., de Gelder, B., Finisguerra, A. and Colzato, L.S., 2018. Transcutaneous Vagus Nerve Stimulation (tVNS) Enhances Recognition of Emotions in Faces but Not Bodies. *Cortex*, 99, 213–223, February. Available from: https://doi.org/10.1016/j.cortex.2017.11.007. Epub 23 November 2017. PMID:29275193.

Smail, D.L., 2007. *On Deep History and the Brain*. Berkeley, CA: University of California Press.

Solms, M.L. 2012. *The Conscious Id, Part I, Neuropsychoanalysis Foundation Lecture*. Available from: https://www.youtube.com/watch?v=s7J1FLZUg3A

Solms, M.L. 2021. *The Hidden Spring: A Journey to the Source of Consciousness*. London: Profile Books.

Steele, K., Boon, S. and van der Haart, O., 2017. *Treating Trauma Related Dissociation: A Practical Integrative Approach*. New York: W.W. Norton.

Thayer, J.F. and Lane, R.D., 2000. A Model of Neurovisceral Integration in Emotion Regulation and Dysregulation. *Journal of Affective Disorders*, 61 (3), 201–216, December.

UNGA Report 75/144, 2020. *Report of the Special Rapporteur on Violence Against Women, Its Causes and Consequences, Dubravka Šimonović, Intersection Between the Coronavirus Disease (COVID-19) Pandemic and the Pandemic of Gender-Based Violence Against Women, with a Focus on Domestic Violence and the "Peace in the Home" Initiative*. Available from: https://documents-dds-ny.un.org/doc/UNDOC/GEN/N20/193/96/PDF/N2019396.pdf?OpenElement [Accessed 19 May 2021].

van der Kolk, B., 2014. *The Body Keeps the Score*. New York: Penguin Books.

3 A Case of Impotence/*Xala*

Impotence focused one of the first cases published by Dr. Henri Collomb and Dr. Moussa Diop in *Psychopathologie Africaine*. The case of Mr. N'D, a 60-year-old Wolof man who had recently married a fourth wife, narrates Mr. N'D's accusations of witchcraft and magic as the cause of Mr. N'D's impotence. The doctors, however, diagnosed neurotic phobia. This 1965 clinical case has compelling parallels with Ousmane Sembène's *Xala*, a widely celebrated 1974 novel and 1975 film. This chapter explores the parallels between the clinical case and Sembène's fictional account of impotence. Sembène's rich and complicated account of the cause of *xala* has compelled audiences since its debut. The rich texture of this fictional account surpasses the case study of Mr. N'D. The clinical case, however, does provide ample documentation of Mr N'D's suffering and of his denunciations of two wives and a marabout for anthropophagic witchcraft. The doctors counter these metaphysical causes with a psychoanalytic approach that settles on neurotic phobia and nervous exhaustion as the root causes of the impotence. Finally, this medical diagnosis is re-evaluated with the aid of polyvagal theory, to introduce consideration of physiological dimensions evident in the case yet not present in the neurotic phobia diagnosis. The doctors' diagnosis exhibits a curious lack of grounding in empiricism while also overlooking details about the wives of Mr. N'D and how their lives featured in the clinical case. Two wives stood accused of anthropophagic witchcraft. Mr. N'D divorced at least one of those. Meanwhile another wife occupied a preferred status. Polyvagal theory provides an alternative explanation of pair-bonding for Mr. N'D's impotence.

Early in Ousmane Sembène's 1975 film *Xala*, in front of her mother and brother, Rama denounces her father, "All polygamists are liars." In this way, Rama argues forcefully against her father, El Hadji's, marriage to a third wife. In reply, her father hits her across the face and knocks her to the ground. Neither brother nor mother make any move to intervene nor to lift Rama, who stays down throughout the scene.

This early scene in *Xala* is consequential. El Hadji falls cursed with impotence on his wedding night to his third wife. He is sure that someone has put a spell upon him. While suspicion falls on his first and second wives, the responsible party declares himself in a surprise ending. Years earlier, El Hadji had stolen this man's inheritance, and in return the man had cursed him. El Hadji's impotence

DOI: 10.4324/9781003112143-4

is finally lifted by this man along with fellow villagers, beggars, and cripples, who gather together to spit upon El Hadji's naked body. This ritualized punishment releases El Hadji from the tangle of theft and retribution in which he was embroiled. El Hadji is humiliated and vastly reduced in status, but also at the same time, he is reintegrated into community among his fellow male villagers.

After the failure to perform on his wedding night, El Hadji confesses to his colleague, the president of the Chamber of Commerce, "I have the x*ala*." Then he walks to gaze out the window of his office and, noticing the beggars and cripples gathered on the sidewalk, he complains: "Can't we get rid of this human rubbish? This is not independence."

The president is quick to help El Hadji. First he calls and arranges the police to pick up the street people, with the excuse that they are bad for tourism. Then the president turns his attention to El Hadji's impotence. "Who do you suspect?" he asks, and immediately supplies the answer, "Your wife, naturally."

El Hadji answers: "Which one? Why? They have all they need. I'm asking you what should I do?"

The president tells El Hadji of his secret and extremely expensive marabout and they agree to go for a cure. El Hadji announces, "No matter the price, I'll pay. I want to be a man." Meanwhile the cripples crawl along the sidewalk outside his office window.

In this scene, Sembène wraps his film about impotence around the unmet needs of the masses, Senegalese national identity, and the kleptocratic tendencies of the ruling class. In Sembène's film, the third wife, who is the nominal threshold upon which El Hadji's impotence is revealed, hardly exists as a person. She does not speak. She does not act. She submits to the marriage ceremony and the marital bed with silent passivity. She is a fulcrum point, but not a personal presence in the film.

In contrast, El Hadji's daughter, Rama, consequent to her early denunciation of her father as a lying polygamist, reappears throughout the film. Rama is the daughter of El Hadji's first wife. She speaks Wolof while her father speaks to her in French. Yet, despite this valorization of her Wolof heritage, Rama also denounces not only the institution of polygamy, but the moral character of polygamists, including her own father.

"All polygamists are liars," she accuses him. In return, El Hadji smacks her so hard that she falls to floor and stays there. It bears repeating that neither her brother nor her mother dare to offer Rama any support or comfort until El Hadji leaves the room. Rama's bold denunciation is deflected throughout most of the movie. Just like the mother and brother who fail to rally to her aid, the plot of the movie turns away from the specifics of Rama's perspective on her father's lying, specifics that are bound up with the suffering of her mother, his first wife.

Instead of looking up-close and personal at the day-to-day lies and denials that sustain a polygamist's marriages, Sembène turns his interest to lies used to secure wealth. Eventually we learn that El Hadji stole in order to marry his third wife, but also, by the end, we learn he even stole to secure financial status for his first marriage as well. "All polygamists are liars," says Rama, and the film leaves us to consider what lies El Hadji told beyond the acknowledged thefts. The dishonesty at the root of El Hadji's high status and ability to take multiple wives blossomed into his impotence. His stealing to pay for a third wife leads him to lose his sex drive, his job, his business, and all his wealth. His failure to pay a marabout leads to further curses laid upon him. At the root of all this misfortune was the theft of a relative's inheritance so that he could set up his first household. Thus, it is the dishonest and malicious theft of another's inheritance, then re-enacted on a national level with the theft of an important shipment of 30 tons of rice, that upends El Hadji's life and sends him spiraling into collapse. Coveting many wives, it seems, is akin to, and even an instigator of, such theft. Impotence figures as the appropriate comeuppance for a man who pretended to status and wives beyond his rightful reach.

Sembène's post-colonial moralism marks a level of personal probity that excites more admiration than emulation. Indeed, the visionary moralist and founding president of Senegal, Léopold Sédar Senghor, banned the showing of *Xala* in Senegalese cinemas. Some 45 years later, Ellen Foley in *Your Pocket is What Cures You*, relates how men commonly marry second and third wives, despite their inability to support them (2010, pp. 119–120). In the words of a woman she calls Faatu, "Here, it isn't even worth it to be against a co-wife, because whether you want one or not you are going to have one" (2010, p. 121). In similar fashion, the first wife of Sembène's El Hadji maintained an implacable veneer of patience as her husband embarked on a third marriage. Indeed, all the misfortune that befalls El Hadji – impotence, loss of wealth, of business, and of status, as well as the loss of his second and third wives – is never because of social disapproval of polygamy. Rama is the only one to denounce the practice. The men in El Hadji's circle are very supportive of his third marriage. Rather, it is dishonest thieving that causes El Hadji's downfall. Polygamy and impotence in the movie figure primarily as allegorical vehicles for these broader messages.

Ten years prior to the debut of *Xala*, Henri Collomb and Moussa Diop published a lengthy study of impotence in the third issue of *Psychopathologie Africaine* (1965). The parallels with *Xala* are striking. In *Xala* the novel (used as a basis for his film), Sembène includes a character named Pathé, who is a psychiatrist and Rama's boyfriend/fiancé. Concerning El Hadji's *xala*, Pathé remarks, "It's purely psychological" (Sembène 1976, p. 42). This reduction of the curse of *xala* to psychology is immediately repudiated by another doctor: "We are in Africa, where you can't explain or resolve everything in biochemical terms. Among our own people it's the irrational that holds sway" (Sembène 1976, p. 42). The person afflicted with impotence, the treatments pursued, and the interpretations offered are explored here to reveal parallels and divergences between the hospital case and the fictional case. In the conclusion we consider the hospital case via the lens of affective neuroscience polyvagal theory. We find clear traces of physiological and behavioral autonomic actions that are narrativized, both by the patient and by the Fann medical team, in a manner that echoes defenses rather than engaging the root cause.

***

Narrating Impotence

A copy of this Collomb–Diop case study on impotence has sat in my files for nearly 20 years. I have hesitated to write about this case for fear of seeming as impolitic, as the eldest daughter character in *Xala*, Rama. In *Xala*, impotence revealed by a new wife carries meaning far beyond the conjugal relationships. In *Xala*, El Hadji's impotence is a broad allegory of the nascent nation that is powerless against kleptocratic governing elites. Indeed, impotence within colonial and post-colonial dynamics implicates national and international politics. In a variety of historical encounters, hyper-sexualization and impotence are twin poles that supported a rhetoric of denigration. Whether the colonized were represented as hyper-sexual and irrational, or as impotent vis-à-vis the French, the metaphorical meanings reverberate strongly (Bullard 2000, pp. 58–59, 2008, pp. 129–131).

However, if we put aside the historian's impulse to politicize and allegorize, discussion of impotence appears as a forthright medical and human exigence. The Drs. Collomb and Diop were full members of the psychoanalytic tradition, which has not been shy of advocating sexual fulfillment. Working together, they diagnosed Mr. N'D with "neurotic phobia" and treated him with talk therapy, two months' sexual abstinence, and three months of anti-anxiety, sedative pharmaceutical (meprobamante, known commonly as Miltown) (Collomb and Diop 1965, pp. 494, 510).

This medical treatment for impotence in 1965 Dakar was straightforward, effective, medical care. The impotence was vanquished and Mr. N'D left the hospital a happier man than when he arrived. However, in Collomb and Diop's case study there is already the very curious denial that Mr. N'D's impotence is related to polygamy. Repeated several times throughout the text, this denial takes little notice of the contrary evidence presented in the text. Indeed, it seems a classic case of denial creating a blind spot and setting off (quasi) magical thinking (for denial as a psychological mechanism see Chapter 7). Some facts are studiously avoided by the doctors even as they advance a theory of neurotic phobia that itself seems in contradiction of the facts. As well, we can point to the extravagant three-month hospitalization for a 60-year-old in order that he recover sufficient sexual potency to maintain multiple wives. The Wolof–Mourid custom which governed his marriages prescribed nightly rotation from one wife to another, so that his time was split evenly among them. Importantly, he owed a duty of sexual satisfaction to each wife. Only in extraordinary circumstances could Mr. N'D suspend this incessant rotation, for example for travel, or, as well, for the interdiction during menses. Collomb and Diop term this religious proscription "a much more beneficent rest for the man than is generally acknowledged" (Collomb and Diop 1965, p. 507).

Thus, despite the obvious circumstance of the onset of impotence upon marriage to a fourth wife, much younger than himself, and despite the open admission that the sexual demand of his wives exhausted Mr. N'D and that the three months he spent in the hospital provided a much-needed recovery from these demands, nonetheless the medical doctors maintain polygamy had nothing to do with his suffering.

How can we now make sense of this apparently anti-empiricist account of the etiology of N'D's impotence? Just as there is a pressure not to impugn the potency of the post-colonial nascent nation, so there was an analogous injunction among the Fann practitioners not to question or impugn the local culture. This is true across all the topics discussed in *Psychopathologie Africaine*. Thus, while many studies in *Psychopathologie Africaine* investigate the psychological implications of polygamous family life, there is a studious avoidance of any statement that might be taken as critical. Perhaps this same pressure led Collomb and Diop to ignore the evidence they had before them and that they included in their essay, in order to claim that Mr. N'D's impotence was unrelated to polygamy and arose instead from neurotic phobia. Indeed, by the simple facts of their account, his impotence is absolutely directly consequent to his polygamous marriages, yet they displace this onto neurotic phobia, as in a parallel move, Mr. N'D displaced his troubles onto *djinns*, *sorciers-anthropophages*, and *maraboutage*.

***

The Clinical Narrative with Comparative Notes

Published very quickly in the wake of Mr. N'D's three-month hospitalization from March of 1965, this case study overflows with vivid material. Indeed, the case study presents much detail – grist for our own understanding – that runs contrary to the claims made by the doctors. Meanwhile Drs. Collomb and Diop obfuscated the cognitive leads, proposed an unexplained dream analysis, and arrived at a happy clinical outcome for the 60-year-old who married a fourth wife. In the end, after three months in the hospital, the monsieur leaves Dakar accompanied by his second wife. Before leaving, she assured the doctors that, yes, her husband was completely restored and conjugally capable.

As told by the doctors, this case of impotence is not about polygamy, despite the fact that it features a man in his 60s with three established wives, who developed impotency suddenly upon marriage to the fourth, a 20-year-old. Collomb and Diop remark categorically, "there is nothing unusual about this" type of marriage among the Mourid Wolof community to which Mr. N'D belonged (Collomb and Diop 1965, p. 487). Later on they wrote: "there is nothing exceptional in Senegal to see sixty-year old men, or even older men, marry virgins or divorced women of 18–20" (p. 509). Thus, they present Mr. N'D's fourth marriage as ordinary, culturally accepted, and religiously endorsed. All of that would indicate that the marriage itself was not the cause of Mr. N'D's impotence.

The case began two years prior to him seeking treatment at Fann Hospital. When he reported to the hospital he also suffered from depression and cénestopathies (odd bodily sensations).

As in *Xala,* the onset of symptoms coincided with Mr. N'D marriage to a 20-year-old as his latest wife.

Mr. N'D traveled to his new wife's village, Thiaré, for the nuptials. He sustained an erection on their first night together, but after falling asleep he had a dream after which he lost his usual sexual ability. Mr. N'D was sleeping together in bed with his new wife when he dreamed that the bolts on their metal bedframe suddenly loosened and fell off. The whole village gathered in the courtyard. Mr. N'D asked them to help with the bolts to put the bed back together. A few people agreed, but others said "'No, let them work it out on their own.' Then he woke up" (Collomb and Diop 1965, p. 488).

After that dream, his impotence set in. First, he could not perform with his fourth wife. This brought on waves of anxiety. Then a couple days later he started having strange feelings in his body (*cénestopathies*). For about a week he could not sleep alone without suffering overwhelming anxiety attacks. The whole time they stayed in her village and even when they left to visit his own parents in the village of N'Doffane, he could not achieve an erection. When the newlyweds finally returned to his own home, suddenly he was able to have sex with his fourth wife, but suffered impotence with his other three wives (Collomb and Diop 1965, p. 489). These wives felt sure that the new wife had put a spell on (*maraboutê*) their husband so that he could only have sex with her.

The husband confronted his fourth wife, and she confessed that she was engaged to a very jealous, non-Wolof *djinn*. In her dreams she and the spirit (*djinn*) had regular sex, which had already ruined her first marriage (at age 17 to a 55-year-old with a first wife). She felt sure, even though she had sought to cure herself, that this fiancé *djinn* would cause impotence in any man she married (Collomb and Diop 1965, p. 489). Mr. N'D nonetheless tried to cure his new wife. He gifted her protective *gris-gris* (spiritual amulets) but each time he gave her a *gris-gris*, the influence of her fiancé *djinn* emerged. Invariably, she would rip off the *gris-gris* while she slept. Mr. N'D felt convinced by his fourth wife's explanation about her *djinn*, and indeed recounted dreams he had a dream of a finely muscled man who looked like a fighter. This dream, he thought, was a dream of his wife's *djinn*.

Still, the husband felt convinced as well that his fourth wife had placed a spell on him, and he demanded that she lift that curse. She, however, explained that this made no sense. Her first marriage was already ruined because her husband couldn't have sex with her. Why would she purposefully ruin another marriage? Mr. N'D considered her explanation, then, perplexed, he sought counsel with his new wife's parents. They swore to their daughter's innocence and suggested instead that it was he, Mr. N'D, who had a "spouse-*djinn*" who, out of jealousy, made him impotent (Collomb and Diop 1965, p. 489). Mr. N'D adopted this explanation as his own. He agreed that he had a spouse-*djinn* who had appeared in his dreams as a young, beautiful woman. He had often dreamt of their marriage, and it was after these dreams started that he became impotent with his other wives.

The fighter *djinn* who appeared in Mr. N'D's dream was the fiancé *djinn* of his fourth wife. The beautiful young woman in his dreams was his own spouse-*djinn*. No explanation could be found for why this spouse-*djinn* had allowed Mr. N'D's new marriage, but the impotence with his other wives eventually led him to divorce his fourth wife while she was pregnant with their child. Collomb and Diop present this impregnation and repudiation of his new wife as a brief aside. However, in the novel version of Sembène's *Xala*, the same events feature as a revenge fantasy. Sembène wrote of El Hadji: "He felt vindictive and was determined to satisfy his urge for revenge. Calculating the expense occasioned by the wedding, he decided his only course of action was to get her pregnant and then repudiate her" (Sembène 1976, pp. 71–72). The doctors make no mention of the vindictive character of Mr N'D's divorcing his pregnant wife. They only note that after their divorce, Mr. N'D was able to manage some sexual relations with his other wives, even though his erections were often soft or subsided during coitus (Collomb and Diop 1965, p. 490).

Mr. N'D described to his doctors at the hospital that whenever he wanted to have sex he would see a flash in the room and hear a dry, metallic clanging. Then he would "feel something indescribable turn in his lower stomach, without causing pain, but his erection would fall" (Collomb and Diop 1965, p. 490). Even when his erection returned it "lacked vigor" and sex was "unsatisfying" (Collomb and Diop 1965, p. 490). After coitus, during the prescribed Islamic purification ritual, he would feel himself "penetrated by a cold wind" (Collomb and Diop 1965, p. 490). This cold wind was the main symptom of his *cénestopathies*. Mr. N'D reported that in his dreams, he still had extremely satisfying sex with his spousal-*djinn*, who took on various female forms (Collomb and Diop 1965, p. 490). However, he also contradicted this claim, stating that in his dreams just as sex was to start, something would happen to interrupt the situation. One paragraph later, Mr. N'D contradicted himself yet again, saying that in his early morning dreams he had very satisfying sex with his spousal-*djinn* (Collomb and Diop 1965, p. 491).

Mr. N'D's *cénestopathies* prompted him to take special precautions. The "cold wind" penetrated his body either via his nostrils or via his feet and, despite itself being a cold wind, it set off an intense heat in his body. He took precautions against this wind by blocking his nostrils and always wearing shoes or slippers. Generally the wind came through his feet when he was indoors and through his nostrils when outdoors. When he blocked his nostrils, the wind sometimes tried to get inside his body via his eyes, which caused him some troubles with his eyesight. But if the wind could not get inside from the top of his body, it would try through his feet and then it would rise up to give him a light erection (Collomb and Diop 1965, p. 491). When he wore boots or thick shoes, the wind could not penetrate his feet, and then it would try his nose. Regardless of how the wind got into his body, it would travel to his lower belly. This happened six to ten times per day, and brought along headaches. Once the wind reached his lower stomach, it would stay several minutes then leave by his anus. However, immediately on leaving his body, the wind would try again to re-enter (Collomb and Diop 1965, p. 492).

Mr. N'D consulted a *marabout* who told him the bizarre internal sensations were linked to his impotence, but N'D came to distrust this explanation and alleged that the feelings came from *sorciers-anthropophages* (*döem* in Wolof) (Collomb and Diop 1965, p. 492). He suspected that his fourth wife, his third wife and her children, and the Fulani marabout he had consulted, were all vampiric witches (*sorciers-anthropophages*) (Collomb and Diop 1965, p. 492). These *sorciers-anthropophages* emitted a violent power from their eyes, "like an electric current," the doctors explained (Collomb and Diop 1965, p. 492). Mr. N'D distinctly sensed this and knew that those people were cannibal-witches.

That *marabout* had performed two rituals in search of a cure for Mr. N'D's impotence. First the *marabout* performed a *listikhar* and then a few weeks later, a *khalva*. The *listikhar* proceeded via a one-day divination that centered on the marabout's dream. He explained to Mr. N'D: "In the night I saw a small female *djinn*. She told me that one day you urinated next to her. For that reason, she became angry and decided to amuse herself by making you impotent"(Collomb and Diop 1965, p. 499). As a remedy, the marabout gave Mr. N'D *safara*, made from water infused with Qu'ranic verses, to wash himself and to drink. The marabout's *khalva*, a five-day process of divination, culminated with a dream in which Mr. N'D went hunting with a rifle and succeeded in shooting an animal, but when he went to find it, he found instead a woman *djinn* with her children. Mr. N'D's gunshot had frightened her and that is why "she made you sick" (Collomb and Diop 1965, p. 499). The marabout explained, "it is the wind that the *djinn* displaced in her flight from the gunshot that penetrates you. It is also this woman *djinn* whom you see in your dreams. She prevents you from having normal relations with your three wives" (Collomb and Diop 1965, p. 499). Again the marabout prescribed water imbued with Qu'ranic verses to be used for washing and drinking. He also directed Mr. N'D to make several sacrificial offerings.

Mr. N'D believed these dream messages, but nonetheless failed to respond to the principle demand of the *marabout*. That is, as with the impotent El Hadji in *Xala*, Mr. N'D failed to pay the marabout. Default on payment to the *marabout*, Mr. N'D explained to the *marabout* as well as to his doctors, arose from the unhappy circumstance that in order to pay he had to sell a horse, but he could not find a ready buyer for his horse. The *marabout* turned a deaf ear to this self-exoneration, and wrote Mr. N'D a menacing letter which said, "You deceived me. You promised to pay me, but you didn't pay me. You will see whether or not I'm a real marabout" (Collomb and Diop 1965, p. 504). The potential for a healing relationship dissolved into animosity.

Such deep distrust and insecurity within long-standing relationships reveals the visceral fear that animated Mr. N'D. Assailed by fear of individuals with whom he had long-standing relationships, Mr. N'D succumbed to waves of anxiety. The failure to pay the marabout which then prompted further curses from the marabout parallels the events in *Xala*. In both the case of Mr. N'D and in *Xala* failure to pay is linked to broader trouble with finances, but the outcomes differ substantially. In *Xala*, El Hadji's dishonest dealings with money reach deep into his past and lie at the root of his difficulties. He has been cursed by a man whom he defrauded in his youth. Mr. N'D, in contrast, suffers a rupture in his personal relationship with the Tidjanie marabout, but no further consequences are noted. Indeed, he escapes that ruined relationship by resorting to hospital treatment. We are reminded of the character Pathé, the psychiatrist, in the novel *Xala*, who remarks glibly of El

Hadji, "his problem is purely psychological." Sembène resists that explanation whereas the doctors Collomb and Diop embrace it.

After about two years of suffering, Mr. N'D came to the Fann Hospital accompanied by his second wife. His three-month treatment regime included two months of abstinence from sex and oral pills of the popular anti-anxiety, tranquilizer, Meprobamate (Collomb and Diop 1965, p. 510). While at the hospital he reported a dream in which a young woman left the home of her new husband. In this dream, Mr. N'D was enlisted by the husband to help bring the young woman back. While at the young woman's parent's house, however, instead of staying in the room to discuss the situation, Mr. N'D went out to urinate. The father followed him and accused him of defecating, which Mr. N'D denied with the justification that he still had his pants on (Collomb and Diop 1965, pp. 500–501).

The doctors Collomb and Diop interpreted the urination in this dream in tandem with that in marabout's dream to indicate a deep prohibition on his relationship with his fourth wife. Despite their several comments that such marriages are common in Senegal, they inexplicably remark that the relationship falls under an incest prohibition as the fourth wife, "about twenty years old" they remind their readers, "could have been the daughter of Mr. N'D" (Collomb and Diop 1965, p. 501). Still, they acknowledge that they have no further evidence for "this hypothesis" (Collomb and Diop 1965, p. 509). To the contrary, such marriages are common and unexceptional, they reported with some accuracy. The emotional account of such sociological data is left out, but implied by the insistence on incest prohibition. The appeal, not explicit but logical, is to natural law, as it appeared in neither religion nor law. Such marriages as they acknowledged were common practice. In 2021 they remain common despite efforts to reform the marriage and family code in favor of women's rights. Proponents of a conservative and patriarchal version of Islamic religious law (*shari'a*) effectively counter and curtail these reform efforts. Later in this chapter we discuss a different understanding of this suggested incest prohibition.

In yet another dream, Mr. N'D recounted, the very young wife leaves her older husband after they argue. Again Mr. N'D is enlisted to help arrange for the wife's return to her husband. In this dream those talks end with failure, after which Mr. N'D walks to his bedroom, but sees ahead of him the young wife about to enter into his own room. He only sees her feet and her shirt, not her face. He reacts to her temerity with a dire threat: "You must not go in my room. If you ever do enter it, I will kill you." At that point he awoke (Collomb and Diop 1965, p. 502). Mr. N'D offered his own interpretation of this dream as a sequel to the preceding one. The young woman, he attested, was his fourth wife. That he only saw part of her – her feet and her shirt – signified her status as a *sorcier*. Despite this dream, he claimed he loved her and stills loves her, but that he cannot maintain a relationship with her. His threat to kill her in his dream signified "that this woman is forever forbidden to him" (Collomb and Diop 1965, pp. 502–503).

The doctors relate Mr. N'D's threat to murder the young wife as a repudiation akin to the urination in his previous dream (Collomb and Diop 1965, p. 503) and link them both to an incest prohibition on father–daughter marriage (Collomb and

Diop 1965, p. 510). This curious assertion of incest taboo for a marital relationship that was endorsed by community and religion must be read as an intentional commentary by the doctors. Instead of focusing directly on Mr. N'D's visceral inability to abide his fourth wife, the doctors turn to an unsubstantiated narrative of incest. Perhaps they intuit that Mr. N'D could not abide his fourth wife, but for some reason needed to maintain silence regarding that antipathy. In this way perhaps they passed over the basic physiological state to an abstract idea, the prohibition on a December–May marriage as evocative of incest, completely foreign to Mr. N'D's own conscious way of thinking. In other words, they are suggesting Mr. N'D is inhibited by an unconscious law.

The susceptibility to psychological impotence, remark Collomb and Diop, is linked to a specific fragility in the organization of sexual functions (Collomb and Diop 1965, p. 506). Collomb and Diop (1965, p. 506) remark:

> Without going into the particularities of Oedipus in traditional African cultures, consider the difficulties of confronting the father and paternal images. The menace of castration only ends with death, which confers definitive status to virility, and definitive power to a man.

After death, man's virility is assured as he assimilates into the unassailable status of the ancestors. Until that end time, however, men live under a constant threat to their sexuality, so that one simple sexual misfire can foster a massive onset of catastrophic anxiety and cascading sexual difficulties (Collomb and Diop 1965, p. 507). Men carry a double duty in their virility: to procreate and to give pleasure to their wives (Collomb and Diop 1965, p. 507). Failure in either these roles throws into doubt their status as a man. Thus, Mr. N'D lamented that each time he failed at coitus, "he became a woman" (Collomb and Diop 1965, p. 508). Conflict with male authority figures, both in his dreams and with the marabout whom he failed to pay, plagued Mr. N'D and rendered his social position insecure. This conflict with male authority figures manifested in the marriage to a very young woman. The impotence, the doctors implied, derived from Mr. N'D acting against the dictates of the fathers to respect the daughter.

Collomb and Diop ascribed Mr. N'D's impotence to psychological causes linked to a disturbed inter-subjective relationship (one prohibited by incest taboo). Added to this was his neurotic phobia of the penetrating, cold, malign wind, which carried its own tendency to manifest in impotence (Collomb and Diop 1965, p. 508). Legible in his impotence, the crime is further punished though the malign wind.

However, his cure, in the opinion of Collomb and Diop, arose as well from the therapeutic relationship with "a psychiatrist of the same ethnicity, younger and with a different training" compared to traditional healers. "From the start, the relationship demonstrated a good quality; not only were the representations of the patient allowed to emerge freely, but they were paid close and sustained attention" (Collomb and Diop 1965, p. 510). In contrast to the troubled relationship Mr. N'D had with the Fulani marabout, "from the moment he entered the hospital he felt relieved. He became less anxious" (Collomb and Diop 1965, p. 510). The young psychiatrist inspired him with confidence to confide his troubles, so that Mr. N'D felt heard and understood, and they had a conflict-free relationship. The ordinary misadventure of sexual failure had elicited a whole series of habitual interpretations, including *djinn* and *sorciers-anthropophages*. These explanations attached to the somatic symptoms of impotence and generalized anxiety handicapped Mr. N'D in his family life, and yet yielded to relatively simple treatment (Collomb and Diop 1965, p. 511).

In sum, Collomb and Diop express satisfaction that the sexual capacity of Mr. N'D was restored and his anxiety diminished if not thoroughly conquered. The importance of complicated narrative explanations faded away with his fading impotence. Both cease to be vital subjects for him as he returned to his home with his second wife. After all, the medical doctor cannot solve metaphysical riddles, but can only promote health to the point where such riddles seem irrelevant, or at least no longer infect day-to-day life with paralyzing thoughts and sensations.

As historical narrative, the case of Mr. N'D lacks the satisfying arc that we find in *Xala*. Sembène's work of art puts into play a surfeit of meaning among which his audience can reflect, wonder, and perhaps find inspiration for new social models. The psychiatric case study, in contrast, supports the healing of Mr. N'D through his successful reinsertion into his own social world. The narrative in *Xala* starts with polygamy, proceeds to impotence and the visiting of marabouts for cures, and then ends in allegorical denunciation of national crimes – the theft of inheritance and of a national shipment of rice. The truth of the opening salvo by Rama, the daughter of El Hadji with his first wife, "all polygamists are liars," spirals outward to include many lies and acts of desperation. "I want to be a man," the suffering, impotent El Hadji pleads for help from the president. Meanwhile, outside his window, beggars and cripples stroll and congregate. This group of men force the viewers to consider: what is a man? If a man loses his sex-caste status when he is impotent, then what actually are all these men on the street whose limbs are twisted, who walk on their knees, or propel themselves with their hands?

Mr. N'D launched a similar signal of distress regarding his manhood. The doctors recorded "each time his erection was inhibited he is no longer a man, he becomes a woman" (Collomb and Diop 1965, p. 508). As discussed above, Mr. N'D's beliefs about manhood vested ultimate power and authority with the ancestors. Any slippage in his own performance of manhood thrust his entire identity into crisis. His claim that he "becomes a woman" reveals his engulfing anxiety. The status of woman is that of legal minor, subjected perpetually to the authority of the male head of household. She is not the one able to make choices and indulge sexual appetite, but the one who must be content to be one among many, to suffer her life in silent obedience. Mr. N'D's fear that he "became a woman" was at best hyperbole and perhaps verged on delusion. None of the actual features of female status applied to him. Moreover, his doctors worked to their best ability and succeeded in restoring him to his full sexual function.

Sembène suggests that the essence of manhood lies elsewhere than in supporting El Hadji's indulgence of lies and ill-gotten gains. Were it not for the impotence,

El Hadji would not have fallen into debt to the marabout, and he could well have continued to enjoy reputation and credit so that his thefts might never have come to light. His impotence, in this sense, exposed his insufficient will. Sembène staged this insight in the scene when El Hadji was voted out his membership at the table of governance. El Hadji's briefcase – which he had received from a white man, stuffed with cash – is seized and given to his replacement. The briefcase is opened to reveal that it is empty except for a phallus-fetish. Everyone laughs at his penis-fetish except El Hadji who angrily declares that his fetish carries the real power. However, he had already proved himself to be an insufficiently empowered, a maladroit robber, one who had lost his verve. His claim to true power is laughed at by those at the table, who quickly welcome his replacement. To close the film, El Hadji is spat upon by the motley street congregation. Their spittle inducts him into a new type of manhood, one based upon membership among the outcast. His first wife and Rama watch this humiliation with tear-stained cheeks, but his second and third wives have already abandoned him.

In contrast, in the medical case study, the fear of becoming a woman is not illuminated by specifics about what sustains a polygamist nor about the lives of his women. The little information recorded about Mr. N'D's wives include their ages, and their children's sex and ages. The first wife, about 45 years old, had two living children, a son who was already married and a daughter, age 11. The second wife, who took on the responsibility of caring for their husband throughout his hospital stay, had three living sons, ages ten, seven, and one year. His third wife was 25 years old and had two daughters, the older was eight years and the young one only eight months. Finally, his fourth wife had conceived a boy prior to her divorce from Mr. N'D, who by the time of the hospital stay was about 18 months old.

The second wife, mother of three sons, accompanied Mr. N'D to Dakar and stayed jn the city, visited him regularly, helped him to tell his story to the doctors, and finally traveled home with him. The second wife's close identification with her husband is revealed in her point of view on his symptoms which was "exactly the same" as her husband's (Collomb and Diop 1965, p. 495). She also testified to the doctors that her husband's virility was restored, his impotence "had totally disappeared," and with that, secured his discharge from the hospital (Collomb and Diop 1965, p. 510).

It is difficult to avoid the fact that compared to lengthy discussions of *djinns* and *marabouts*, the references to Mr. N'D's wives, even the wife who was there at the hospital with him, are extremely minimal. This obfuscation of the women in the impotent patient's life points to underlying assumptions on the part of the doctors that seem intended to mirror those of the patient and his social milieu. Essential among these assumptions are: the subordinate status of women, women's interchangeability, and the minimal power of pair-bonding for the man as compared to the power of sexual novelty. The doctors focused on Mr. N'D's conflict with male authority figures and then proposed an incest prohibition for which they openly acknowledged they have no proof. They wrote that "this woman represents a prohibition (incest) for Mr. N'D. Unfortunately, we have no further reasons to confirm this hypothesis" (Collomb and Diop 1965, p. 509).

Meanwhile the doctors follow social convention when they largely overlook the personal presence of Mr. N'D wives in his life, in particular the one with him at the hospital. The second wife was clearly strongly bonded with her husband as is evidenced by her opinion that was "exactly the same" as his. That type of absolute inter-subjective congruence is achieved and maintained out of visceral loyalty and an internalized duty of obedience. Mr. N'D., the master of his household, was equally supposed to be master of his wives. His second wife plays this subjugated-wife role to perfection, while wives three and four fall under suspicion as insufficiently subjected to his will, to the extent that Mr. N'D portrayed them as acting as *sorciers-anthropophagiques*. The visceral pair-bond between wife two and Mr. N'D thus worked in opposition to the visceral repudiation of wives three and four.

At a minimum, it is clear that these denunciations indicate failed relationships. The viscerality of the fear – implicating the dorsal vagal neural system – is explicit. *Sorciers-anthropophages* compulsively eat the souls and liver of other people and can provoke actual physical death. No one is safe from their nocturnal predations. That Mr. N'D denounced his third wife and her two daughters, one age eight and the other not yet a year old, is a significant fearful repudiation of a long-standing and central alliance. The Fulani marabout who treated him was also someone he had known well for 30 years. The doctors do not recount, and likely did not know, the social reverberations of Mr. N'D's denunciations of these individuals as *sorciers-anthropophages*. In an early time, Père Boilat recounted instances of such suspected individuals sold into slavery in Mauritania (Boilat 1853, p. 316). Well into the twentieth century such vampiric witches among enslaved Black Mauritanians in Mauritania could fall victim to further suspicions and mortal rough justice (Acloque 2013; Bonte 1998; McDougall 2001; Pettigrew 2016).

Case Discussion: Affective Neuroscience and Autonomic Evidence

In general we recall that the shortcomings of mental health practices are not peculiar to the transcultural situation, but rather characterize mental health practices, in all probability, in most situations. Mental health care, especially for the broad public, is notably under-funded, stigmatized, and led by medical knowledge that is fragmented by specialization and priorities in research funding. This reminder is meant to level the field. Moreover, in 2021 the treatment for erectile dysfunction (commonly called ED) is almost exclusively biomedical, with well-known prescription drugs widely deployed. These drugs are common and subject also to recreational use. Where the drugs fail, mechanical interventions step in with penile pumps and implants.

Despite the over-abundance of meaning-generating explanations recorded in this case study there are many unknowns and many broad avenues left unexplored and unexplained. To focus on the most glaring: loyalty, compassion, bonding, and generally interpersonal affection and disaffection do not feature in the discussion. Even when Mr. N'D accused his fourth and third wives of being *sorciers-anthropophages*, the topic of love or its opposite, antipathy, remains obscured. The divorce of Mr. N'D from his fourth wife is entered into the case study almost as an aside, whereas in *Xala* the novel, as we have remarked, that same type of divorce features as vindictive behavior. No remark is inserted considering the fate of his marriage to his third wife, nor of her children with Mr. N'D, all of whom he accused of being *sorciers-anthropophages*. We might presume he divorced this third wife, but that is not stated.

The doctors worked with care not to replace Mr. N'D's voice with their own. Nonetheless it is remarkable that no place in the case is there overt discussion of sexual attraction. The displacement or projection of such feelings onto *djinns* and *maraboutage* is examined as a social convention, but not in terms of what such defenses accomplished personally for Mr. N'D. Sexual pleasure – or, more specifically, lack of sexual pleasure – is raised in relation to Mr. N'D's impotence, but this is not investigated further in what would have been a short and relevant step of inquiry: what is absent or present that provokes this lack of pleasure. Thus, his complaint of lack of sexual pleasure is accepted as a product of his impotence rather than a cause of his impotence. An implicit assumption seems operative. That is, it seems to be assumed that Mr. N'D should be capable of accepting any woman as a wife. The complicated physiology of sexual attraction and pair-bonding is now, in the twenty-first century, more clearly understood. Porges explains the affective neuroscience of love in which the ventral vagal complex, the dorsal vagal complex, the sympathetic nervous system, oxytocin and vasopressin are deeply involved (2011, pp. 167–185).

The sexual unavailability of both wife number four and Mr. N'D is demarcated on their first night sleeping together. Rather than directly discuss this sexual refusal of Mr. N'D's new wife, he and the doctors focus on his projections and defenses. Thus, they make much of the *djinns*, the possibility he was bewitched or perhaps attacked by a vampiric witch. The fourth wife has a fiancé *djinn* and Mr. N'D has a spouse-*djinn*, thus neither of them are sexually available to the other. The doctors Collomb and Diop turn from the *djinns* to incest prohibition to explain this sexual unavailability. Their reasons for this explanation have left no trace in their writing. Such an incest prohibition would put into doubt the ethics of numerous older husband – younger wife pairs in the region. Considered from the perspective of how frequently such marriages were (and are) contracted in Senegal, this assertion of an incest prohibition regarding them is a monumental statement. Moreover, what they never emphasize is even more curious, the strong emotional bond between Mr. N'D and his second wife. The entitlement of men to more than one wife seemingly renders the woman's emotions irrelevant with respect to other women her husband might marry. A correlative presumption is that the husband's own emotions simply disregard the emotions of their existing spouses. That is, if the wife feels upset, abandoned, threatened, or betrayed, in order for the husband to proceed with carrying out a subsequent marriage, he must disregard his existing wife's (or, wives') emotions. Women's emotions faced with polygamist behavior from their husband can vary widely (Martins 2015). The novel *Xala* describes the emotions of the first and second wife with words such as "like an angry sea, her resentment welled up" (Sembène 1976, p. 14), "painful bitterness," "loneliness," and "abandonment" (Sembène 1976, p. 21). About five years later Mariama Ba explored the sentiments of a similarly betrayed wife in *So Long a Letter* (Ba 1979). Moreover, the polygamist man's emotions might not necessarily conform to his behavior. The choice to take a new wife might be motivated by social obligation or status seeking, more than by emotional considerations. For example, in *Xala*, El Hadji interrogates his own reasons for his new marriage, had he "been in love," or "was it simply old age," or his wealth, his weakness? Was he a libertine, a sensualist? Had his married life been intolerable? (Sembène 1976, p. 39). Hatred gripped him (Sembène 1976, p. 39). His new wife "seemed to be the embodiment of mental and physical torture" (Sembène 1976, p. 59). Finally, El Hadji admits to himself that his new wife's aunt had pushed and manipulated him into marriage (Sembène 1976, pp. 70–71).

In contrast, Collomb and Diop never openly consider that perhaps Mr. N'D could not manage his emotions with respect to a fourth wife. This attitude exemplifies traditional deference to senior male authority. "*On ne touche pas au père africain*" (Kesteloot and Gounongbé 2009, p. 211). Perhaps he actually cared too much for one or more of his existing wives, and that was why he could not successfully take up a life with a new wife. Overlooked by Collomb and Diop, such considerations can only be discussed as limited by the fixed data of the case. There is no possibility now to pose questions to Mr. N'D nor pursue unexplored therapeutic avenues. We can only take account of facts recorded and left without satisfactory examination.

Mr. N'D complained of specific physiological symptoms, including a seizing up of his gut and a cold wind that passed through him and induced intense heat throughout his body. The stomach contractions and cold wind combined to deflate his erection or to soften it to the point where penetration could not be achieved.

The dorsal vagal nerve system is implicated in Mr. N'D's feelings in his gut and penis (Porges 2011, pp. 178–179). The anxiety-inducing wind that came in cold and then turned Mr. N'D's body hot describe autonomic physiological state changes that veered from the extreme dysregulation by dorsal vagal complex neuroception to a semi-regulation by the sympathetic neural fight or flight response. Under the sway of dorsal vagal complex arousal, his extreme anti-social physiological state provoked anti-social, anti-bonding behavior, and then, to narrativize this inability to bond with his fourth wife, he projected his own anti-social physiological arousal onto the supposed *djinns*, and onto those he alleged were *sorciers-anthropophages* or sources of *maraboutage*. Once Mr. N'D convinced himself he was enmeshed in these threatening metaphysical forces, his fear increased, generating more dorsal vagal complex arousal and more anti-social behavior. Cut off in this way from secure social relationships, Mr. N'D suffered repeated anxiety attacks in the form of the cold wind that continually tried to penetrate him.

The root cause of Mr. N'D's impotence and anxiety, according to the doctors, is a neurotic phobia expressive of incest prohibition. We must, however, consider the primary trigger of his dorsal vagal neuroception which caused a cascade of physiological and behavioral outcomes. Here we need to distinguish between curiosity about Mr. N'D's actual emotions and thoughts behind his conventional behavior, and satisfaction at the relief he obtained. His medical doctors aimed primarily to relieve his suffering. Thus, if relief could be obtained without disturbing the deeper conditionality of his persona and social position, the doctors had no need to dig deeper. Nonetheless, specific reference to the original source of neuroceptive danger alert is a more precise rendition of his condition. From the perspective of Porges' polyvagal theory, the key dimension of the onset of symptoms was overlooked. Dr. Collomb and Dr. Diop focus on the dream of bolts falling off the bed and the onlookers' refusal to help Mr. N'D put his marital bed back together. This transparent representation of an unhappy nuptial night, interpreted with the aid of polyvagal theory, points to the significance of Mr. N'D spending the night asleep with his new wife. It is the act of sleeping together, according to Porges, that triggers the masculine pair-bonding mechanism (Porges 2011, p. 184). For women, the pair-bonding neural mechanism is triggered in the act of sex and is fortified by sleep. For men, however, the more active sexual posture impedes the release of neural mechanisms that promote pair-bonding whereas relaxation in sleep after sex triggers male neural ability to pair-bond. Thus, when Mr. N'D had sex with his new wife he was still acting outside the influence of pair-bonding vagal neural mechanisms, but when he fell asleep the pair-bonding mechanism would have kicked in. In his case, massive visceral hostility prevented the pair-bonding and gave rise to his dream of marital-bed disaster. Thus, the polyvagal theory provides a means of more directly accessing Mr. N'D's conflict. What is allegorized by Mr. N'D and his family as *djinn*, *maraboutage*, and *sorciers anthropophagique*, from the polyvagal perspective is a dorsal vagal neuroceptive (a visceral) rejection of his new wife. His body refused the pair-bond. The most direct explanation for why his body would reject a pair-bond is that it was already tightly bonded with someone else. Thus, in this polyvagal analysis, his mind was willing to betray his deeply loyal second wife, but his body was not.

Here, however, we must abjure further speculation and acknowledge the intransigent opacity of this case study. Unlike Sembène's fiction, which overflows with meaning-laden parallels and metaphors, the case of Mr. N'D portrays his own recuperation against a canvas composed of barriers and blank spots. We do not know what happened when the patient left the hospital with his second wife to return to their village. We do know that he had already divorced wife number four, but we know nothing of how she struggled with the opprobrium of this failed marriage (her second failed marriage), along with the suspicion that she had bewitched her second husband and/or tried to suck his blood. What Mr. N'D did regarding his third wife, whom he also denounced as a *sorcier-anthropophage*, is not mentioned, but if he made that accusation outside the confines of confidential hospital treatment, we can presume they divorced and that she too had to struggle to regain spiritual equilibrium and social status for herself and her daughters. Meanwhile, thanks to the hospital cure, Mr. N'D seemingly continued to occupy a position of absolute authority, as befit a traditional Wolof husband, with respect to his first and second wives.

****

Works Cited

Acloque, B., 2013. Accusations of Remote Vampirism: The Colonial Administration in Mauritania Investigates the Execution of Three Slaves. *In*: A. Bellagamba, S. Greene and M. Klein, eds., *African Voices on Slavery and the Slave Trade*. London: Cambridge University Press, 282–304.

Ba, M., 1989 [1979]. *So Long a Letter*. M. Bodé-Thomas, trans. Chicago: Heinemann.

Boilat, P., 1853. *Esquisses sénégalaises*. Paris: P. Bertrand.

Bonte, P., 1998. *L'émirat de l'Adrar: Histoire et anthropologie d'une société tribale du sahara occidental*. Thesis (Ph.D). Paris: École des hautes études en sciences sociales.

Bullard, A., 2000. *Exile to Paradise*. Palo Alto, CA: Stanford University Press.

Bullard, A., 2008. Sympathy and Denial: A Postcolonial Re-Reading of Emotions, Race, and Hierarchy. *Historical Reflections/Reflexions historiques*, 34 (1), 122–142.

Collomb, H. and Diop, M., 1965. A propos d'un cas d'impuissance. *Psychopathologie Africaine*, 1 (3), 487–511.

Foley, E. 2010. *Your Pocket is what Cures You: The Politics of Health in Senegal*. New Brunswick NJ: Rutgers University Press.

Kesteloot, L. and Gounongbé, A., 2009. *La recherche féministe francophone: Langue, identités, et enjeux*. Fatou Sow, ed. Paris: Éditions Karthala, 205–215.

Martins, C., 2015. Polyphonic Disconcert Around Polygyny: Riwan ou Le Chemin de Sable. *Cahiers d'études Africaine*, 220, 787–810. Available from: https://doi.org/10.4000/etudesafricaines.18305.

McDougall, E.A., 2001. Slavery, Sorcery and Colonial "Reality" in Mauritania, c. 1910–1960. *In*: C. Youé and T. Stapleton, eds., *Agency and Action in Colonial Africa: Essays for John E. Flint*. London: Palgrave Macmillan, 69–82. Available from: https://doi.org/10.1057/9780230288485.

Pettigrew, E., 2016. The Heart of the Matter: Interpreting Bloodsucking Accusations in Mauritania. *Journal of African History*, 57 (3), 417–435.

Porges, S.W., 2011. The Polyvagal Theory: Neurophysiological Foundations of Emotions, Attachment, Communication, Self-Regulation . New York: W.W. Norton.

Sembène, O., 1976 [1974]. *Xala, a Novel*. C. Wake, trans. Chicago: Chicago Review Press.

Xala, 1975. Film. Directed by Ousmane Sembène. Dakar: Filmi Domireve SNC.

4 The Man Who Makes Trees Cry

A Healer's Art

***

El Hadji Ba was a highly reputable Fulani healer. Charles de Preneuf worked in collaboration with Henri Baro and Henri Collomb to give a detailed portrait of this healer and his practices. The clinicians were on friendly terms with this healer, whom they called Ousmane. However, in this discussion, we retain the more formal honorific and surname. El Hadji Ba instructed de Preneuf in his healing methods via an extensive practicum. Several times in this case study from 1969 we find reservations about any ability to do justice to El Hadji Ba's teachings. De Preneuf reiterates that translating Ba's mystical knowledge into psychological and biomedical terms empties it of essential metaphysical dimensions. This chapter presents Ba's narrative in summary fashion, but hews closely to his words and beliefs. Minimal historical commentary is reserved for the chapter's concluding section. The intent is to allow direct appreciation for El Hadji Ba's outlook and healing practices.

El Hadji Ba employed a mixture of mystical recitations and plant-based treatments to effect his cures (de Preneuf and Baro 1969; Kerharo and Adam 1964). These cures operated primarily on the metaphysical level, taming or eradicating the *sétanyé*, *sukuñabé*, *djinn*, or *maraboutage* (magical curses) that afflicted his patients. If that metaphysical cure proved effective, his patient obtained relief. Ba's cures involved the recitation of charms and prayers, laying on of hands, spitting, ingestion of medicinal plants and fumigation with the medicinal plants. These treatments often caused vomiting, coughing, diarrhea, and overall weakness that necessitated bedrest for several days. Purgatives that did not cure the first time were repeated until the patient was freed of the affliction. Another common cure involved daily washing with water infused with mystical properties, variously via recitation of prayers, charms, or Qu'ranic verses, or via powdered plant material, or some combination of these.

Troubled individuals also sought protection against magic via carefully worked *gris-gris*. These are braided and knotted cords, made with the recitation of specific charms and prayers chosen according to the desired efficacy. The cord is worn as a type of protective amulet, tied around the waist, ankle, or wrist. Generally,

DOI: 10.4324/9781003112143-5

the magic worked via knotting, so that counter-knots could ward off magic, and unknotting could undo magical curses.

At the conclusion of this case study, Dr. Henri Collomb published a short remark that admonished psychiatrists to make an effort to understand, if not outright collaborate with, such magical healers as El Hadji Ba. Collomb reasoned that in general people do not understand biomedicine and sometimes they repudiate it outright. "Indeed, who can replace the observant magician," reflected Collomb, "who has deep roots among his people, who he frees from fears before those fears can ravage them, and who comforts them through the grace of the only language that they truly understand, the language of the marvelous?" (de Preneuf and Baro 1969, p. 458).

Common dimensions of folk medicine populated this Fulani healer's toolkit. Viewed from the global human species perspective facilitated by polyvagal theory (PVT) (Porges 2011, 2017a, 2017b), we can appreciate the inter-subjective physiological state regulation achieved by Ba, as well as how narrative of physiological states formed shared beliefs. Charms, amulets, curative water, mystical plant-based cures, all of these are found the world over. The healer possesses an ability to channel fear, anxiety, hope, and well-being into these sacred objects. On an abstract level, the emotions that work between individuals and within individuals animate meaning that is fixed to stories and beliefs about metaphysical beings, whether good, evil, or mischievous. The meaning created through these specific cultural inflections adds to our global open civilization (Diagne 2019). The sincerity of this religious faith-healing calls for our compassion as witnesses to such pervasive terrorized suffering and longing for relief. Nonetheless, this appreciation acknowledges as well the purgative and sometimes violent methods of El Hadji Ba, as well as the inevitable limitations on his art. Ba's healing worked via strongly hierarchal relationships, which compares indirectly to contemporary psychotherapeutic relationships.

El Hadji Ba participated in the suffering of the sick, and hence took up and enacted the patient's projections and/or the projections of the patient's family members. Such a healer wields power to shape the symbolic order and thereby to sanction social status and meaning attributed to the patient and to the patient's distress or symptoms. The patient is healed to the extent this re-ordering of the symbolic is effective. His curative power relied on the ability to mobilize various spirits and magical forces. Communing with the spirits, in turn, furnished Ba a strong foundation for on-going spiritual rituals and high social status.

El Hadji Ba's Word: To Make Trees Cry

El Hadji Ousmane N'dombo Ba, a Fulani healer, told de Preneuf how he approached the trees whom he wanted to question: "I call them, and they answer me; I hit them until they cry and tell me their use (*a quoi ils servent*)" (*de Preneuf and Baro 1969*, p. 415). Ba made trees cry out to him their healing powers as well as the powers of the dependent plants that grew among their boughs. His technique was straightforward, but relied for its results on his powers of perception and interpretation that were superior to most mortals. *Leki*, spirit-trees, and the medicinal plants hosted by them each have a family name and a first name.

> When going to see them, we greet them just like a person. If you try to collect *leki* without greeting the plant by its full name, then what you collect isn't *leki*. *Bilédjo* [a person who can hunt and trap malevolent spirits] really know how to flatter *leki*, just like a *griot* flatters people. They flatter the *leki* until they divulge all their uses.
>
> (de Preneuf and Baro 1969, p. 415)[1]

After greeting the *leki* but before touching it, El Hadji Ba took care to recite a prayer specific to the type of disease he sought to heal. Each spiritual presence – *djinn*, *sukanabé*, and *seytané* – possessed its own *tcifol* that they themselves recited when taking flight. Only after reciting those words of flight, did Ba touch the plant to access its healing forces. In El Hadji Ba's own estimation, no other Black between Diaba and Dakar equaled his detailed knowledge regarding the healing forces of plants.

El Hadji Ba's healing knowledge was anchored in a cosmology composed of seven worlds, with humanity occupying the "world of Adam." The six other worlds include the world of angels (which is the largest world), the world of *djinns* (Islamic spirits), and a world with one angel who takes up the entire world, whose sole purpose is to glorify God.[2] The world of Adam is the smallest of the worlds. The *seytané* live on the world of Adama, alongside humanity. Only humanity and the *djinns* have autonomy. The *seytané* are parasites on humanity (de Preneuf and Baro 1969, p. 396).

Regarding the *sukañabé* (*döm* in Wolof, and often translated into French as *sorcier*, or into English as witch), the healer related that the original term was *iarobidédian* or "drinkers of blood." According to him the *sukañabé* originated when an army during the original Islamist expansion beheaded so many people that rivers of blood flowed through the land. Then came a torrential rain, so that the blood mixed with water. A troop of very thirsty warriors passed by and drank from this water mixed with human blood. Later on they found pure water, but they had developed a taste for bloody water and so they refused pure water and continued to seek out human blood. Ever since that time, when they see people bleed, they come to suck the blood. When they sleep, their soul goes to attack people to suck their blood. Their appetite was aroused by blood, and soon they wanted to eat the flesh as well (de Preneuf and Baro 1969, p. 397).

Ba explained that Black Africans and Arabs have *sukañabé* among them, but that he is uncertain whether Europeans have them too. However, without a doubt, the Black *sukuñabé* are afraid of European souls and do not attack them (de Preneuf and Baro 1969, p. 399). When an innocent soul is attacked during the night by *sukuñabé*, that soul returns to its body, but bears the marks of the attack in what is called the disease of *sukañabé* (de Preneuf and Baro 1969, p. 397). The *sukuñabé* are born from mothers who descend from the original *sukuñabé*. Any child of a female sukuñabé will be a *sukuñabé*. If a male *sukuñabé* has a child with a non-*sukañabé*, then the child will be a *tciolgodo*, a half-*sukañabé*. This creature cannot attack the soul of others, but does nonetheless attack people and give rise to an illness very difficult to heal. Children of *tciolgodo* are called *noxos*, and are indistinguishable from normal individuals. If two *sukañabé* have a child, then that child will be a "reinforced" *sukañabé*. If a child is born of non-*sukuñabé*, but is attacked prior to birth by *sukuñabé*, then that child will be born with teeth. Without proper healing, that child will go mad. At night the baby with teeth will be terrified by the sight of *sukuñabé* and *djinns*. Such a child, if she or he is healed, bears gifts of exceptional intelligence and even genius, and can become a gifted healer.

El Hadji Ba revealed that he, himself, was born with teeth, but that his father knew how to heal him. Thus, he can see the *sukañabé* and knows how to "break their wings" and remove their power (de Preneuf and Baro 1969, p. 398).

Evil Parasitic Spirits from the Underworld, S*eytané*

The *seytané* all originated from Iblis, the father of them all. Iblis was an angel who adored God throughout thousands of years, but he was a soul destined, prior to birth, for damnation. When God created Adam, He ordered all the angels and Iblis to adore His new creation. Iblis responded, "Me, I am more real than a ball of earth, I will not prostrate myself before it."

God responded to Iblis: "Because you refuse, you are damned." However, Iblis had already worshipped God for thousands of years. Even though he was damned, he received compensation. Thus, Iblis was granted the right to have children. While he dwells in hellfire, he does not suffer from those flames. However, those who follow Iblis do burn in those flames. In this hellfire he is able to eat the souls of the good who have fallen into his power (de Preneuf and Baro 1969, p. 399).

The *seytané* are neither male nor female, but rather have a male thigh and a female thigh. Each time those thighs rub together ten *seytané* are born. The *seytané* can only live within people or within trees. They prefer termite hills and baobab trees. They give the energy to anger.

Iblis and *seytané* seek to draw the loyalty of people, and anyone dominated by them is damned. The *seytané* also collaborate with *sukuñabé*. Souls that are captured by *sukuñabé* are sometimes delivered to the *seytané*, who then eat half the soul. Even if a person escapes or is rescued by a healer, he will carry the marks of this attack (de Preneuf and Baro 1969, p. 400).

Seytané *Illnesses*

A soul attacked by *seytané* is frequently half eaten, which causes paralysis on one side. A small child attacked by *seytané* will develop periodic convulsions causing him to fall. He seizes and contracts, bites his tongue, becomes rigid as though someone knocked him out. This can lead to insanity if not properly treated (de Preneuf and Baro 1969, p. 410). *Seytané* can also make someone crazy, and incite theft and anger. The *seytané* is a damned being, and thus the person attacked by this spirit becomes intolerable, like it. He is aggressive, assaults people, throws stones, hits. Especially on Fridays, he is given to running about and insulting people. "People were created to adore the Lord, not for this type of behavior," remarked Ba (de Preneuf and Baro 1969, p. 410).

The victim, Ba assured, is not responsible. All crazy people are innocents, like children, they will all go to paradise. What makes people responsible is conscience (de Preneuf and Baro 1969, p. 410).

***

Sukuñabé

A *sukuñabé* can attack via numerous methods and easily uses intermediaries. Their attack can come through the bite of a reptile, the horn of a cow, a dog bite, or the prick of a pin (de Preneuf and Baro 1969, p. 406). They prefer to attack only sons and pregnant women. *Sukuñabé* can attack the stomach of a woman, and if her flesh tastes good, it returns, and this prevents her from having children.

The *sukuñabé* only eats the soul, not the actual flesh of a person, but this can make the body perish. The person attacked can have vertigo, frequent uncontrollable nose bleeds, or dreams of attack by all sorts of wild animals. Pains in the throat, heart palpitations, these symptoms repeat and can lead to insanity (de Preneuf and Baro 1969, p. 408). The person can become delirious. When he wakes up, he thinks he is still dreaming. He feels he is attacked and menaced. He sees *seytané*, who attack him like scavengers seize on carrion (de Preneuf and Baro 1969, p. 408).

If a *sukuñabé* attacks and does not confine the *xux* (soul) to the *seytané*, then sickness ensues. The victim falls as though dead. Sometimes he cries out. He cannot speak nor respond to questions. The recitation of a *tcifol* (prayer) and spitting in his ear will lend the victim's voice to the *sukuné* (a person host to *sukuñabé*) who will then reveal his name (de Preneuf and Baro 1969, p. 408). But if the individual is not released from the *sukuñabé*, then he can deteriorate into complete loss of sanity. He speaks incoherently, stares like an animal, without understanding what he sees, and his body goes soft. He is not violent or agitated (de Preneuf and Baro 1969, p. 408).

Attack by *sukuñabé* can happen extremely easily. El Hadji Ba explained, for example, "if he meets my eyes when I am about to take a bite of food, I will have a very serious illness that can kill me without the proper *léki* to make me vomit" (de Preneuf and Baro 1969, p. 409). This *léki* could be given right away, or even after years, to cause the vomiting of the illness. In all that time, if the sick person vomits without the *léki*, they will not be cured (de Preneuf and Baro 1969, p. 409).

Djinns

El Hadji Ba recounted how the *djinns* are second only to the angels in terms of size and length of life. In former times, the *djinns* were numerous and powerful, but since the time of Souleymane/Solomon, their presence in the world of Adam has been vastly reduced. Even though few in number, the *djinns* are more powerful than humans. Even the *seytané* and *sukuñabé* are afraid of the *djinns*.

Like humans, the *djinns* can be good or bad. They prefer to live in termite hills and baobab trees. According to Ba, they are like the Chinese in Africa, found only infrequently, but when they are present, they cause mischief. They are faster than Apollo XIII (American lunar rocket), and can travel vast distances in a blink of an eye (de Preneuf and Baro 1969, pp. 400–401). Ousmane himself sometimes collaborated with *djinns* when his own healing power is too weak. Ba offered the *djinns* a gift of money, and the *djinns* would help his healing efforts.

Anyone who sees the *djinns* loses sanity, unless that person is fortified with esoteric knowledge. Adults who go out into the forests, or herders who sleep out in the fields, can go completely crazy. *Djinns* can come on the wind, or as a disembodied voice that calls out to you, or as a huge eye, or an enormous arm that moves around. Indeed, *djinns* can take on any form they desire. Perhaps the form of someone you know, to do you harm, or as a horse, to scare you.

If a *djinns* attacks, but cannot eat you because your flesh tastes too bitter, then the victim is "*naskada*," which is a diminished individual. A *naskada* is not a crazy individual, but an imbecile, who can only speak a language no one else can understand (de Preneuf and Baro 1969, p. 412). If the flesh of the victim is not too bitter, then the *djinns* devour it completely, with death following, sometimes quite quickly, either by illness or by accident. "It is as though when the roots of a tree are severed. At first the tree remains green, but then it dries up and dies" (de Preneuf and Baro 1969, p. 413). Gifts are used to entice the *djinns* to relinquish their prey. "For everything God created, he created a remedy" (de Preneuf and Baro 1969, p. 413).

Magic/Bandanal/Maraboutage

To *badanal* someone means to work to bring them troubles or afflictions. This can be accomplished without any of the spirits El Hadji Ba discussed, but rather arises directly from the healer's knowledge. Ba viewed *bandanal* with disdain, because he thought it forbidden by Islam, but he also acknowledged that if a *seytané* inspired prayers to God to give the power of *bandanal*, that can be effective. If harm comes to people through these prayers inspired by *seytané*, then the healer will burn in hell in the afterlife. Good *bandanal* is a precise science that is practiced using water that has washed Qu'ranic tablets. Evil *bandanal* is worked by *bilédjo* who use *tciéfi*.

Two goals of *maraboutage* are particularly prominent: insanity, and a type of pain that roves about the body but which has no clear cause (de Preneuf and Baro 1969, pp. 411–412). Magic can make a person crazy or imbecile. It can make a person spout nonsense in court, or make them leave the country when they are supposed to receive an inheritance (de Preneuf and Baro 1969, p. 411). If magic is used to attach a person to a bird, then every time that bird flies, the person moves as well.

El Hadji Ba maintained that anyone who has been magically worked upon knows it without fail. Magic is always commissioned by a person against another person. It follows that the person afflicted can intuit who among her or his relations has reason to ensnare them in magic.

***

El Hadji Ba's Practice as Healer

El Hadji Ousmane Ba's status bore numerous marks of privilege. In addition to being born with teeth, and hence biologically marked as a healer, he held pilgrim (*hadji*) status, had several wives, numerous children, and was widely sought after for his healing prowess. He presented himself as widely renowned for his esoteric knowledge and healing powers.

Born with Teeth: Bilédjo

As a healer born with teeth, El Hadji Ba possessed the ability to see the *djinns* and *seytané* within his dreams. He claimed that no one could deny this reality. According to Ba, all babies born with teeth and who are properly healed, become a *bilédjo*. A *bilédjo* is a type of "net caster" who can ensnare malign spirits and counter-act at least some of their harms (de Preneuf and Baro 1969, p. 401). A child born with teeth who is not healed properly by the age of between seven and ten will go mad (de Preneuf and Baro 1969, p. 407). Normally a soul grows along with the body, but for a child born with teeth, his soul flies at night and, terrified by the spirits it sees, the soul returns each day diminished (de Preneuf and Baro 1969, p. 407).

As a *biiledjo* himself, Ba served as the protector of human souls. At night, he could see the blood-suckers and flesh-eaters, and then, the next day, he could tell if an individual had been attacked. He could recognize at glance if someone had their throat slit by a *sukuñabé* (de Preneuf and Baro 1969, p. 403).

For Night Soul Flight: Ba believed

El Hadji Ba's tcifol, For Night Soul Flight:

Ba believed that people, *djinns* and *seytané*, each possess souls (*xux*) that travel during the night. Animals, in contrast, do not have such souls. Those who know that God wants their souls to fly at night should recite a prayer to ensure that their soul is stronger than any *seytané*, *djinns*, or *sukañabé* they might encounter.

The prayer he offered was as follows:

> In the name of God, I lay myself down on the side of my head. With the compassion of God, I lay myself on the side of my head. I hit the heads of others, but no one hits me. If anyone hits my head, whosoever it might be, his head bursts, his brain seeps out. He is overwhelmed. His head is covered. He is tied. He is contained. He spends the hot season with the squirrels. He spends the wet season with the rats. I am the bull of God. The bull of God has flown.
>
> (de Preneuf and Baro 1969, p. 402)

"No one can lasso the bull of God," Ba remarked. To fight the blood-drinkers, the flesh-eaters, the evil spirits, you don't need a club or a gun. It is prayer that will protect you. "Say the prayer when your *xux* (soul) is in you, and this will protect you if you have to fight" (de Preneuf and Baro 1969, p. 403).

Ba's Healing of a Slave

Ba recounted a story regarding a *sukuné* who he freed by "breaking his wings" and hence releasing him from the nighttime compulsion to fly abroad and eat human flesh (de Preneuf and Baro 1969, p. 411). As Ba told the story, he was young, very well dressed, and extremely handsome on his resplendent horse, when he passed a slave whom he greeted. The slave was deeply impressed by Ba's pristine clothing, his beauty, and his horse, and offered his hand in greeting. Ba noticed right away that this slave had the mark of a *sukuné*, that is, he was a man who hosted *sukuñabé*.

Ba introduced himself and the slave invited him to rest through the heat of the day at his house. The slave took good care of Ba, providing him with food, and caring for his horse. Ten days later, the slave came to visit Ba, saying, "I learned you just recently married." The marriage was indeed very recent, so recent that the bride, Assisata Seydou, was still living with her father. The two set off together to visit Ba's new wife. That night Ba and the slave shared a bed. In the morning Ba left quite early to go about his business, but the slave stayed for breakfast. After that meal, the slave "shook Assisata Seydou's hand and took her with him" (de Preneuf and Baro 1969, p. 420). "When I came back that night," El Hadji Ba recounted: "my wife cried, 'the guest wants to cut my throat!'" Ba mounted his horse and rode to find the slave, who was asleep in his own home. He punched the slave and threatened him with a gun: "'if you make even one gesture, if you say even one word, you will get it.' I put him on my horse and brought him back to my house. I said to him, 'You attacked my wife. If you don't let her go, I will kill you.'"

The slave answered, "'it's true, but it was not because I wanted to attack her. I might have attacked my own son or mother. I would prefer to eat nice fat cows, because human meat has a bad tast. As for Aissata Seydou, today I left her flesh.'" The slave pleaded with Ba, "'I swear to you by the name of God, I left her flesh.'" To Aissata he said, "'It was involuntary that I took you. Your husband is my friend." Then the slave took Ba aside and asked the healer to make him vomit and "to break his wings." The slave explained how he had been accused before, "'People have told me that I killed so and so, but these are my great friends, and I am attacked. Now the same thing has happened with you.'"

Ba administered a *leki* to the slave who then turned deep red, sat on the floor like a dog, and stared with very red eyes. Ba related, "I pushed on his side and he vomited chunks of red meat until he couldn't vomit any more. I broke his wings'" (de Preneuf and Baro 1969, p. 420). Ba checked on the slave a few days later to see how he was getting on. The slave greeted him and thanked him, "Now I am at peace, thank-you. I don't fly during the night anymore. I don't fight anymore and I no longer live in fear" (de Preneuf and Baro 1969, p. 421).

El Hadji Ba's Victory over Sukuñabé *in Rufisque*

Ba recounted another time he "broke the wings" of the *sukuñabé* who had infested a whole neighborhood in Rufisque. His hostess warned him not to spend the night because the powers of the Lebou *sukuñabé* have stronger spirits than the *bilédjo*. Ba responded with pride, "No, I will stay here overnight. I have no *gris-gris* with me, but what I have in my head and in my heart, you will see tonight." The *sukuñabé* arrived in the form of carrion birds in the dark of night. Ba worked his healing power via *leki* burned over a small fire. The birds grew excited and flew away. The next morning when the people came out they were in disarray, dazed because the *sukuñabé* had fled (de Preneuf and Baro 1969, p. 421).

El Hadji Ba's Wife, Also Born with Teeth

Ba's personal power is revealed in numerous healings viewed and recorded by de Preneuf. Ba's first wife, Aissata, was one among his numerous patients. She was "born with teeth" and suffered fearful visions of "things above her own power." Her father enlisted Ba to heal her when she was a child, and then later on gave her to him as his wife saying, "You cared for her since her childhood so that she has developed into a normal person, so now I am giving her to you."

> The attitude of Aissata toward her husband was an undefinable mixture of respect, submission, reserve, and abandon. She grew suddenly radiant when Ba hugged their son. . . . She did not meet his eyes, but nonetheless between them there was a sort of exchange of looks, a complicity of tenderness but in an infra-verbal language of a surprising intensity.
>
> (de Preneuf and Baro 1969, p. 447)

Ba smiled at his wife, and Aissata in response "sat immobilized in a type of serene adoration." According to de Preneuf, this worshipful pose did not last long, "After a moment she left, discretely, with her child."

***

Reflections on El Hadji Ba's Narrative

The dynamics between the healer, his first wife, and the flesh-eating slave reveal so much more than de Preneuf spells out for us. Above all, we are impressed by the exalted status of the healer, and the healer's license to threaten the life of the slave. This license to kill underwrites the slave's confession to involuntarily eating Aissata as well as other people. He has experienced repeated accusations from his "great friends" and desires, above all, to be free of such accusations. Hence he subjects himself to Ba's authority and to Ba's violently purgative medicine and, finally, to have his wings broken by this celebrated healer. In this way the slave secured for himself respite from the repeated accusations that he was (involuntarily) attacking the soul and flesh of other people.

Indeed, it is difficult to see what option the slave might have had, once this renowned healer accused him at gun point, other than to conform to the healer's point of view, to act with contrition, and to let himself be freed of the *sukuñabé* that possessed him.

Aissata likewise has very low status in comparison with her husband. She was one among three wives. While she shared with her husband the status of "being born with teeth," in her case the healing she endured did not also turn her into a *bilédjo*. Rather than transform from healing into a powerful healer, she remained a supplicant to the one who healed her, her husband. In each other's presence, he acts freely while she "freezes" into a pose of adoration and submission.

The status differential in these relationships – wife and slave to the healer – finds no mirror in current therapeutic relationships. Contemporary psychotherapy as well as clinicians at Fann Hospital in the 1960s emphasize above all the will of the patient as the driving force to regaining health. Indeed, the emphasis on hierarchical status in the traditional West African societies as well as in colonial societies contrasts sharply with the doctrine of equality that rules in twentieth- and twenty-first-century therapeutic milieux. Even so, it would be naive to accept the therapeutic doctrine of equality as absolute, as the mental health practitioner is always assumed to have expertise and authority that to some extent exceeds that of the patient. Indeed, why otherwise would the professional be paid for his or her service? Thus we should consider with care the nature of the relationship and the assumptions about the patient's status and potential autonomy.

The power of such hierarchal relationships should not be overlooked, nor should it be unduly minimized. Rather we should weigh the relevance of such hierarchy with clear eyes. The subjugated status of the slave and the wife that we find in El Hadji Ba's healing exploits was normative in Pular society. Indeed, a similar story lies at the historical roots of the historic Pular uprising against Mandinge rule in the Sene-Gambia region (N'Gaïdé 2012). Malal Coulibaly, a servile-status Bambara from Mali immigrated to Soulabaly as a warrior. He was welcomed by a rich and noble Pular by the name of Samba Egge. In Egge's household there lived a slave possessed by *djinn* whom Coulibaly healed. Egge then gifted that healed slave to Coulibaly as a wife. From this union was born the man who led the Pular freedom campaigns, Alfa Moolo, as well as his brother Bakari Demba. Alfa Moolo, like his father, grew up to possess considerable charismatic power that granted him a magical and mystical aura capable of attracting intense loyalty as well as healing capacities (N'Gaïdé 2012, pp. 74–75). Even after prolonged warfare to secure liberty of former slaves, strong nostalgia for the master–slave relationship reasserted itself among educated elites among the Pular (Fulani) in the Foota region (N'Gaïdé 2012, note 134, pp. 92–93).

Within the context of highly hierarchical relationships, in which a healer can be "gifted" the patient, the meaning of what it is to be "healed" clearly does not mean that the healed individual is autonomous, makes his or her own decisions, and/or follows his or her own desires in order to obtain gratification and self-directed life achievements. Rather, as Fann Hospital clinicians so often reflected in their case studies, traditional healing offered a means of reintegrating the suffering individual back into family and social relationships. This is true, as well, in liberal societies, but the social relationships in the liberal societies differ to some important degree by the emphasis placed upon individual liberties and the presumption that an adult person makes his or her own decisions upon his or her own reasoned decision-making. However, even within the liberal-rights idiom, some individuals claim the right to voluntary enslavement or proclaim pride in their slave-status (Woolfe 2016).

The individualistic society, into which Western therapeutic methods reintegrate the suffering individual, enables and limits lives in distinctive manners. Successful psychotherapy enables success in such arenas as education, work, and wealth-building opportunities. However, limits on individual success can be overwhelming, arising as they do from multifaceted domains, including industrial-capitalist inequalities, exploitation, and pollution, as well as systematically disfavored identity markers (*e.g.*, sex, race, age). Thus, the patient returned to "reason" is returned as well to the relative function and dysfunction of the wider hierarchical and exploitative society in which she or he makes their life.

Authoritarian relationships, in which the man commands and the wife or slave must obey, are still common throughout West Africa. Neither is authoritarianism difficult to find in liberal states such as France or the United States. Particularly in the United States, there is pronounced taste for authoritarian religious figures, who speak in tongues and perform faith healing among their adoring acolytes. The phenomenon of Trumpism, still in full flower in 2021, runs on charismatic authoritarianism, magical thinking, and gut-level loyalty rather than rational appraisal and choice (Lee 2017).

On the other end of the spectrum, mental health practitioners who encourage autonomy offer to their patients an extreme existential vision of the individual in which the stable feature in their life is the ever unfolding essence of self-hood (Frederickson 2021). To a certain degree, this is its own form of mysticism, one that is sustained via a secularized encounter with myriad mystical traditions, including Buddhism and progressive Christianity. The emphasis on compassion and love as the center of meaningful life, as we find for example in the work of the neuroscientist Porges, certainly shares deep roots with mystical traditions even if it is voiced in the language of secularized science (Porges 2011, pp. 167–185, 2017b).

Indeed, mental health professionals who focus on self-realization without due deference to loving and compassionate affective basis can produce significant malformations. The power of corrosive or negative emotions cannot be discounted, nor can we discount or overlook the ever-present efforts of some to manipulate or coerce in order to control the vulnerable.

When the individual continues in a mind-body state that enshrines hatred and anger, and hence is incapable of social engagement and loving social bonds, Porges emphasizes the strong role of the unmyelinated vagus nerve and consequent "reptilian" anti-social behaviors (Porges 2017a, pp. 49, 107, 162). That individual will continue to suffer and to be viewed by others as a more or less outcast, mentally unstable or impaired. Health is obtained via love and compassion, radical acceptance, and secure and gratifying status within the species community. These are carried as a truth in many religious and mystical practices. PVT, however, overlooks hierarchy and subjugation as human norms, even though hierarchy is a strong characteristic throughout human societies and institutions. Porges would contend he has now put ancient spiritual truisms on scientific footing (Porges 2017a, 2017b). He combines the deep breathing, musicality, and mammalian life-course dependence on social bonds as central parts of healthy physiological balance. However, hierarchy and subjugation are left unaccounted by PVT.

The healing offered by El Hadji Ba created an approved status for the healed individual. The healed slave no longer had to contend with allegations he was a blood-sucking sukuné. Ba's wife similarly escaped terrorizing visions of dangerous spirits by entering a protective relationship with Ba. These strongly hierarchal relationship provided safety for the wife and for the slave. Thus, while accepting subjugation to the healer, both wife and slave secured on-going protected status. Such subjugating healing techniques are not a contradiction to PVT, but rather operate via mystical intuition to exploit mechanisms that PVT discusses in scientific language.

Notes

1 A griot is a musician, which is a caste-based inherited status, who sings songs of praise and eulogy for their patron. Griots perform at festivals, celebrations, weddings, and other social events. Refusal to pay the griots can provoke long dissonant songs that quickly change tune when the pay is given.
2 The other three worlds are not described.

Works Cited

De Preneuf, C. and Baro, H., 1969. L'Homme qui fait pleurer les arbres, El Hadji Ousmane N'Dombo Ba, therapeute et magicien. *Psychopathologie Africaine*, V (3), 395–459.

Diagne, S.B., 2019. *Postcolonial Bergson*. L. Turner, trans., J.E. Drabinski, foreword. New York: Fordham University Press.

Frederickson, J., 2021. *Co-Creating Safety: Healing the Fragile Patient*. Kensington, MD: Seven Leaves Press.

Kerharo, J. and Adam, J.G., 1964. Plantes médicinales et toxiques des Peulh et Toucouleur au Sénégal. *Journal d'Agriculture Tropical et Botaniques appliquée*, XI, 384–444, 543–588.

Lee, B., 2017. *The Dangerous Case of Donald Trump*. New York: St. Martin's Press.

N'Gaïdé, A., 2012. *L'esclave, le colon et le marabout; le royaume peul du Fuladu de 1867 a 1936*. Paris: L'Harmattan.

Porges, S.W., 2011. *The Polyvagal Theory: Neurophysiological Foundations of Emotions, Attachment, Communication, Self-Regulation*. New York: W.W. Norton.

Porges, S.W., 2017a. *The Pocket Guide to the Polyvagal Theory: The Transformative Power of Feeling Safe*. New York: W.W. Norton.

Porges, S.W., 2017b. Vagal Pathways: Portals to Compassion. *In*: E.M. Seppälä, E. Simon-Thomas, S.L. Brown, M.C. Worline, C. Daryl Cameron and J.R. Doty, eds., *Oxford Handbook of Compassion*. New York: Oxford University Press, 187–202.

Woolfe, Z., 2016. A Composer and His Wife: Creativity Through Kink. *New York Times*, 24 February. Available from: www.nytimes.com/2016/02/24/arts/music/a-composer-and-his-wife-creativity-through-kink.html [Accessed August 2021].

5 Witch Narratives

Stolen Souls and Aggression

***

We naturally anticipate that the Fann Hospital personnel approach the symptoms and narratives of their patients from a biomedical and psychological perspective. However, it is fair to say that their perspective is very distinctive, particular to the early post-colonial history of Senegal. We distinguish it from both later post-colonial perspectives on the paranormal and witchcraft, and the colonial. In particular, we ask about the nature of the reality which we can infer or assume regarding such activities as *sorcellerie*, spirit possession, and magic. The Fann personnel psychologized these Senegalese practices. This chapter discusses the process and weighs the costs of such psychologizing. The Diola witch trials of the 1920s are contrasted to the modernist perspective of the Fann personnel. Yet the modernist assumption that witchcraft will fade away with the advent of technological urbanism is not documented. Rather this chapter concludes with a portrait of Senegalese futurism that weaves relational identity into both technological modernity and the persistence of the paranormal.

The psychologizing practiced at Fann Hospital is particular not just to the clinicians' professions – in various fields of mental health practice – but particular to their professions in a particular time and place. What they viewed as psychological events and beliefs, others viewed as spiritual. The emphasis on physiology that characterizes earlier French psychiatry, meanwhile, seems to fall away. The Fann case narratives focus on cultural beliefs, practices, and rituals. The biomedical treatments are used without remark on how exactly they impact the body or the mind, or how they disrupt the terrorized narratives. Yet intense physical experiences, including autonomic physiological states over which an individual has little conscious control, figure prominently in the various states of fear, anxiety, and persecution. Such physicality is irreducibly located in the individual's body. At the same time, the bodily experience takes form within social relationships, and can be grasped by all of us embodied individuals. Thus, affective neuroscience once again shifts the perspective, this time away from spirit-displacing psychology to neuroception, physiological state, and the polyvagal perspective on narrativizing that itself accounts for physiologically induced behavior and beliefs. Accounting

DOI: 10.4324/9781003112143-6

for spirit crises, also known as mental illness, makes more sense when we agree that it does not, in fact, make sense. Rather, it makes narratives of life and death.

Psychopathologie Africaine Cases

The first substantive grappling with *sorcellerie* in *Psychopathologie Africaine* was in a 1965 article by Moussa Diop and Henri Collomb. They examined witchcraft in relation to the impotence of a 60-year-old man upon marrying his fourth wife, a 20-year-old divorcée. As we discussed in a previous chapter, this impotence was ascribed variously to spirit possession, *maraboutage* (magic), or *sorcellerie* (witchcraft). Diop and Collomb explained that *sorciers-anthropophages*, or "*döm*" in Wolof, are the "eaters of men." They appear like ordinary humans, but they can act in the invisible world, attacking individuals and causing death within a few hours. *Sorciers-anthropophages* can also cause chronic suffering once they have stolen the *fit* (vital force) of their victim and delivered it to bad spirits (*seytanés*). Cure from the attack of a *sorcier* depends on engaging the aid of a *bilédio* (a witch chaser) to identify the *sorcier*.

Another patient treated by Diop was Yaya, a student with a seemingly promising future as a teacher, whose symptoms began when he dreamed of two people who attacked him with hatchets (Ortigues 1984, pp. 205–216). "I'm going to die," Yaya screamed, "they've come to kill me" (Ortigues 1984, p. 207). From that time, Yaya suffered recurrent anxiety attacks. He was convinced that he was about to die and that a *sorcier* was eating him.[1] In the worst attacks, he endured extremely painful and agonizing sensations of someone drinking his blood and eating his heart and liver.

Marie-Cécile and Edmond Ortigues proposed a psychoanalytic explanation for Yaya's symptoms – and those of others suffering witchcraft – seeing them as evidence of pre-genital, oral aggression. According to the Ortigues, the phantasmic dual relationship is characterized by ambivalence and repeated alternations between active and passive states. The devouring and incorporating figure of the *sorcier* is also shape-shifting (metamorphic), changing shapes as it changed skins from human to animal. The body is imagined as destroyed from the inside, with the contents devoured. This body is a containing body rather than a phallic (obtruding or penetrating) body. The victim experiences massive, undifferentiated anxiety that puts life itself (not this or that possibility in life) at risk. Specific symptoms of the anxiety include difficulty breathing or a feeling of heaviness on the chest, a vivid sense of emptiness, fear of being alone, fear of losing oneself if one loses *l'autre*, and an anorexic reaction in which the victim is seized by vomiting of "bad" or infecting food (Ortigues 1984, p. 204).

As observed by Diop and Collomb, cure for the bewitched relied on identifying the *sorcier*. Witch-hunters pursue their vocation by identifying *sorciers* and freeing the bewitched. The Ortigues emphasize the peculiar focus on discovering the *sorcier* as a means to cure, which is distinctive for witchcraft as opposed to magic. "As always observed in such cases," they write, "the anxiety of the patient is mobilized by an urgent need to discover who is eating him" (Ortigues 1984,

p. 210). This obsession leads to the inference that the victim's chief means of feeling alive is to feel him or herself being devoured by an unknown assailant. The victim – ceaselessly on the verge of death – demands to know, who is it, who is it? Marabouts and healers, in such situations remark the Ortigues, seem to function in order to make the devoured/devouring couple exist (Ortigues 1984, p. 210).

The Ortigues interpreted Yaya's bewitchment as a case of anxiety at becoming an adult, which anxiety provoked regression to a pre-genital stage. His identification with his father was stymied because his father favored his ne'er do well brother. His identity was then split between a powerful, phallic mother and society, which figured as the "bad mother" that sought to destroy its infant. Yaya eventually tamed his anxiety, with the help of Équanil tranquilizers over a six-week stay at Fann, and was able to continue his schooling even if not at the previous competitive pace.

This prolonged struggle with bewitchment is itself a sign of a cultural struggle. Normally a bewitched individual fell dead within days or even hours of being struck by a *sorcier*. Yaya's long struggle prompts overt reflections on his own situation. If he were really bewitched he would already be dead (Ortigues 1984, p. 209). As his anxiety lessened, he developed a vacillating view of his illness. He continued to attribute it to witchcraft, but also expressed doubt about that. Finally, as he returned to his studies with his anxiety largely assuaged, he simply declared that he did not know. He let the topic fall away in favor of stronger interest in his education and in dating girls (Ortigues 1984, p. 216).

The Ortigues drew heavily on British anthropologists, especially E.P. Evans-Pritchard, in developing an understanding of witchcraft. They cite with approbation his declaration that witchcraft is a psychic act. They also rely on the French anthropologist Denise Paulme's interpretation of animist religions as mechanisms to control and protect from witchcraft (Ortigues 1984, pp. 201–202; Paulme 1962, 1954). The dissolution of traditional culture allowed anxiety to proliferate unchecked, they reasoned, with consequent rise of witchcraft accusations. Prophets in Africa, Paulme observed, choose fighting witches as their chief task. As summarily expressed by the Ortigues, "witchcraft translates the anxiety of the individual in the face of his or her individuality and in the face of others' individuality. Witchcraft finds its antidote in institutions that regulate the relationships of each individual with all the others" (Ortigues 1984, p. 202). In general, Fann practitioners accepted expressed beliefs without judging or condemning. But they were able to do so only by laying a psychological interpretation on top of the fervent convictions of their patients.

Weighing the Wider Scholarship

The outlook adopted by the Fann personnel was far from universally accepted, and indeed it seems to rely on a highly distinct secular, psychoanalytic subculture. Their modernist perspective assumed that witchcraft beliefs would fade as Senegal embraced Western education and Western individual rationality. This projected abandonment of belief in witchcraft has receded in more recent years. Renewed grappling with witchcraft and other occult forces continues to preoccupy scholars, who record compelling insights (Ashforth 2005; Bernault 2009; de Rosny 1992, 2005; Geshiere 1997; Hamès 2008; Kiernan 2006; Pelgrim 2003; White 2000). Common among this scholarship is the demand that witchcraft, including the fear and excitement associated with it, must be taken seriously with no attempt to reason it away nor to reduce it to other terms (Geschiere 1995, p. 21). *Sorcellerie* closely mirrors power, according to Peter Geschiere, and needs to be approached from a non-moralizing perspective. Too often, he remarks, moralizing relegates *sorcellerie* to the domain of evil. His fieldwork revealed much fascination and excitement associated with *sorcellerie*. Good as well as bad could arise from cultivating this power. The individual, remarks Geschiere, is held responsible for cultivating his *djambe* to promote his individual goals, and yet *djambe* is embroiled in mystery, rumor, and innuendo. In the realm of *sorcellerie*, the extent of an individual's power is unknowable and mysterious; the contours of the individual are blurred (Geschiere 1995, pp. 41, 216, n.16). Luise White (2000), meanwhile, dwells at length on the role of rumor and hearsay in witchcraft, and how the reality born of rumor has an elusively powerful character. Adam Ashforth's work on post-apartheid Soweto, anatomizes the spiritual insecurity that is unavoidable in a society ridden with fears of witchcraft. Combined with this spiritual insecurity is epistemic anxiety produced by the competition between religions and world views. Epistemic anxiety is particularly relevant in relation to ancestor worship, explains Ashforth, because in some churches ancestor worship is likened to devil worship, whereas in animist practices, ancestor worship is a central ritual and is the most exemplary of behaviors (Ashforth 2005, p. 127). Ashforth illustrates this epistemic confusion in the life of a young woman who could not decide whether the ancestral spirits that haunted her were forces to conciliate, or demons. He reflected: "this I call epistemic anxiety, a sense of unease arising from the condition of knowing that invisible forces are acting upon one's life but not knowing what they are or how to relate to them" (2005, p. 127).

It is difficult to discuss *sorcellerie* in any depth without at least pondering the nature or extent of its actual powers. Geschiere points the way in his remark that *sorcellerie* can be fathomed only once the distinction between fantasy and reality is abolished (1995, p. 21). Such a bridge between fantasy and reality was built in the late nineteenth-century Durkheimian tradition of "collective representations." Just as mind is irreducible to brain, Durkheim argued, so collective ideas exist in and of themselves and form the animating social spirit, the *conscience collective* (Durkheim 1898 cited by Bullard 2000, p. 280). Both collective representations and *conscience collective* surpass the sum of their parts, creating a hyper-spiritual social life. Human sentiment and reason are transformed and raised to a new degree of complexity in the hyper-spiritual social realm. Social life thrives through the bridged dualities that unite individual minds within a collective world that grows, changes shape, and in turn shapes individuals (Bullard 2000, pp. 280–281). This Durkheimian social theory acknowledges the collective and interpersonal dimensions of witchcraft, as well as expressing its contagious dimensions. Emotions and beliefs are extremely sharable. Durkheimian conscience collective informs crowd theory and the psychology of the masses (Barrows 1981). But even if Durkheimian innovations allow us to bridge the fantasy-reality duality, even if *conscience collective* accounts for the contagious dimension of witch fears, we need to still consider such dualities as: material–spiritual, physical–metaphysical, and objective–subjective.

The Fann group freely resorts to discussion of Durkheimian collective representations, but there is more at stake here than understanding the cultural idioms of the Senegalese. While the Ortigues and others practicing at Fann resorted to cultural and psychoanalytic interpretations, their perspective contrasts with dominant views in the colonial era which expressed a more literal understanding of at least some aspects of *sorcellerie*, and contrasted yet again with the expressed religiosity of their patients.

Colonial Perspectives

In the colonial era, witch hunting provoked the ire of authorities much more than did acts of bewitching. Colonial-era legislation prohibited witch hunting and prosecuted those accused of it. This had the perverse effect within Senegalese cultures of leaving the broad population exposed to bewitching and yet without recourse to witch-hunters, or *bilédios*. Prosecutions of those accused of witchcraft, including the eating of the bewitched, were rare (Labouret 1935). Baum writes:

> Until the 1920's, however, French intervention in Diola religion had been limited to a prohibition of poison ordeals in the searching out of witches, a phenomenon that had become increasingly common during the years immediately following the French occupation of the Casamance.
>
> (2004, p. 209; Maclaud 1907)

Arrest, imprisonment, fines, and even execution could befall the unlucky healer apprehended by French authorities (Baum 2004, p. 208; Meunier 1913; Buell 1928, vol. I, p. 1101).

A system of native courts, first organized in 1903, adopted the difficult goal of allowing local customs to flourish while also upholding the ideals of French civilization (Mbodj 2017). Originally local chiefs were granted jurisdiction over lesser offenses, but reforms put in place under Governor William Ponty reorganized the courts, and empowered the lieutenant-governor of each colony to establish special courts. The judges in these courts served as well as administrative officials, so that the same individuals responsible for implementing laws and policies held the power to try and convict members of the colonized population. Subdivision officials presided over the lower court, the tribunal du premier degrée, while the Commandant du cercle presided over the higher court, le tribunal du deuxième degrée. There was also a court of appeals. The courts did not have peer juries, but rather used local officials to decide guilt or innocence.

In general, authorities brought legal action against practices that threatened (or appeared to threaten) French authority and against practices that shocked the authorities' sense of humanity. Each court was aided in its determinations by two native assessors, who were selected for the trial from a list approved by the lieutenant-governor. The native assessors were supposed to be drawn from the same ethnic group as the parties in the suit so that cases were adjudicated, to some degree, according to the customs of the parties (Opoku 1974; on indirect rule see Conklin 1997, pp. 122–128; see Baum's description of tribunals used in Diolan witch trials, 2004 p. 206, Buell 1928, vol. II, pp. 133–134). Muslim qadi (judges) could also be called upon to aid the courts (Lydon n.d., p. 8). The toleration for local customs, however, stopped short of most dimensions of *sorcellerie* and healing.

The practices most abhorrent to French sensibilities included ritual murder, divination using poison, cannibalism, and witchcraft accusations. Cannibalism, it must be remembered, was linked intimately to witchcraft, as is indicated by the term *sorcier-anthropophage*. Unlike the doctors, psychologists and sociologists at Fann Hospital, many colonial authorities understood such cannibalism to be a physical act. In 1910, during the governorship of William Ponty, it became obligatory for officials to prosecute such "abhorrent practices" (Joucla and Desvallons 1910, p. 84). In 1955, A. P. Robert published a critical assessment of the degree to which French criminal prosecutions changed African society in the years before 1946 (Robert 1955, pp. 57, 86, 147, 191, 202–216).[2] The obligation to prosecute "abhorrent practices" seemingly carried with it a mandate to view cannibalism as a physical rather than metaphysical act. The reorganization of the penal code in the early 1940s, that eventually extended the reach of French courts to all criminal cases in French West Africa (A.O.F.), reaffirmed the French opposition to "shocking" practices. The new code outlawed divination through the administration of poison (even in cases where the parties consented), calumnious denunciation (which would include accusations of witchcraft), and sorcery, magic and "charlatanism" (Anon. 1941, pp. 31, 38–39; Saar 1974, p. 115). In 1946 the French courts in the AOF took over all criminal prosecutions. On November 19, 1947, the A.O.F. published a renewed law against cannibalism and in 1952 legislation on practicing medicine without a license became applicable in the A.O.F. (Bouvenet 1955, p. 51).

In his 1957 publication on how jurists should enforce French colonial laws, René Pautrat reasserted the colonial practice dating from the early twentieth century, that in cases where customary law "deeply shocks our sense of humanity" it should be contravened (Pautrat 1957, p. 92). Pautrat's standard applied, for example, to divination by administration of poison, to accusations of witchcraft, and to cannibalism. These practices are all related to witchcraft and witch hunting. Rituals practiced to heal spirit possession, such as *ndöep*, and magical practices of Islamic *marabouts* are not mentioned in this catalogue of "shocking practices," and yet nonetheless were sometimes prohibited.

Among the array of Senegalese healing practices, French colonial authorities concerned themselves mainly with the detection of witches by witch-hunters (see discussion of Balanta and Diola witch accusations in Maclaud 1907). Identifying witches was vital to family and village health, since a witch who ate the soul of someone caused serious illness and eventual death (as discussed by Geschiere 1997, p. 263, n.5). Protection from witches, thus, formed an essential part of local practices. However, from the French perspective, the supernatural powers ascribed to witches did not really exist. Thus, equally from the French perspective, no one needed to be protected from witches, because, as they held, witches did not really exist and certainly had no metaphysical powers. As Robert Baum explained, "Since the vast majority of colonial administrators did not believe in witchcraft, their response was to outlaw witchcraft accusations and to punish those who made such accusations" (Baum 2004, p. 201). When colonial authorities got wind of accusations of witchcraft, there was no thought of providing broader assurances of safety to the people. Rather, the accusers were subject to prosecution for defamation. Or, if divination proceedings had been employed, the so-called witchdoctor might be subject to prosecution either for witchcraft or for poisoning. Or, if the accused witch had succumbed to the witchdoctor's divination potion or subsequent ritual murder, the diviner might be prosecuted for witchcraft and murder. In Senegal in 1909 there were 15 convictions of witchcraft; four in Casamance, seven in Diourbel, one in Dagana, and three in Thiès (Senegalese Archives, Sous Serie 6M, dossier 055). These convictions compose only a small percentage of the overall number of criminal cases in 1909. Other cases of medical-magic may have been prosecuted as fraud or swindling, defamation, and in the case of divination through the ingestion of harmful substances, poisoning or murder. Casamance, which had four sorcery convictions, also had 19 swindling convictions.[3]

The colonial justice system aimed to repress witch hunting and accusations of witchcraft more assiduously than it concerned itself with straightforward witchcraft. This is because according to French perspectives, witchcraft did not really exist whereas the negative impact of witch accusations and witch hunting – in the forms of trial by ordeal that resulted in injuries, poisoning, and even murder – were all too visible. However, one aspect of witch's behavior drew a stern response, the practice of devouring one's victim. According to various sources, witches ate their victim's heart and liver. They devoured their soul and thereby killed them. Or, they killed them and then dug up their fresh cadavers to feast on the meat. Depending on what sources are judged credible, this cannibalism was strictly metaphorical and spiritual: that is, witches ate the soul of the victim. The body consumed was the metaphysical double of the material body of flesh and blood. Or, witches actually, physically ate the flesh of their victims. Mid- and late twentieth-century scholars – including, for example, Baum (2004), Geschiere (1997), Simmons (1971), Ames (1959) – generally accept the soul-cannibalism thesis. Geschiere also maintained that in the Maka region of Cameroon, physical cannibalism existed as a part of warfare, if not as part of witchcraft practices (1997, p. 33).

During the colonial era, there was ample documentation of the metaphysical nature of cannibalistic-witchcraft (*sorcellerie-anthropophagique*). One Wolof legend, for example, published in a prominent work by the nineteenth-century métis missionary, Père Boilat, explained both the origins of *sorciers* and of soul cannibalism (Boilat 1853, pp. 315–317). According to the legend, witches originated in the early times of human history when, after the fall of Babel, humanity was dispersed. As people fled the fallen tower, they grew desperately thirsty. They came upon a lake, but it was filled with blood. Most people refused to drink from the lake of blood. They fought their thirst until they reached a second lake of pure water. However, some did not wait to arrive at the second lake. They drank their fill from the lake of blood. These people became *sorciers*. Boilat recounts that "immediately they gained the power to leave their skins during the night, to fly through the air clothed in their stripped flesh, and to eat the souls of their near ones" (1853, pp. 31–316). Boilat explained that all the peoples of West Africa believe in *sorciers*, and that they understand *sorciers* to be "people with the power to eat human souls." According to his Wolof sources, witchcraft is found among all people, although it can be difficult to know who is a witch, since they appear to be normal individuals. Also, since witchcraft was believed to be inherited, even the witch him or herself might not be aware that he or she was a witch. Only a diviner, a witch hunter, could discover who among a group was a witch. The detailed account by Boilat compares substantially to late twentieth-century and twenty-first-century accounts (Baum 2004; Simmons 1971; Ortigues 1984).

In 1907 Dr. Ian Maclaud, on the other hand, published a long description of diverse ethnic groups in the Casamance region in which he testified to numerous trials by ordeal, mob murders of those suspected of witchcraft, and the urgent need to guard cadavers so that villagers did not dig them up and eat them (pp. 183, 187, 191–92, 195–96). Maclaud opined that civilization has led to the decline of the peoples of the Casamance. He noted that the rise of material standard of living had done nothing to assuage the overwhelming terror provoked by their superstitions (1907, p. 200). Their habits, described by Maclaud as "vicious, revolting, and barbaric," could only be changed by a "civilizing process" that confronted and overcame these superstitions.

The Diola Trials

Overlooking the spiritual dimension to cannibalism described by Boilat – that is, that witches were reputed to eat the souls of their victims not their bodies – and echoing instead Maclaud's perspective, colonial laws wrote cannibalism into the physical world. Legislation in 1923 tightened laws against cannibalism, aiding widespread prosecutions from 1924–1927 in the region of Casamance (Anon. 1926). Baum links this witch hunt to a desire by one local faction to stamp out the power of local priests. He evoked a situation in which the local chief, appointed by the French, held no real power. Meanwhile "another occult power – the békine – powerful in the practice of sorcery" exercised "an absolute authority" that extended to "all important issues concerning the community" (Baum 2004, p. 205, n.15).

The legal troubles started in 1924 with the report that a young boy had been exhumed and eaten in the village of Seleki. The Diola chief of the province, Benjamin Diatta, lead the research into this and other reported cannibal crimes. The secret sect of the Koussanga[4] occupied center-stage in these trials. The Koussanga was a group that was reported to meet secretly at night for cannibalistic feasts, dancing, and orgies. This administrative description of the Koussanga contrasts with Boilat's opinion that such secret societies originated out of philanthropic goals. Admittedly, as a staunch Catholic priest, Boilat was suspicious of the influence of Islam and pagan religions in these sects, which he identified with demon worship. However he never hinted at such vast crimes as the Koussanga allegedly committed (1853, pp. 457–462). By 1927, 161 Diola had been arrested for cannibalism. This included 59 arrests in 1926 in the canton of Seleki, and 102 arrests after inquires in the province of Ousseuye in March of 1927. Mr. Darand and Chef Benjamin Diatta oversaw the trials of those arrested in Osseuye. The Governor of Casamance (new to his post in mid-1927 and not involved in the arrests of 1926) viewed these trials as particularly important politically. Indeed, the consolidation of French authority in Casamance was pursued through these trials (Anon. 1927a).

The archival records from these trials are riveting and sometimes grotesque. They plunge us into a Francophone world which leaves little hint of the actual words spoken by the villagers. Those on trial adamantly denied the allegations of horrifying crimes. Robert Baum's admirable history of these trials features interviews with one of the court interpreters, a man named Teté Diaddhiou. According to Diaddhiou, "It was not flesh . . . it was the soul . . . it was witchcraft that we transformed into cannibalism . . . in witchcraft, it is the soul that one eats" (Baum 2004, p. 26). According to Diaddhiou, in order to take advantage of French courts of law, the accusers transformed a widespread belief in cannibalism of the spirit into a fictive cannibalism of the flesh. The accusations arose from a desire to oust animist and anti-French villagers from positions of power in the community. The French court documents, however, present only the accusations of cannibalism and the futile defenses. The court documents do not reveal the double or triple meanings of these accusations. The univocal character of these trial records is emphasized in a special report to the Governor of Senegal in which the administrative head of Casamance expressed unquestioning conviction that many of the Diola were cannibals, stating as an indisputable fact that there existed "in lower Casamance a vast secret association whose members exhume the dead in order to eat them" (Anon. 1927a).

Our interest in this troubling moment in colonial Senegal is limited to the gaps between Senegalese and French understandings of health and healing. These trials reveal a topsy-turvy world of misunderstanding and deception. The political motivations of the accusers, possible distortions by court interpreters, and the French desire to consolidate power in this rebellious province, combined forces to create a series of trials that yielded death sentences, but little in the way of truth. These events reveal a readiness to believe horrendous accusations, as well as a readiness of local administrators to ignore knowledge of West African cultures that formed part of the French canon from at least the mid-nineteenth century. The French did not believe in witches and they did not consider themselves to be prosecuting witchcraft. Indeed, a separate law applied to those accused of witchcraft and it was comparatively very little used. The Diola did believe in witches, and they believed that witches could eat the souls of certain victims. Hence the word for "cannibal-witch." However this witchly cannibalism is usually explained as occurring exclusively in the spirit world. The French did not believe in witches, yet it consented to try 161 people for cannibalism. In essence, they were trying people for alleged crimes committed in a spirit world they did not believe existed.

The 1927 report from Casamance to the Governor of Senegal makes plausible the existence of this "necro-anthropophagic society" by explaining it in terms of ritual cannibalism that had degenerated in confrontation with French colonization (Anon. 1927b). The report explains that "in the beginning the [K]oussang only engaged in cannibalism on the occasion of the demise of a notable person, someone with truly remarkable qualities" (Anon. 1927b). On those rare occasions, the body was exhumed two days after burial, a tiny portion taken and added to the preparations of a huge feast shared by all the Koussang. During the exhumation a ceremony recalled the strengths of the deceased, "the macabre communion had for its goal the acquisition of these same qualities" by the members of the [K]oussang. *L'idée primitive* was, then, to make the past live again, in so far as it was good, and to give each person a part of this past" (Anon. 1927b, p. 4). As we have seen already, Dr. Maclaud, writing in 1907, had given a very similar explanation for cannibalism among the Diola, explaining that a local person had told him that "this practice is a vestige of a forgotten rite through which the survivors inherit the soul of the deceased" (p. 200).

Although they were qualified as macabre and primitive in this report, the origins of the Koussang rituals appear somewhat respectable insofar as they were understood within tradition of ritual incorporation of virtuous qualities. Indeed, such ritual cannibalism resonates with the Christian practice of communion as discussed in ethnographic literature (Bullard 2000, pp. 276–278). This restrained and ritualized cannibalism, according to this official report, had become completely deformed, retaining only a remote connection with ritual communion, and giving way to a naked desire to eat human flesh. Ceremonial gatherings no longer sufficed to sate the hunger of these adepts. Indeed, the report claimed that, "the Koussangas do not hesitate to sacrifice individuals when they have no cadavers to eat," even going so far as to sacrifice family members in order to provide meat to fellow Koussangas (Anon. 1927b, p. 4). The report concludes with the claim that rooting out this vast organization which had spread terror throughout the region augmented French prestige and authority (Anon. 1927b).

The colonial authorities seemed to defer to a general ethnographic knowledge, such as expressed in Maclaud 1907, while also evoking a widely accepted view that superficial or incomplete colonization could provoke adverse reactions. The more specific knowledge of spirit-cannibalism in West Africa, however, was conspicuously absent from the Diolan witch trials. In sum, the officials attributed this epidemic of necro-anthropophagie to a pathology of the civilizing process, thus making it more plausible since social scientists widely evoked such pathologies. Psychiatric examples of pathologies in the civilizing process include Dr. Meilhon's 1896 study, "L'Aliénation chez les Arabes; études de nosologie comparée," and Dr. Donnadieu's, "Psychose de civilization," published in 1939. Indeed, the provocation of mental illness by civilizational processes emerged as a major theme in psychiatry, which for many years tried to establish the relation of mental illness to civilizational processes (Heaton 2013, pp. 42–43; Keller 2007, pp. 124–150).

The ethnographic record of the colonial era is cloudy with the same types of confusion that one finds in the court records. For example, Henri Labouret, a colonial military man and respected ethnographer, seemed thoroughly convinced that West Africans practiced orgiastic cannibalism (Kambou-Ferrand 1993 provides a biography of Labouret, Friedman 1996 discusses Labouret's correspondence with Marc Bloch). Writing in 1935, Labouret clarified the distinction between the material body and the body's double. Labouret explained: "that which explains all the superstitions concerning witchcraft, is the power of the double (or, shadow image) to leave the sleeping body, to lead its own existence involving pleasure, pain, and exposure to dangers" (1935, p. 463). Witches operate by leaving their bodies behind and using their "doubles" to travel about in the night. Despite Labouret's clarity on this subject, he nonetheless fell prey to the temptation to literalize and materialize the night world of doubles. Indeed, he produced a line of argument worthy of inclusion in William Arens, *The Man-Eating Myth* (1979): not exactly here, I've not seen it personally, but I have it on good authority that in the next town, in times in the not too distant past, cannibalism was common. Labouret's own words run as follows,

> It seems that in times past associations of witches existed who gathered in the night in hidden locations to eat human flesh, perform magic, and dance. It is not questionable that, in isolated areas of the Soudan region, certain groups still occasionally do these things, but only with the greatest secrecy and in times of duress, such as famine, epidemics, or some other cataclysm. But these associations are becoming more and more rare and it is difficult to find information about their actions.
>
> (1935, p. 470)

After this demonstration of evidence that titillates and enthralls rather than convinces, he mentions recent court cases in which individuals belonging to a witch's coven were convicted of eating human flesh. Although he locates these cases in the Ivory Coast, he could as well be referring to the Diola trials in the Casamance.

***

Fann Hospital and *Sorcellerie*

This detour into witches, cannibalism, and judicial prosecutions might seem rather wide of the mark for a book on transcultural psychiatry and globalization. The role of spiritual beliefs in Senegalese medical cures, however, requires that we consider these dimensions to the colonial past. The partial and distorted historical records on illness and healing reveal that the effort to gain acceptance for Western medicine was also an effort to gain headway for French civilization.

The administrators regarded the Diolan trials as an effort to stamp out barbarous practices and to extend the reach of French standards of civility. As reinterpreted by Baum, however, the trials served aspiring local Muslim elites in their efforts to solidify their status by undermining that of their animist rivals. At any rate, these trials effectively established to French authorities the presence of endemic cannibalism in the Casamance. In 1958, in an official publication of the University of Dakar, E. Rau contended that

> the most solid proof that cannibalism remains active in all of West Africa, is that in 1947 the French parliament was led to legislate against it, "to be punished by death anyone who is judged guilty of a murder committed with the intent of cannibalizing the body."
>
> (Rau 1958, p. 180)

Rau himself followed the tradition of Labouret rather than Boilat, and wrote with a firm conviction that cannibalism and *necroanthropophagie* were endemic in West Africa.

This colonial physicalization of *sorcellerie anthropophagique* was only tempered during the 1950 legislative session when proposals were advanced that sought to strengthen the prohibitions on witchcraft. The administrator-ethnographer Marcel Griaule successfully intervened against this proposal, arguing that in an area with one doctor for every 45,000 inhabitants, healers were needed. He argued that true healers should be allowed to practice and only charlatans should be prosecuted: "only our ignorance of the local sociological and philosophical systems sustain our belief that most of reported actions are actually legally watertight cases of witchcraft" (Griaule 1957, p. 91). As with the Fann doctors, Collomb and Diop, Griaule does not describe how to distinguish a "true healer" from a "charlatan."[5] He leaves intact the label "witchcraft" for the charlatan while removing it from the "true healer," and ignores entirely how to distinguish between *sorcellerie* and healing. This leaves us in a confusing labyrinth, in which good healing and bad witchcraft are confounded even if still said to be different.

The practitioners at Fann followed Griaule's lead, and sought to build bridges between distinct cultural norms. Not surprisingly, the bridge the Fann personnel built emphasized a psychological and psychoanalytic interpretation of *sorcellerie*. They do not discuss the dangers of witch hunting, and even in the case of the murder of an alleged witch (the case of S.C.), the offense of homicide is de-emphasized while the psychological dimensions of anxiety and reassurance via a *bilédio* are emphasized. Writing in the 1960s, Maric-Cécile and Edmond Ortigues demonstrated the psychoanalytic significance of spirit-cannibalism. The Ortigues accepted the metaphorical nature of cannibalism, and thereby were able to work with this cultural artifact to gain access to the psychic lives of their clients (1966). Such psychoanalytic and cultural analysis of the Fann researchers stands in marked contrast to the legal order of the (by then defunct) colonial world, and also against the religiosity of their clients. Perhaps, for those thoroughly convinced of psychological truths, there is no essential difference from religion.

Yet within the realm of religion, the metaphysical, and the spiritual there reside mysterious powers that are incommensurable with mere psychology. Polyvagal theory accounts for the persistence of narrativized beliefs regarding the inexplicable, which persists even when science is fully engaged. The autonomic nervous system, the ancient neural mechanisms from long extinct evolutionary ancestors, neuroception, and interoception, all of these bodily forces that continually reassert themselves in a complicated dance with beliefs and narratives, this will never go away. Such forces arise through our living bodies.

The Fann approach, we could say, drained the spiritual terror from *sorcellerie*, whereas PVT allows for science, psychology, and terror. In saying to themselves and to their patients that is "merely psychological," that is "individual," that is "existential anxiety," that is "not terror in the face of evil," they were able to distance themselves from the dangers of witchcraft. The American anthropologist, William Simmons, did not obtain such a distanced perspective on witchcraft during his fieldwork in the 1960s and 1970s among the Badyaranke of the Casamance region of Senegal (Simmons 1980). His Durkheimian interpretation of the social tensions that witchcraft seeks to dissolve apparently conformed with Fann-style analysis, but Simmons was much more alive to the destructive power of witchcraft accusations and counter-accusations. He discusses deaths and severe beatings, and individuals within extended families who escaped with their lives only by extreme good fortune. Simmons' analysis presents witchcraft as largely dysfunctional, casting blame on kin and close neighbors for misfortunes and accidents far beyond the powers of those accused (Simmons 1980, pp. 456–458). Modernizing forces, according to Simmons, have lessened the power to control witches among the Badyaranke and increased the power of the witches, hence increasing the pervasive fear of accusations and terror of bewitchment (1980, pp. 461–462). Simmons emphasizes that witchcraft accusations are destructive, not functional, in their social consequences. Again, to be concrete, by destructive Simmons means that people accused of witchcraft are beaten, forced to flee their homes, or are killed. The fear and violence associated with witchcraft are similarly emphasized by Ames (1959), Lallemand (1988) and Ashforth (2005).

Adam Ashforth, reflecting on rampant *sorcellerie* in post-apartheid Soweto, arrives at hatred as a fundamental dimension to the phenomena (2000, pp. 217–225). Witchcraft is a nightmare, Ashforth concludes, composed of hatred and fear for one's life in the face of malice (2000, pp. 248, 253). Drawing on his ten years of living in Soweto and his experiences helping his friend, Madumo, find effective treatment for a bewitching, Ashforth reflects on the philosophy of *Ubuntu*, "a person is a person through other persons." He adds to this a negative corollary, "because they can destroy you"(Ashforth 2005, p. 86). Sorcery's destruction of people's lives, he reflects, inevitably prompts claims for justice, which claims are also constitutive of healing. This inter-subjective dynamic is rendered with greater metaphysical weight by Eric de Rosny, who describes *sorcellerie* as rooted in the perennial perversity of humanity as they seek to harm those close to themselves (2005, p. 29). Even if we were to get rid of *sorcellerie*, de Rosny reflects, this perverse desire to harm those close to us will endure.

Such dysfunctional and threatening dimensions to witchcraft and witchcraft accusations largely escape discussion by Fann Hospital personnel. The psychoanalytic and cultural analysis they developed voices a post-colonial apologetic dedicated to proving respect for erstwhile colonial subjects and enjoining the discussion of dysfunction. Even more important was the opposition among Fann personnel to the colonial conviction that actual cannibalism was endemic in West Africa. At Fann Hospital, the nature of *sorcellerie*, as well as possession and magic, was fundamentally psychological. The Fann clinicians explored the link between the psychological and spiritual, and yet, as professionals dedicated to mental health, the primary allegiance at the hospital was to the psychological. The social fear and dread of bewitching was transformed at Fann into individualized anxiety, a transition which the medical professionals viewed as a salutary psychological step on the road to modern individualism. Sandwiched between fears of the colonial past and the contemporary grappling with resurgent witchcraft, the outlook of the Fann practitioners has a distinctive hue. Tenaciously engaged with understanding how the cultures of Senegal work to foster harmony and healing, how they manage spiritual crises and control *sorcellerie* in their midst, the Fann practitioners paid homage to cultural processes their colonial forbearers sought to suppress.

Conclusion: Senegalese Futurism

The expectation that magic and witchcraft would decline and eventually vanish with the arrival of modern social conditions has proven to be mistaken. Instead, the conditions of neo-liberal capitalism, steep economic inequality, and globalized networks layer new technologies and increasing urbanization, upon the enduring forces of magic and witchcraft.

Abdoulaye Elimane Kane, a philosophy professor the University of Dakar and later on a government functionary, portrayed such a milieu of magic, witchcraft, and technological modernism in his novel, *Les magiciens de Badagor* (1996). Notably, this futurist novel – which touts the wonders of computer science as well as that of futuristic architecture and urban planning – is utterly infused with magic and witchcraft. Pathé, the main character, is an architect and city planner who turned away from Leninist-planning to focus on fostering mid-sized cities in order to secure the well-being of humanity. Pathé is brilliant, daring in his thinking, and over the course of the novel, his career reaches global importance. Pathé is also obsessed with his computer, which he has named Everything-Machine because he puts into it everything he can no longer remember. A mysterious ailment, indeed, attacks Pathé's memory, so that he is more and more dependent on his imagination, while the machine guards his memory (Kane 1996, p. 108). Nafi, his lover, operates the computer with mysterious clairvoyance, so much so that her mind can control the machine without any physical intermediary. Thus, while Pathé is more and more dependent on his computer, Nafi is more and more in control of the computer. Their identities are intertwined via their love and via the computer. Pathé, however, remains reluctant to marry Nafi, and instead devotes himself more and more to his futuristic city planning. The fever-dream events of the novel spiral to ever-more grandiose levels and far-flung geographies, encompassing rural Senegalese villagers, rival traditional healers with magical powers, ministers of the national government, the president of the Republic, a previously unknown love-child from Canada, a professor and a mayor from the U.S.A., and the distinguished representative of an 800-year-old oracle society from Athens, Greece.

The power of divination and magic thrums through the disparate networks in which Pathé is enmeshed and from which he gains strength and identity. Nonetheless, after a long interior struggle, Pathé rejects marriage to Nafi in favor of his career and global fame. She disappears from his life, marries a magician-healer, and herself becomes a powerful diviner. The cataclysmic conclusion involves a celebration of futurist amenities brought to a small village. "Read the Future" is the motif for the event. The celebration culminates when Nafi arrives. Dressed like a bride, she abruptly plunges off the balcony, taking Pathé with her, to their mutual deaths.

The murderous end to Nafi and Pathé's relationship exemplifies the "all or nothing" struggle of witchcraft. The jealous and angry aggression of Nafi against her former lover is wrapped in occult powers that magnify her emotional injury, her physiological dysregulation, and her ability to harm. "Read the Future" is the closing message of this novel. It is difficult to interpret the outcome of the tragic deaths of Nafi and Pathé as other than an allegory that repudiates the separation of memory and imagination from love and the fecundity represented by marriage. The theme of Pathé losing his memory and losing his relationship with Nafi, along with the hypertrophy of his imagination and ambition, echoes entrenched themes of madness and identity. Pathé's obstinate refusal to unite the disparate parts of his life, his determination to pursue his own future without memory (Nafi), even despite his utterly entwined identity with Nafi and his computer, spells his downfall. The repudiated Nafi re-emerges in Pathé's life as an irresistible, murderous spirit. Kane's novel shows a highly technological Senegalese future that is only attainable by balancing diverse forces, including magic, witchcraft, and identity based in relationships. Within the history of psychiatry, such endurance of magic and witchcraft is explicable via PVT and the inevitable ancient autonomic dimensions of life.

Notes

1 I retain the French word *sorcier* because in English a "witch" is presumed to be female. As this discussion develops the gendered dimensions of *sorcier* are explored.

2 While not the object of this present history, it should be noted that imposing French as the language for judicial decisions of Muslim courts, in 1911, had far-reaching consequences for the colonization of West Africans, perhaps more so than the suppression of specific rituals of healing (Lydon n.d., p. 9).

3 These archives give only the French view of events and brings to mind Frantz Fanon's eloquent denunciation of the power of the colonial interpreter (embodying the authority of the regime toward the non-French speaker, intimidating and often motivated by

personal desires other than transparent representation of speech). African voices are present in these documents, but they are recorded only in French, through the filter of an interpreter. See Lawrence *et al.* 2006. Saliou Mbaye, chief archivist at the Senegal National Archives, and Dr. Tamba M'Bayo, from Michigan State University, are both working on interpreters in Senegal. For an account of the role of the interpreter of the documents concerning the Diola cannibalism trails see Baum 2004.
4 Koussanga is also spelled as Boussanga in documents. I will uniformly use Koussanga.
5 Protocols for distinguishing charlatans from healers were developed alongside the post-colonial legalization of (some) healing in Senegal in the 1970s. This is not without its ironies, as recounted by Eric Fassin and Didier Fassin, "De la quête de légitimation à la question de la légitimité: les thérapeutiques 'traditionnelles' au Sénégal," *Cahiers d'etudes africaines*, 28: 110 (1988), pp. 207–231, see pp. 214–215. See also Joseph Tonda's update of these dynamics, "Le syndrome du prophète: Médecines africaines et précarités identitaires," *Cahiers d'etudes africaines*, 41: 161 (2001), pp. 139–162.

Works Cited

Ames, D., 1959. Belief in 'Witches' Among the Rural Wolof of the Gambia. *Africa*, XXIX (3), 263–273.

Anon., 1926. *Territoire de la Casamance, Rapport sur la Situation Politique de la Casamance et Programme de Désarmement et de Mise en Main de la Population, Archives Nationales du Sénégal (ANS)*, 2D5-3455. Available from: https://halshs.archives-ouvertes.fr/halshs-00705436/document.

Anon., 1927a. *L'Administration Supérieur de la Casamance à M. le Lieutenant-Gouverneur du Sénégal à Saint Louis*, 11 juillet, Sous serie 6M 329. Available from: https://gallica.bnf.fr/ark:/12148/bpt6k5454478x/texteBrut.

Anon., 1927b. *Territoire de la Casamance, Rapport Politique générale annuel, 1926*, 42, 17 February, Signed, L'Administration Superieur, Signature Illegible. ANS 2 G26-66. Available from: https://www.sas.upenn.edu/~cavitch/pdf-library/Anderson_et_al_Unconscious_Dominions.pdf.

Anon., 1941. *La Justice indigène en Afrique occidentale française*. Rufisque, Senegal: Imprimerie du Haut Commissariat.

Arens, W., 1979. *The Man-Eating Myth: Anthropology and Anthropophagy*. New York: Oxford University Press.

Ashforth, A., 2000. *Madumo: A Man Bewitched*. Chicago: University of Chicago Press.

Ashforth, A., 2005. *Witchcraft, Violence and Democracy in South Africa*. Chicago: University of Chicago Press.

Barrows, S., 1981. *Distorting Mirrors Visions of the Crowd in Late Nineteenth-Century France*. New Haven, CT: Yale University Press.

Baum, R.M., 2004. Crimes of the Dream World, Robert Baum's Crimes of the Dream World: French Trials of Diola Witches in Colonial Senegal. *The International Journal of African Historical Studies*, 37 (2), 201–228.

Baum, R.M., 2009. Concealing Authority: Diola Priests and Other Leaders in the French Search for a Suitable Chefferie in Colonial Senegal. *Cadernos de Estudos Africanos*, 16–17, 35–51.

Bernault, F., 2009. De la modernité comme impuissance: Fétichisme et crise du politique en Afrique équatoriale et ailleurs. *Cahiers d'études Africaines*, 195 (3), 747–774.

Boilat, P.D., 1853. *Esquisses Sénégalaises*. Paris: P. Bertrand.

Bouvenet, G.J., 1955. *Recueil annoté des textes de Droit Pénal applicables en Afrique Occidentale Française*. Paris: Editions de l'Union française.

Buell, R.L., 1928. *The Native Problem in Africa*, vol. 2. New York: Palgrave Macmillan.

Bullard, A., 2000. *Exile to Paradise*. Palo Alto, CA: Stanford University Press.

Conklin, A., 1997. *A Mission to Civilize*. Palo Alto, CA: Stanford University Press.

De Rosny, E., ed., 2005. *Justice et sorcellerie: Colloque international de Youndé*. Yaoundé, Cameroon: Presses de l'Université Catholique d'Afrique centrale.

De Rosny, E., 1992. *L'Afrique des guérisons*. Paris: Karthala.

Diop, M. and Collomb, H., 1965. A propos d'un cas d'impuissance. *Psychopathologie Africaine*, I (3), 487–511.

Donnadieu, A., 1939. Psychose de Civilization. *Annales Médico-Psychologiques*, 97 (1), 30–37.

Friedman, S.W., 1996. *Marc Bloch: Sociology and Geography*. Cambridge: Cambridge University Press.

Geschiere, P., 1997 [1995]. *The Modernity of Witchcraft; Politics and the Occult in Postcolonial Africa*. P. Geschiere and J. Roitman, trans. Charlottesville: University of Virginia Press.

Griaule, M., 1957. *Conseiller de l'Union Française*. Paris: Nouvelles Éditions Latines.

Hamès, C., 2008. Problématiques de la magie-sorcellerie en islam et perspectives africaines. *Cahiers d'études Africaines*, XLVIII (1–2), 81–99.

Heaton, M., 2013. *Black Skin, White Coats; Nigerian Psychiatrists, Decolonization, and the Globalization of Psychiatry*. Athens, OH: Ohio University Press.

Joucla, E. and Desvallons, G., 1910. *Afrique occidentale française, Justice indigène: Jurisprudence de la chambre d'homologation publiée sous le patronage de M. William Ponty, gouverneur général*. Gorée: Imprimerie du gouvernement général.

Kambou-Ferrand, J.M., 1993. Guerre et résistance sur la période coloniale en pays lobi/birifor (Burkino Faso) au travers des photos d'époque. *In*: M. Fiéloux, J. Lombard and J.M. Kambou-Ferrand, eds., *Images d'Afrique et sciences sociales: Le Pays lobi, birifor et dagara (Burkino Faso, Côte d'Ivoire, Ghana)*. Paris: Karthala, 77–99.

Kane, A.E., 1996. *Les magiciens de Badagor: Roman*. Saint-Maur, France: Éditions de SÉPIA.

Keller, R., 2007. *Colonial Madness: Psychiatry in French North Africa*. Chicago: University of Chicago Press.

Kiernan, J., ed., 2006. *The Power of the Occult in Modern Africa*. Berlin: LIT Verlag.

Labouret, H., 1935. La Sorcellerie au Soudan Occidental. *Africa, Journal of the International Institute of African Languages and Cultures*, VIII (4), 462–472.

Lallemand, S., 1988. *La mangeuse d'ames: Soycellerie et famille en Afrique*. Paris: L'Harmattan.

Lawrence, B.N., Osborn, E.L. and Roberts, R.L., eds., 2006. *Intermediaries, Interpreters, and Clerks: African Employees in the Making of Colonial Africa*. Madison, WI: University of Wisconsin Press.

Lydon, G., n.d. *Obtaining Freedom at the Muslim's Tribunal*. Leiden Conference Paper. Available from: www.ascleiden.nl/Pdf/paper-Lydon.pdf [Accessed 9 July 2021].

Maclaud, 1907. Le Basse Casamance et ses Habitants. *Bulletin de la Société de la Science de Géographie Commerciale de Paris*, XXIX, 176–202.

Mbodj, H.H., 2017. *L'organisation de la justice pénale en Afrique occidentale française: Le cas du Sénégal de 1887 à l'aube des indépendances (1887–1960)*. Droit: COMUE Université Côte d'Azur (2015–2019).

Meilhon, Dr., 1896. L'Aliénation chez les Arabes; études de nosologie comparée. *Annales Médico-Psychologiques. 8ème série*, III, 17–32, 177–207, 365–377 and IV, 344–363.

Meunier, P., 1913. *Organisation et Fonctionnement de la Justice Indigène en l'Afrique Occidentale Française*. Saint-Brieuc: Imprimerie de F. Guyon.

Monteil, C., 1931. *La Divination chez les noirs de l'Afrique occidentale fran aise*. Bulletin du comite des tudes historiques et scientifi ques, 14 (1), 27–136.

Opoku, K., 1974. Traditional Law Under French Colonial Rule. *Verfassung und Recht in Ubersee*, 2 (1), 139–155.

Ortigues, M.C. and Ortigues, E., 1984 [1966]. *Oedipe Africain*, 3rd ed. Paris: L'Harmattan.

Paulme, D., 1954. *Les gens du riz*. Paris: Plon.

Paulme, D., 1962. *Une société de Côte d'Ivoire, hier et aujourd'hui, les Bété*. Paris: Mouton.

Pautrat, R., 1957. *La justice locale et la musulmane en A.O.F.* Rufisque, Senegal: Imprimerie du Haut Commissariate de la République en Afrique occidentale française.

Pelgrim, R., 2003. *Witchcraft and Policing: South Africa Police Service Attitudes Towards Witchcraft and Witchcraft-Related Crime in Northern Province*. Leiden: African Studies Center.

Rau, E., 1958. Le juge et le sorcier. *In*: *Annales Africaines*. Dakar: la Faculté de Droit et des Sciences Economics, 179–204.

Robert, A.P., 1955. *L'évolution des coutumes de l'Ouest Africain et la législation française*. Paris: Éditions de l'encyclopédie d'outre-mer.

Saar, D., 1974. La Chambre Spéciale d'Homologation de la Cour d'Appel de l'Afrique Occidentale Française et les coutumes pénales, 1903–1920. *Annales Africaines*, I, 101–115.

Saar, D. and Roberts, R., 1991. The Jurisdictions of Muslim Tribunals in Colonial Senegal, 1857–1932. *In*: K. Mann and R. Roberts, eds., *Law in Colonial Africa*. Portsmouth, NH: Heinemann, 121–145.

Simmons, W.S., 1971. *Eyes of the Night, Witchcraft Among a Senegalese People*. Boston: Little Brown.

Simmons, W.S., 1980. Exploitation and the Soul Eating Witch: An Analysis of Badyaranke Witchcraft. *American Ethnologist*, 7 (3), 447–465.

White, L., 2000. *Speaking with Vampires: Rumor and History in Colonial Africa*. Berkeley, CA: University of California Press.

6 Devoured by Fear in Childbirth and Haunted "No-Good" Children

***

Introduction

The terror that frequently directed Senegalese lives is evoked in this chapter via devouring fear in childbirth and the alternating promise and terror of "no-good" children (*l'enfant nit ku bon*). These cases draw us close to significant life events and the disequilibrium that too frequently arose. The physiological PVT perspective is emphasized with respect to mental illness in relation to pregnancy and the *nit ku bon*. Childbirth and children figure in this chapter as crucial vectors for ancestral spirits or other metaphysical forces to enter and disrupt lives. Childbirth, governed by autonomic physiological processes, figured as a moment of significant peril for many Senegalese women. The supreme social significance of motherhood opened the woman to the spirit world. If her post-partum body did not close properly, women suffered on-going torment and persecution. Social insecurity – difficulties with husband or co-wives – figured prominently in these case studies as did intense physiological dysregulation. The cases exhibit disturbances of interoception (*cenestopathie*), feeling that animals lived under the skin (*zoopathie interne*), and feelings of being eaten, and burned. Ideation included persecution by witchcraft, magic, and (less frequently) spirit possession. The case of Khady Fall transitions this chapter from a focus on childbirth to a focus on children. Spirit crises heavily marked Khady Fall's two pregnancies and sent her on a path to becoming a priestess in possession rituals. The perils of childbirth sometimes produced "no-good-children" (*l'enfant nit ku bon*). The "no-good child" is viewed with deep ambivalence – either as exceptionally promising or outrageously dangerous. Such a child is characterized by its ability to choose death at any moment; the child seems to belong more to the spirit world than to the world of humans. A *nit ku bon* might bring unexpected good fortune to the family or might endanger the whole family and community. Spells and rituals forced the child to declare its true identity, encouraged it to stay among the living, or made it return to the spirit world where it belongs. This chapter concludes with a summary of Binta's case. On the verge of adulthood, this young woman was struck down

DOI: 10.4324/9781003112143-7

in the marketplace by spirit crisis; the case illustrates Binta's illness and Fann personnel views on this crisis.

Mental Illness Related to Pregnancy and Childbirth

Pregnancy and childbirth figured centrally in the lives of Senegalese women and mental health troubles, or spirit crisis, frequently followed in the wake of this pivotal life event (Guena *et al.* 1970, p. 111). Giving birth, indeed, figured as a woman's supreme achievement. Infertility created intolerable stigma, a catastrophic failure of one's life purpose (Guena *et al.* 1970, p. 120). Throughout childhood, a girl was prepared to become a mother. The marriage dowry was paid based on reproductive promise. Successful birthing created the most valuable dimension of a woman's life (Guena *et al.* 1970, p. 120).

Childbirth poses physical dangers for all women. The process, especially for first time mothers, is normally long and painful. The body's processes in birthing are unlike any other life experience. Even for individuals educated in the details of biological reproduction, giving birth is mysterious process. The powerful interior forces of the body seize control. Intense muscular contractions, bleeding, panting, sweating: all these create an intense physiological state that in many ways mimics intense fear reactions. Even women in modern hospitals experience psychological disequilibrium, some become intensely fearful, some dissociate and refuse to accept the reality of the moment. For those women who inhabit a metaphysical world of spirits, magic, and witchcraft, childbirth is a moment of exceptional spiritual openness and peril. Welcoming new life into the world is an ages-old and perennial miraculous moment that ties women intimately to the portal between being and non-being, life and death.

In 200 case studies collected from 1965–1970 at Fann Hospital, we see that pregnant and post-partum women experienced terrifying persecution delusions (Guena *et al.* 1970). The attending doctors classified these deliriums variously as *bouffées délirantes*, depression, or mania. Persecutory delusions formed a common theme. The terrorized minds of these women are portrayed vividly in their delusions. Lack of safety in the home – arising from difficulties with husband, co-wives, or perhaps the mother-in-law or other member of the household – figured prominently in these case studies. Physiological dysregulation provides a powerful lens by which to appreciate these troubling episodes. Case after case these women exhibited disturbances of interoception (*cenestopathie*), feeling that animals lived under the skin (*zoopathie interne*), and feelings of being eaten, and being burned. These physiological disturbances prompted culturally rooted ideation regarding persecution by witchcraft, by magic, and (less frequently) by spirit possession. These women's symptoms were subdued with pharmaceuticals and electro-shock, after which they returned to their families. This litany of cases evokes the prevalence of such illnesses.

Anta, a 24-year-old Wolof woman, returned home after a successful birth of her fifth child, and promptly accused her maid of being a *sorcière*. Anta claimed that at the hospital she acquired special insights into the spirit world (*xam-xam*) and a new mission. She complained her maid wanted to attack and eat her and that the maid now wanted to eat her baby (Guena *et al.* 1970, p. 126). Anta wanted to protect her sleeping baby from witches who could steal and eat it while it slept. So she prevented its sleep by shaking it incessantly and violently so that it would wake up and cry. Anta's family reacted by first dismissing the maid, and then bringing Anta to the hospital. The doctors treated her with electro-shock therapy and "she rapidly improved" (Guena *et al.* 1970, p. 126).

Fatou, a 21-year-old Wolof woman, fell ill the day her new baby was baptized, the eighth day after giving birth. She gesticulated wildly, and laughed inappropriately and without emotion. She took off all her clothes, walked around nude, and confronted anyone who tried to approach her. Her baby no longer interested her; she refused to care for it. Abruptly weaned, the baby soon sickened and died. Seven months after this brutal onset of symptoms, Fatou's family brought her to the hospital. In the meantime they had sought cure through a series of *marabouts* and traditional healers, none of them successful. She presented to the doctors as incoherent, given to hallucinations and delirious speech. "Ants are eating my breasts," she said, "my family speak the language of the birds." She was treated with electro-shock and anti-psychotic drugs and soon regained her equilibrium (Guena *et al.* 1970, p. 127).

Aminata, a Bambara woman age 23, was hospitalized during her difficult pregnancy. After hospitalization she developed psycho-sensory hallucinations. She told her doctors that she had a spirit-vision and that the neighboring patient was a *sorcière* who wanted to devour her. This *sorcière* appeared to her surrounded by roosters and pearls. Then a male voice spoke to her with insulting immodesty as she watched a crowd of children undergoing circumcision. After the usual treatment, she too quickly regained her health (Guena *et al.* 1970, p. 128).

Oumou, a 31-year-old Bambara woman, entered the hospital after a spontaneous miscarriage in her sixth month of pregnancy. This would have been her fifth child. After the miscarriage she became agitated, refused to eat, and insisted that she was a saint and that someone wanted to kill her. She accused her co-wife of placing a spell on her (*maraboutage*) in order to kill her baby. At the hospital she insisted that she was not ill but rather that she had been cursed in an attempt to kill her. In her words, "it is the co-wives and the lovers of my husband who did it because my husband, who loves to run after women, prefers me above all others." Oumou then insisted that a neighbor by the name of N'Diaye had taken on the form of her husband and with his wives had plotted against her. The very day of her miscarriage, Oumou said, she had traveled into "the other world; I was dead, the midwives could not see me, they could only hear my voice." Oumou received sedatives and after two months left the hospital to return to her life with her "unfaithful husband" ((Guena *et al.* 1970, p. 130).

Aissatou, a 20-year-old Wolof woman, gave birth to a healthy baby but on that same day fell into a delirious state marked by persecution. She complained of *maraboutage* and *sorcellerie*. "My whole body hurts," she complained, "the *sorcières* want to kill me and eat me." She accused her half-sister, her mother-in-law, and the co-wife of her mother. Anxious, fearful, and agitated, Aissatou tried to run away several times. She wanted to go join her friends "in the water of the river." She refused to accept that she had been pregnant and refused to take care of her baby, treating it with hostile aggression so that her family had to take it away (Guena *et al.* 1970, p. 131).

Fatou, a 26-year-old Toucouleur, began experiencing odd, disagreeable, and abnormal internal sensations during the end an unusually long pregnancy. She felt her body burning. She felt animals walking about underneath her skin. After a successful birth Fatou continued to suffer, which her family explained as the birthing-blood rising up into her head. The traditional post-birth massage, designed to close the body to the spirit world and re-establish equilibrium, failed to alleviate her distress. In the hospital she expressed ideas about persecution, accusing her aunt in particular. "My aunt is burning my stomach," she said, "the smell of the fire is coming out of my nose. Flames are coming out of my eyes." Fatou then accused her mother and her doctors, "who removed her spine and put broom straw in her skin" (Guena *et al.* 1970, p. 131).

Another woman named Fatou, a 15-year-old Wolof woman, fell ill upon the birth of her first child. In the maternity hospital she developed signs of agitation, insomnia, and refused to eat. Upon transfer to the Fann Hospital, she was delirious and hallucinating. "These cats want to steal my baby," she said, "don't eat me, I don't want to die. Everything I had in my belly has been killed. I've had 20 pregnancies, and 20 miscarriages." She drummed on her stomach and genitals saying "my mother spoiled my stomach, she made the baby die." She chanted praises to powerful *marabouts*, hid her face in her aunt's lap, lumped together the sandy soil of the courtyard and offered it as a present. She approached the nurse, imploring her, "Grandmother, grandmother, please nurse me, please nurse me, teach me to walk." The family explained Fatou's behavior as a *maraboutage* by a co-wife. After the usual treatment, Fatou too was cured and returned home (Guena *et al.* 1970, pp. 133–134).

N'Deye, a 22-year-old Wolof woman, began exhibiting disturbing symptoms in her second month of pregnancy. She would cry without motivation and refused to answer her husband's questions. He took N'Deye back to stay with her parents, where her health improved. However, once back in her husband's house, she became agitated, chanted and danced, laughed and then abruptly cried, and tried to burn her clothing. A second stay with her parents did not help her. She made numerous attempts to run away, reporting that she could hear a voice telling her, "You must leave, you must go into the water, you must go to Sangomar." Sangomar is the place where the spirits (*rab*) live. These auditory hallucinations came from an old, dark man with a menacing face and big beard. N'Deye's husband explained:

> When the old man is present, she is completely crazed, her heart begins to heat her up, she is very mean with me, and hits me when I want to stop her from going into the ocean. I think this man is a *rab*.

N'Deye also self-harmed. She frequently hit her belly and demanded a knife "to open her stomach and to remove the baby in there." The old man-rab told her,

"The baby is not good for you. If you take the baby out, you'll be healed." The family took N'Deye to several healers and *marabouts*, each with a different opinion, whether *rab* or *maraboutage* caused her illness. Finally her father decided that the pregnancy itself lay at the source of N'Deye's troubles, and they waited expectantly for a cure when she gave birth. As it happened, N'Deye did experience a reprieve upon the successful birth, but the next day she again suffered agitation, with screaming and crying. She refused to nurse her baby and treated it aggressively. Then she began trying to steal other newborn babies. Transferred to Fann Hospital, N'Deye presented a perplexing case for the doctors. She seemed relatively lucid, but her mother explained that N'Deye was never "there" on Fridays, on that day the spirits always took her away. N'Deye replied to this, "I want to leave to see my mother, my mother who is white and is in the ocean. Samoury wants me to go." Samoury was the old man, a *rab*, who lives in Sangomar. N'Deye recovered in a "spectacular manner" after the normal treatment (Guena *et al.* 1970, pp. 135–136).

Fatou K., a 24-year-old Toucouleur, married at the age of 13, suffered a breakdown during the birth of her fifth child. Shortly before the baby was due she was out walking and was hit by a wind. Then she dreamed that someone told her, "Hurry up and give birth. Afterward, I'll devour you." Next she dreamed that her baby was a boy, but that instead of her carrying the boy, the boy was carrying her. About a month after the birth, Fatou started to isolate herself. Her husband wanted her to start up her normal housekeeping chores, but she said she couldn't because she no longer knew anything. After that she developed insomnia, inability to eat, confusion, loneliness, a fixed regard and random crying. She finally fell into complete mutism. Failed treatment by a *marabout* preceded hospitalization. A series of electroschock treatments brought her quickly back to health.

Aminata F., a 23-year-old Lebou, fell ill one month after a difficult birth. She suddenly took extreme fright of her child and ran from the house to her mother where she explained that the baby had transformed into a terrifying giant. She refused to touch the baby for three days, but on the fourth day her health improved and she began nursing again. That same night she woke up screaming that her "baby was a menacing giant." Her mother-in-law, who was sleeping in the same room, had also transformed into a giant. Panicked, Aminata hid under the bed then fled, undressed, out into the street. When her family brought her to the hospital, Aminata was agitated. She sang, she imitated the gestures of everyone around her, grimaced, repeated questions posed to her, and laughed at her own behavior. She took on erotic and humorous poses, played with everything, demanded people hug her, displayed her genitals, caressed them, and showed the injury from the difficult birth. When interviewed by the doctors, she spoke of menaces and danger. She feared her young daughter, her mother-in-law, and her husband. A few days later she became convinced that she had not given birth yet and that she had to incessantly give birth, but that the nurses did not want her child to be born. Treated with anti-psychotics and electro-shock, Aminata's health steadily improved (Guena *et al.* 1970, p. 143).

***

Becoming a Priestess of the Rab: Khady Fall's Births

The life events of Khady Fall unite the metaphysical dangers of pregnancy with spirit possession of the young child. Fall's earliest memory, from when she was two or three, involved her unintentionally breaking some pottery in a Serer neighbor's domestic shrine (Zempleni 1977, p. 103). The uproar that ensued involved the Serer household shouting, Khady Fall fainting, and her mother running to her rescue. Fall's father, who arrived somewhat later, was resigned to his daughter's death. When she revived, he went to the local Serer chief's home and accused him of attempting to eat his daughter. The chief denied this accusation of witchcraft, instead alleging that Fall was possessed by *rab*.

The *rab* continued to pursue Fall throughout her life, so that *rab* marked both of her own pregnancies. Fall gained release from her symptoms only when she embraced her role as a messenger of the *rab*. She was not able to do this until she reached her 30s (as recounted in Chapter 8, Ancestors). Married already at age 16, a *marabout* foretold that her first pregnancy would produce twins, a human child and an amorphous "companion," that is, a *rab*. Fall had consulted the *marabout* because she had dreamed of the death of an important man in the village. Prior to the dream, she had seen this noble man tie a young *griot* boy to a tree and beat him mercilessly (Zempleni 1977, p. 104). Within days of Khady's dream, the man was seized with vomiting and quickly died. Fall then told the village of her dream, and people agreed that the man was a witch. However, after telling her story, Fall became mute. This mutism arose, so the *marabout* explained, because she had betrayed the secret knowledge the *rab* had granted to her. When the time came for her to give birth, Fall delivered a "normal boy" and "the second is not quite a human being (*nit*). Both are stillborn" (Zempleni 1977, p. 105).

Fall's second pregnancy produced a healthy young girl. However, when the girl was still an infant, Khady and her husband encountered several snakes while working in the fields. The husband killed the snakes, who in retrospect Fall understood to be *rab*. Just days later, a man fell on her child, instantly killing her (Zempleni 1977, pp. 105–106). On the very day her daughter died, Fall felt the *rab* "cut her bowels." From that day forward she was sterile. She reflected on this event that she knew she had to accept her heritage as conduit of the *rab* but nonetheless she continued to resist (Zempleni 1977, p. 106). Over the years, Fall continued to experience interventions by the *rab* until she finally became a priestess of the *ndöep* possession rites.

***

Nit ku bon

L'enfant nit ku bon describes a syndrome recognized among the Wolof and Lebou as documented by Andràs Zempléni and Jaqueline Rabain. The Serer had a similar concept which they called *o kin o paher*, or "the bad person" ["*la personne qui est mauvavaise*"] and *o kon o paf* or "death that passes by" ["*la mort qui passe*"] (Zempleni and Rabain 1965, p. 332). The odious name for this syndrome, however, sometimes is construed as the opposite. That is, the "no-good child" is actually sometimes the prized and exceptionally gifted child. Thus *nit ku bon* (bad person) could actually mean *nit ku bax* (good person). The inversion of the meaning in the name aims to deter jealousy. An exceptionally beautiful child, with large eyes and preternatural wisdom, might be called *nit ku bon* to help hide the child from malicious forces, whether arising from a jealous neighbor's *maraboutage*, *sorcellerie*, or directly from evil spirits (Zempleni and Rabain 1965, p. 357). This interpretation, however, is not exclusive. Deep ambivalence characterizes the family and social attitude toward the *nit ku bon* child.

The *nit ku bon* child usually could be recognized at a very young age. Thus, wise old women and those gifted with vision (*borom xam-xam*) might notice a peculiar type of cry, the clarity of facial expression, refusal to nurse, rapid growth or rapid loss of weight, early walking, or being born without a prepuce (Zempleni and Rabain 1965, p. 333). The *nit ku bon* was normally very good looking, with large eyes and a solemn demeanor. However, they also frequently refused to meet other people's eyes, "he looks inside himself" or "he looks into the void, somewhere else" (Zempleni and Rabain 1965, p. 334). Such a child frequently hides her face and keeps her eyes averted or downcast. Their speech is infrequent. They do not confide in others. They prefer to isolate themselves. Or, if they join in the games of other children, they behave oddly and do not respond to casual interactions. They are frequently sick. Their behavior can be changeable, from hour to hour or day to day, first laughing and playing and then suddenly withdrawn and solemn or crying in a corner. Extreme reserve is coupled with extreme sensitivity. A *nit ku bon* who is reprimanded might cry and refuse to eat for days on end. They hide and efface themselves, as though embarrassed. They are "a being which is wrapped into itself, which has no relationships with others" (Zempleni and Rabain 1965, p. 335). At social events, they hide or cry.

These behaviors, which are tempting to compare to autism spectrum disorders, lead family to believe that the *nit ku bon* does not love them. They say that "its heart is ugly" (Zempleni and Rabain 1965, pp. 334–335). They say that the child is mean. He stays alone, is never happy or content. Above all, such a child reacts with passion when she is disciplined or feels anger coming from another. The child can fall into a fit of screaming and crying that lasts for days. Such fits can even lead to death (Zempleni and Rabain 1965, pp. 335–336). These diverse symptoms are summed up in phrases such as *xon bi dafa naw* (his heart is ugly, or, he is mean), *dafay faglu* (he is sad or angry), or *dafay sis* (he is asocial) (Zempleni and Rabain 1965, pp. 334–335). The *nit ku bon* is a child who can die from one moment to the next. This close relationship with death is the key to this culture-bound syndrome (Zempleni and Rabain 1965, p. 336). Usually these children die young, before puberty. The rare *nit ku bon* who survives into adulthood, however, is considered an admirable person, a good worker, and a desirable spouse.

The affected child might leave for the other world at any moment. This is because of their relationships with the spirit world. They are thought to be an ancestral spirit (*rab*), or a human person possessed by a *rab*, or a reincarnation of a recently deceased relative, or a child of a *yaradal*. A *yaradal* is a mother who lost several children one after the other. The succession of children is considered, in fact, the same child who keeps coming back. The one who survives is the "child of a *yaradal*" and is likely also, though not necessarily, a *nit ku bon* (Zempleni and Rabain 1965, p. 349). This type of child has a clear penchant for dying, indeed is capable of dying at its own will. All the *nit ku bon* die easily and can choose to die. Self-willed death, in effect suicide, is their final defining feature (Zempleni and Rabain 1965, p. 349). Their privileged relationship with the spirit world gives them knowledge and power beyond their years (Zempleni and Rabain 1965, p. 350). As a child, they act with a freedom reserved for adults, for example by making independent decisions. Within the Senegalese context, this age-defying independence up-ended the normal family relationships. A child who does not obey, who refuses to respond when called or given a task, is a child "not long for this world" (Zempleni and Rabain 1965, pp. 422–423). The usual repression of behavior outside the norm of an age-class, however, in the case of a *nit ku bon* is suspended. Responsibility lies with the *rab*, not with the child.

Dr. Moussa Diop clarified the nature of *rab*, who assume such a central role in the *nit ku bon* diagnosis. *Rab* generally means an ancestral spirit, but Diop's origin-story of the *rab* refines the relationship between them, humans, and ordinary ancestral spirits. Zempleni and Rabain summarized Diop's account (1965, p. 340) as follows: The original grandmother gave birth, whether to a girl or boy, and the placenta transformed into a snake. This snake then made a home, perhaps in the crook of a tree or in the roof-beams. One day the village suffered a disaster and the snake saved the village – by providing water, fecundity, happiness, or good luck. In return, the people gratified the snake with ritual offerings of food. In this way the *rab* became attached to the land. Thus, the *rab* is a type of twin-spirit to the human, born not from a deceased person, but from a placenta transformed into a snake. Like humans, *rab* procreate and develop lineages, so that the spirit worlds of human ancestors and *rab* ancestors continues to proliferate in parallel, twin-like manner (Zempleni and Rabain 1965, p. 340, n.16). Diop emphasized the blurry boundary between human and *rab*; every birth has the possibility of birthing both human infant and placental *rab*.

The attitudes and conduct toward the child, explain the investigators, are organized by collective representations – a Durkheimian phrase indicating shared beliefs rooted deeply in shared emotions – that are also the same as available to the child (Zempleni and Rabain 1965, p. 379). In this way the status of the *nit ku bon* is established and grows more powerful as the child develops. Processes and customs of caring for such a child arise in and through these collective representations, which carry a powerful ability to alienate the family from the child, and the child from the family. Calling someone *nit ku bon* not only denotes a perturbation of family relationships, it further produces profound disruptions. This feedback loop operates from an early moment of the child's life so that "it is impossible to isolate the initial trouble from the ensuing collective representations." This circular escalation of alienation, they remark, is commonly recognized among Western-trained therapeutic communities (Zempleni and Rabain 1965, p. 379).

Zempleni and Rabain recorded numerous curative rites designed to help conciliate the *nit ku bon* with its family. This unknowable being in their midst launches the entire family into distress. The rites seek out the true identity of the child, commune with the *rab*, and ensure proper social order. Magical verses and practices, as detailed by Zempleni and Rabain, served to help the young child bear the powerful presence of the *rab*, or to reveal the true identity of the *rab* (Zempleni and Rabain 1965, pp. 343–355). A successful integration of the *rab* into the life of the child could produce a powerful healer, a leader for the village. However, the negative valence of the *nit ku bon* child appeared in the belief, for example, that a woman *nit ku bon* who touched a pregnant woman would cause a miscarriage. Some thought it necessary to "attach" or "tie" the *nit ku bon* child with powerful magic in order to gain protection from his or her bad wishes. The *nit ku bon* might also be a young *sorcier*, thus a very bad person, sucker of blood and eater of souls (Zempleni and Rabain 1965, p. 358). These threatening potentials intensified family dynamics that sought to ascertain the identity of child via mystical practices. Special spells existed for when the family was even more deeply disconcerted, suspicious of hidden plots with heavy consequences, or gratuitous cruelty (Zempleni and Rabain 1965, pp. 360–361). The ambivalent attitude to *nit ku bon* children is evident as well in magical spells to make the child stay among the living, and other spells to rid the family of the child by forcing it to return to the spirit world (Zempleni and Rabain 1965, pp. 368, 373–374).

The healer chants the *jat* rhythmically, melodically, and repetitively. This rhythmic sing-song repetition recalls Porges' emphasis on the strong role of prosody in establishing social bonds (2017, p. 23 and *passim*). As the child is enveloped in the rhythmic incantation, the healer swings about, lifts the child, and caresses his body (Zempleni and Rabain 1965, p. 343, n.22). For a young person such a ritual would present a strong moment of physiological co-regulation. In response to tender and conciliatory *jat*, the child's physiology might stabilize so as to augment an ability for social engagement. A healer with an aggressive manner or a *jat* that cast suspicion on the child, however, seems likely to induce a panic reaction, thus shutting down the child's social engagement. Estimating the impact of the ritual on the child can be only a mental experiment, but a balanced perspective should also consider the possibility of the child's neural atypicality. Some *nit ku bon* demonstrated extreme sensitivity, with startle responses that triggered much more easily than for others in their families. Thus, even a gentle *jat* might have provoked a negative physiological response.

Here is a rough paraphrase of a flattering *jat* designed to elicit the *nit ku bon*'s esoteric knowledge:

> Bissimilahi, I turn my back on Allah who created you and I turn away from his prophet by whose grace you were created, because, for myself, you suffice, in all manner of ways. To me, I seized you with fifteen hands; I do not

> know for what you are insufficient, but to me, you suffice. I do not know who you don't please, but you please me. You, Moussa, I ask you to remember that at each moment, someone needs you. I need your fathers. I need your grandparents. Moussa,[1] I need you.
>
> (Zempleni and Rabain 1965, p. 352)

This same *jat* continues with a heightened plea for whatever information the child has about witches or magic. Notably to receive this information the healer renounces Islamic fundamentals, as above in the renunciation of Allah and Muhammad. In an act of radical trust, the healer declares allegiance only to the *nit ku bon*. Thus the healer chants,

> Nothing escapes me concerning the *djinns*, the *seytãne*, or the angels. If you know something about witches, the evil eye, the evil tongue, the poison pen, well, you know that I need you. I know nothing of writing [i.e., the *Qu'ran*]. Moussa, tell me to come directly to you each time that I am upset, or when I am afraid. Be me! I am you! Be my everything. I'm your everything.
>
> (Zempleni and Rabain 1965, p. 353)

Indeed the unifying trust in this *jat* is so strong that the healer and child become one. One more time in this *jat* the healer declares loyalty only to the *rab* and its world,

> I do not believe in Islamic mystical science. I believe only in *rab* and the forces of your world. I'm selling my faith in God, buy it! Moussa, from today forward, all that you tell me, that's all that I need. If you call me, I will answer.

After establishing a union based in radical and exclusive loyalty, the healer makes his final request: "Me, I ask only one thing: that I can know all that is not human and all that these beings do. Make it so that I know all that has happened, and so that I know all that will happen" (Zempleni and Rabain 1965, p. 353). After this rhythmic recitation, the healer "spits the *jat*" into curdled milk. He passes the milk bowl around the child's head eight times. Then, he has him drink the milk" (Zempleni and Rabain 1965, p. 352).

The strong threat to a stable family relationship for the *nit ku bon* creates on-going anxiety which then further disrupts the child's need for inner safety. Zempleni and Rabain write that the rituals designed to integrate the child more securely into the family "are inserted into a situation where the relationships are already disrupted" (Zempleni and Rabain 1965, p. 363). Family turn to the rituals blindly, out of fear the child might die any moment. The collective representations, in which the child lives and grows, are polarizing, according to Zempleni and Rabain. This polarization of identities and interests – the child is seen as an outsider, whether for better or for worse – structures the family's inter-subjective reality and continues to reshape it. The *nit ku bon* is not overlooked or allowed to fade into the background. Rather such a child poses an urgent promise or threat from the spirit world, and so is of central importance for the family. Tense, anxious, and sometimes fearful relationships organize around the child. Zempleni and Rabain remark that "without the [collective] representations about the child's origins and desires, the attitudes and conduct toward the child would not be what they are. But without the [collective] representations, the child himself would not be whom he is" (Zempleni and Rabain 1965, p. 363).

One of the most common aids for the *nit ku bon* was to "attach it" in order to restrict its movements and confine its will. One such ceremony called for cutting tree roots to the measure of the child's right hand, left foot, then left hand and right foot. The healer also measures wood to the size of the face, the nose and the forehead. He circles this cut wood three times around the child's head. He takes a bit of sand from nearby footprints made by the child and puts it into a pot into which he places the bundle of roots, tied together with a string. This pot is then hidden under the child's bed. In this way, the child "will not budge from where he is" (Zempleni and Rabain 1965, p. 365). The "tying" *jat* implores the *nit ku bon* to leave behind his fellow *rab* and to stay in the world of humans. The healer promises the child a peaceful life and the best of welcomes in this world. He tells the child, "I know that you do not need those whom you've left [in Sangomar]. Moussa, you came here. This is where you want to be. This is where you are loved" (Zempleni and Rabain 1965, p. 367). The healer's flattering reassurance in this *jat* aims to placate and ingratiate the child. If, however, the *jat* provokes a crisis – such as frozen immobility and falling to the ground – the healer takes a few grains of sand wetted with urine and places them in the child's nostrils (Zempleni and Rabain 1965, p. 368). Zempleni and Rabain are puzzled by this introduction of "dirt" into the ritual, all the more so because the *rab* reputedly prefer the cleanliness of Sangomar to the unpleasant world of human dirt. Viewed from a physiological perspective, the child's rigid immobility and fall indicate an extreme dorsal vagal stress reaction. This is an ancient reptilian autonomic response to fear. Porges, as discussed in Chapter 2, dwells at length on how this unmyelinated vagal neural reaction launches individuals into physiological states from which humans have difficulty returning. Unlike the "flight or fight" response, which deactivates comparatively easily, the dorsal vagal feigning of death is itself characteristically rigid and unresponsive. Peter Levine writes of the physiological tactic of "shaking off" such a torpor (2005, p. 29). The acrid smell of urine, akin to smelling salts, might provoke exactly the type of shudder and shake needed to return to a more regulated physiological state and to greater social engagement.

A relatively aggressive ritual and *jat* designed to force a *nit ku bon* to declare its true identity prescribed as follows:

> You take a cord and you wrap it around a bit of cloth to form a whip. Each night, at two in the morning, you wake the child. . . . You use water to dissolve the ashes of wood from a tamarind tree [a preferred habitat for spirits] and you soak the whip in this water. After grabbing the child's big toe, you hit his

> head eight times. You do this as many nights as necessary for the *nit ku bon* to show his true character.
>
> (Zempleni and Rabain 1965, p. 359)

This procedure is accompanied by an invocation,

> *Bissimilahi*, I discover he who is hidden in a person. Moussa, I swear that today you will know that an experienced witch has returned from the nightly hunt, and no one can subject him to witchcraft without a great struggle. So, Moussa, I tell you to take off this appearance of someone else that you are wearing. Put on your own appearance. Abandon the character of the other that you have borrowed and take on your own character. Stop hiding yourself and disclose who you are.
>
> (Zempleni and Rabain 1965, p. 359)

The *jat* continues:

> Moussa, your mother said she is tired of you. Your father said he is tired of you. Moussa, you, I think that if people are tired of you, you could do something for yourself. Moussa, your father is a *rab*. Your grand-father is a r*ab*. Your great-grandfather is a *rab*. Moussa, you can't hide yourself from me, because I know you. Moussa, we have been following you, but, we will not follow you anymore because we don't want anything to do with you. Moussa, you, you have wronged those who have sent you. Why have you changed your character, as though the character of your ancestors isn't enough for you? Me, I think that the person who changes their gifts, it's because their gifts do not satisfy them. Moussa, why do you change your appearance, you manners, and your desires?
>
> (Zempleni and Rabain 1965, pp. 359–360)

This incantation was delivered at two in the morning, night after night, with a wet whip tapped eight times to the child's head, sought to demand the child's identity, to find out if it is truly an evil spirit or an auspicious rebirth. Zempleni and Rabain include many such Wolof and Lebou incantations in their study, which creates a remarkable record of the rites as practiced in the early 1960s. These *jat* included many diverse aims: to prevent the child from visiting with spirit friends, to discover what deceased family member had returned, to discover the child's secret spirit-world knowledge, to discover the child's true character, to hold the child among the living and, to encourage the child to depart again for the spirit world. Techniques alternated between "gentle caresses, imploring, and tenderness" and "annoyance, distrust, and rejection" (Zempleni and Rabain 1965, p. 377). Zempleni and Rabain remark that the child "who wears the clothing of another" is in reality clothed by the family. By this they evoke the family relationships, expectations, and interpretations, in and through which the child forms an identity. The *nit ku bon* is called into existence via the family's narrations. The search for the child's true character, they remark, risks producing only a reflection of those who seek so desperately (Zempleni and Rabain 1965, p. 377).

When the family feels compelled to force the *nit ku bon* back into the spirit world, the following *jat* might be used:

> Have the child go to sleep on top of a sieve or strainer. Place other strainers next to each hand, each foot. Under each strainer place three roots from the tamarind tree and a bit of earth from a termite mound. Then I [the healer] put my *lar* [fetish stick made from a bull's tail] on the strainer that is under the child. To the right of the child's head, I write the father's name in the sand. To the left, I write the mother's name. At the top, I write the child's name. I treat the child at six in the evening. At midnight, he leaves. In performing this, I circle the child forty times. When I'm finished, I go home no matter how far away my house is. The child who hears the noise of the *nit ku bon* who leaves [the world of humans], will be deaf for life. He would be extremely difficult to heal.
>
> (Zempleni and Rabain 1965, pp. 373–374)

This *jat* demands to know,

> Who are your parents. Talk to me about your family! Moussa, tell me, where did you come from? Moussa, leave this family where you have come. Leave this mother to whom you came. Leave this father to whom you came, and return to Sangomar which is your native land.
>
> (Zempleni and Rabain 1965, p. 374)

The healer invokes an Islamic blessing, then says he is going to Sangomar to make war on Sada, the king of the *rab*s' world. The healer then recites King Sada's lineage and where each spirit lives, and reminds him to take back his grandchild, the *nit ku bon* (Zempleni and Rabain 1965, p. 375). "*Rab*, open your eyes and look at your child! Allah Akbar, *Rab*! Come with your hands empty and do not leave with your hands empty! . . . I take that which is not mine and I give it back to those to whom it belongs" (Zempleni and Rabain 1965, p. 376). In contrast to other *jat*, which focus on the child, in this one the child hardly appears at all. The focus is on the *rab* and compelling them to repossess their child. The impact of such a ceremony on a child could be extremely physiologically destabilizing. Fann case studies to routinely report how extreme fears could provoke death. In this situation, that would have been the sought-for outcome.

Such a *nit ku bon*, destabilized and alienated, appeared to family and to healer as a dangerous foreign being, a spirit whose home was Sangomar rather than among humans. Senghor's expression that "I give birth to the other by knowing them" here demonstrates a dreadful outcome (1964, p. 259). Considered not just strange and unknowable, but also dangerous, such a child indeed becomes just that. The polyvagal theory of Stephen Porges explains the inter-subjective process of achieving physiological safety. Without that perception of safety, the young child floods with anxiety. When the child cannot feel a subjective (interior) sense of safety in the home with his primary caregivers, this will in turn produce an attachment disorder, from which any number of psychological problems can develop (Fisher 2017, pp. 35–36; Porges 2017, pp. 137–151; Steele *et al.* 2017, pp. 3–34). The hydra-like manifestations of primal lack of safety are evoked by Fisher, who writes of a conglomeration of dysregulated autonomic system, disorganized attachment patterns, and structurally dissociated parts (2017, p. 29). The trauma of a child's disrupted bonds drives a re-enactment compulsion that leads to myriad forms of re-victimization and self-victimization (Fisher 2017, p. 36 citing van der Kolk). In contrast, in the *jat* that invoke a type of extreme compassion, self is dissolved in the safe arms and identity of another. The *jat* that evoke a split child, part *rab* and part human, might evoke an internal alienation, a type of divorce of mind from self. Less extreme than the *jat* calling for the child's death, nonetheless this could call forth a lost self, a condition in which the self is so fragmented that it appears only via identification with an other. Such a condition tends toward soul theft, in which the fragmented individual falls under the control of someone covetous or malicious. This results in a type of extreme subordination, shared with the psychology of enslavement. In the terms of polyvagal theory (Porges 2017), in soul theft, the visceral nerves are controlled not through self-regulation, but through an external covetous agent.

Even just a single instance of de-mobilizing fear, according to Porges, suffices to establish within a person a habitual default to unmyelinated visceral reaction (2017, p. 162). Such extreme anxiety, dissociation, freezing, flat affect, and feelings of emptiness or even of impeding death, can produce delusions, psychosis, and death itself. Controlling another can be achieved through manipulating such "trauma reactions" – both by intentionally creating the trauma and then by offering a supposedly safe haven against repeated trauma in return for obedience. Unlike Porges, who expresses only optimism regarding the implications of his PVT, we must understand the intense neural reactions, and consequent impact on social bonds, are susceptible to various influences and formations, some increase human capacity and well-being, and some increase vulnerability, fragility, and exploitation.

In her later research, Rabain discovered that the *nit ku bon* was only one type of spirit possession identifiable in Wolof children (Rabain 1979, pp. 161–212). Rabain describes the child-voyant, or seer, who is kept blindfolded, bound and gagged because she sees and talks to much about witches (*dëmm*), "but during the night, the *rab* untied everything" ["*quand il était enfant, on lui attachait les mains, les pieds, la bouche pour qu'il ne parle pas, il voyait trop, il parlait des dëmm, mais la nuit le rab détachait tout*"](Rabain 1979, p. 209). These magical ties responded to the threat of metaphysical danger. The potential for the child's experience of harm or fear is by-passed, as Rabain keeps a steady focus on how the adults are trying to control the world in which they live, a world peopled by spirits of diverse sources and diverse powers, the likes of which a mere child should not be seeing or revealing.

Father Gravrand, a contributor to *Psychopathologie Africaine* but not a member of the hospital staff, described in less veiled terms the fate of abnormal children born into Serer families. In a prolonged investigation of the life cycle among the Serer, Gravrand described the initiation of the baby into the community after eight days of life. Such initiation, however, was denied to infants who suffered deformities. In cases of doubt whether a child was defective, it could be allowed to live up to the age of five years at which time a definitive judgment was made, resulting in the killing of the child who failed to appear normal (Gravrand 1965, pp. 296–297).

By now, in the third decade of the twenty-first century, the Western social scientific insouciance toward the spirit world, and most especially toward witchcraft, can be bracketed between the fear and outrage of the colonial era and fear and concern in the present. Rising awareness of the rights of children, inscribed in international law via the 1988 United Nations Convention on the Rights of the Child, and promoted via diverse international and local civil society and non-governmental organizations, acknowledges the suffering of children accused of harboring demons and killing their parents via witchcraft. Senegal is not a primary source of such reports.[2] Moreover, there is of course a distinction between the child who hosts an ancestral spirit and a child witch. The salient point is the plight of the child implicated in perceived metaphysical danger or evil. Whether inept host to an ancestral spirit, or possessed by an Islamic or Christian "demon," the metaphysically dangerous child is a child in danger. Such a child was thought to bring on the death of his or her parents and/or siblings. While Rabain remains silent on the reaction of parents alive to such a danger in their midst, Gravrand – as discussed above – presents in detail the fate of children deemed, for a wide variety of reasons, unable to find a place in society (Gravrand 1965).

Henri Collomb added his own reflections on such issues in an essay exploring the meaning of death in African cultures. Comparing Bantu cultures with the Serer, Diolan and Beudik of Senegal, Collomb writes:

> the child belongs still for some time to the world of the dead (of the ancestors); world from which he comes, in which he participates, and world which he recalls often and to which he wants to return. His future is uncertain; sometimes it is only after several attempts that he remains in the world of the living. . . . Baptism is only performed on the eight day, when the child has demonstrated by not dying in the first days, that he does not desire to leave again. Weaning is another time of life-death dialectic: the child definitively leaves the order of the ancestors to enter in the order of its age-group. He or she loses the wisdom and knowledge [of the ancestors] at the same time he acquires social language.
>
> (Collomb 1970, p. 832)

The sacredness of death, meanwhile, has become unthinkable and indefensible in Western culture.[3]

***

Binta's Choice

We conclude this chapter with the case of a girl on the cusp of adulthood who fell victim to the spirits in the marketplace. This case illustrates yet another type of illness in women's life-cycles. The case portrays as well how Fann clinicians viewed the suffering individual as caught between the culture of spirit crises and that of mental illness.

Binta was a 16-year-old girl, born of a Wolof mother and a Toucoleur father (for Binta's case study see Ortigues *et al.* 1966). She was one of ten children her mother had. Her father had four wives and 32 children. Binta lived with her mother, her older sister, and several younger children in a government-sponsored housing development in Dakar. One day, when Binta's older sister was out of town, her mother also had to go out and she assigned all the household tasks to Binta. Normally the housework was done by the mother, the older sister, and a maid, so this responsibility was new to Binta. Staying at the housing complex without her mother filled her with fear, as she had the impression that many witches lived nearby. She took her younger sister and went to buy food at the local market. There, her sister bumped into an old woman and earned her reproaches. Binta tried to intervene, but the old woman told her she was too young to converse with her. Then a man offered them kola nuts, and Binta accepted even knowing that her mother would disapprove. Upon biting into the kola nut, Binta fell to the ground, mute, limbs flailing about, and unresponsive. She arrived at the hospital as an emergency case. She was totally mute, her arms flailed about uncontrollably, her wide-open eyes roved about rapidly and at random. A barbiturate administered via an intravenous line soon calmed these symptoms, and Binta regained an ability to respond to simple questions. However, her parents' visit a few hours later set off a new crisis, which only ceased after her parents left. The next day Binta was able to speak but was still haunted by a vague sense of anxiety and fear. Within two more days, her symptoms had ceased.

Binta explained this episode as a case of bewitchment, likely by the old woman her sister had bumped into at the market. Binta's mother suggested that Binta was possessed by a *rab*, just as she and her sisters were, and she went about securing a ritual healing for this possession even before Binta left the hospital. Binta's father meanwhile rejected both explanations, saying that this was a simple case of illness, to be treated by the doctors and forgotten.

The interpretive choice that confronted Binta was characterized by Ortigues, Martino, and Collomb as an option to maintain a traditional position, or to evolve into a more personally responsible view of her illness and of her conflicts (Ortigues *et al.* 1966, p. 449). Despite their self-consciously circumscribed roles as white doctors rather than local healers, the Fann personnel viewed their roles in this and other illnesses as not just calming the individual, but also assisting, when possible, with this transition to personal responsibility within the illness. About Binta's case they comment: "not only is Western nosography put into question, but also the definition of family relationships and social adaptation must be reconsidered" (Ortigues *et al.* 1966, p. 449). The outcomes of such a reconsideration depended on the outlook and choices of the patients as much as on those of the hospital staff.

Notes

1 All the *jat* in this chapter use the name Moussa for the child's name. Moussa is an arbitrary choice. In actual practice, the given name for the child would be used.
2 Senegal has not featured in international reports on child witches in the way that the Democratic Republic of Congo and Nigeria have. See for example reports on Christian evangelical witch-hunter, Helen Ukpabio, of Nigeria, "On a Visit to the U.S., a Nigerian Witch-Hunter Explains Herself," *NYT*, Saturday, May 22, 2010, p. A11 and the 2008 film by Mags Gavan and Joost van der Valk, "Saving Africa's Witches," produced by RedRebel Films and Oxford Scientific Films.
3 The controversial rise in the West of the right to end one's life via assisted suicide does not signify a renewed sacredness of death so much as its continued secularization. Paradoxically the Holocaust (the term denotes a burnt sacrifice offered to God) is the most prominent modern enshrining of the sacredness of death. This term itself generated controversy among Jews, many of whom resisted the sacralization of the systematic murders carried out during the Second World War.

Works Cited

Collomb, H., 1970. La mort en Afrique. *Revue de Neuropsychiatrie infantile*, 18, 10–11, 827–836.

Fisher, J., 2017. *Healing the Fragmented Selves of Trauma Survivors: Overcoming Internal Self-Alienation*. London: Routledge.

Gravrand, R.P., 1965. Aux sources de la vie d'apres les traditions serer du Sine. *Psychopathologie Africaine*, I (2), 286–302.

Guena, R., de Preneuf, C. and Reboul, C., 1970. Aspects psychopathologiques de la grossesse au Sénégal. *Psychopathologie Africaine*, VI (2), 111–146.

Levine, P.A., 2005. *Healing Trauma: A Pioneering Program for Restoring the Wisdom of Your Body*. Boulder, CO: Sounds True.

Ortigues, M.-C., Martino, P. and Collomb, H., 1966. Intégration des données culturelles Africaines à la psychiatrie de l'enfant. *Psychopathologie Africaine*, II (3), 441–450.

Porges, S.W., 2017. *The Pocket Guide to the Polyvagal Theory: The Transformative Power of Feeling Safe*. New York: W.W. Norton.

Rabain, J., 1979 [1994]. *L'enfant du lignage: Du sevrage à la classe d'âge*. E. Ortigues, Preface. Paris: Payot.

Senghor, L.S., 1964. *Liberté I*. Paris: Le Seuil.

Steele, K., Boon, S. and van der Haart, O., 2017. *Treating Trauma Related Dissociation: A Practical, Integrative Approach*. New York: Norton.

Zempleni, A., 1977. From Symptom to Sacrifice: The Story of Khady Fall. *In*: V. Crapanzano and V. Garrison, eds., *Case Studies in Spirit Possession*. New York: John Wiley, 87–139.

Zempleni, A. and Rabain, J., 1965. L'enfant nit ku bon; un tableau psycho-pathologique traditionnel chez les Wolof et Lebou du Sénégal. *Psychopathologie Africaine*, I (3), 329–441.

Zempleni-Rabain, J., 1966. Modes fundamentaux des relations chez l'enfant Wolof du sevrage à l'intégration dans la class d'âge. *Psychopathologie Africaine*, II (2), 143–178.

7 Trauma Defenses

Denial, Dissociation, and Magical Thinking

***

Introduction

Denial suppresses the sense of vulnerability to that which occasioned fear; the altered version of reality that is achieved via denial is an exemplar of magical thinking. There is, among educated Westerners, the strong compulsion to deny our own magical thinking. The compulsion itself points to a disowned affective center, one that has been obfuscated or fractured because of a previous trauma. The endurance of that fractured or obfuscated desire is notable. Physiology helps us to survive, recounts Stephen Porges, so that death feints, dissociative compliance, somnolent indifference, or even refusal to accept the reality of a situation should be considered valuable evolutionary mechanisms designed to ensure the individual's survival of extreme danger (Porges 2017, p. 151). The dorsal vagal autonomic response to fear, a legacy of long extinct reptilian ancestors, allows the individual to survive. Dissociation – the feigned death – is prime among the dorsal vagal autonomic responses.

Humans, however, ceaselessly adopt their physiological state into their emotions, their perceptions, and from thence into conscious narration. Within that rich, complicated process, we focus for the moment only on the narration. Denial and dissociation promote stories of elision. That which is left out of the story is the denied. Metaphysical content of such narration has stood as a dividing ground from the scientific, rational narratives. This chapter, however, emphasizes the common ground of physiological autonomic dorsal vagal states that give rise to denial, dissociation, and magical thinking. This physiological process is universal even if narrative differs among individuals, and between groups. Equally true, denial conditions narrative scope, perspective, and modality. Consciousness arises in interaction with physiological state and feeds back into the neurobiological mechanisms. Affective perception of external stimuli and interoception of the body itself might share common qualities with a larger or smaller group, or might be idiosyncratic. Dysfunctional idiosyncratic perception and ideation characterizes mental illness.

DOI: 10.4324/9781003112143-8

In no event, however, can an individual be free of affective dimensions to consciousness for the simple fact that physiological processes are the conditions that permit human life. Similarly, each individual experiences even the most common events on the physiological level of the individual organism. This organism-centered perspective is shared by all of humanity. Consciousness of one's own life as that of one organism within our species makes evident that all others also possess their own perspective. The engagement with denial and magical thinking is similarly shared across all humanity, arising inexorably, as it does, from our ancient evolutionary physiology. These physiological mechanisms ensure that humanity cannot escape occult or magical thinking.

***

On the Endurance of the Occult and Fear of Witches

In 2015 the former president of Senegal, Abdoulaye Wade, accused Macky Sall, the sitting president, of having a family of slaves and *sorciers-anthropophagiques*. Notably this calamitous denunciation met with rebuke from Wade's erstwhile allies as well as from his opponents (Ba 2015). Wade's denunciations of Sall themselves were denounced. Thus, even his own cohort opined that his accusation was itself a "moral failing," undignified of a former president, and the act of a "delinquant" (Ba 2015). In comparison, in the United States, Donald Trump's repeated accusations of witch hunting – a clear inversion and projection – echoed in press accounts without any repudiation from those among his allies. His credulous followers exhibited increasingly fervid attachment to his fantastical statements. His unreason obtained willing echoes, until the crescendo of violence on January 6, 2021. Nonetheless, his party continued in 2021 to feed delusional beliefs and to support his unfounded accusations. In contrast to Senegal in 2015, in the U.S.A. in 2021, no unity arose to effectively denounce Trump's hysterical and delusional accusations, even though lives were lost in the January 6, 2021 mob violence. Consider as well the words a twenty-first-century American mother wrote regarding her son: "Can you imagine being desperately afraid because your son, twice your size, with eyes that are dark and wild, tells you to get away, because you are a witch, a devil, a vampire?" (Clark 2018).

Witchcraft continues to haunt us. The widely accepted prediction by the early twentieth-century sociologist Max Weber held that modernity would inexorably lead to the disenchantment of the world and the widespread adoption of rational *persona*, but Weber was wrong (Stuart Hughes 1958, p. 332). Witchcraft and magic endure. Consider, for example, the Houston, Texas-based medical doctor, Stella Immanuel, who claimed demon sperm causes COVID-19 and that it can be cured with hydroxychloroquine. Immanuel, who was born in Bali, Cameroon, earned her medical degree at the University of Calabar in Nigeria. Immanuel also claims that many ailments of the womb arise from sexual intercourse with demons. Immanuel's views, unorthodox in the accredited biomedical community, nonetheless demonstrate the persistence of ancient metaphysical beliefs in the twenty-first century. Immanuel is a member of a Pentecostal Church established in Nigeria, the Mountain of Fire and Miracles Ministries. Her fiery version of Christianity fits neatly with other charismatic religious sects prevalent in the evangelical movement, just as her support for the 45th president's re-election fits neatly with the general evangelical belief that the president was anointed by God to fight demons and to free the world of the international cult of pedophile predators (Gagné 2020). The QAnon conspiracy figures here as another powerful reminder of the ineradicable power of unreason, magical thinking, and crowd hysteria (Bloom and Moskalenko 2021).

Witchcraft in our globalized world is everywhere and nowhere. It is everywhere because all individuals are susceptible to unreason, fear, anxiety, and narratives of malicious forces. Nowhere are we free of the physiological polyvagal dynamic that generates emotional and contagious unreason. Within that pervasive human susceptibility, "[s]pecific forms of witchcraft follow the cultural migrations of communities that observe practices of the occult. One may find vodou witch-doctors in urban settings in New Orleans as readily as in remote regions of Haiti" (Nagle and Owasanoye 2016, p. 567). Witchcraft is nowhere because the metaphysical narratives informed by physiological states of extreme fear are optional. Such metaphysical narratives are not necessary. Nonetheless, insofar as initiates and dabblers believe and seek to bring harm to fellow sentient beings, and insofar as individuals believe they can fall victim, there is a real identifiable power of witchcraft. Certainly the physiological need for safety is real, and lack of safety provokes physiological fear states that induce a range of troubling ideation, dissociation, flat affect, vacant stares, episodes of rage, or other symptoms common to hysteria. Moreover, via neuroception, such physiological fear reactions are contagious, so that groups of people can collectively de-stabilize and collectively narrate their experience of unreason. The various techniques for conjuring and healing – chants, dances, recitations, inhalations, aspirations, fumigations, burials, rebirths, casting out of spirits, worship at altars – aim to dissuade maleficent spirits and powers, and to calm and regulate physiological fear responses. Mindful regulation of physiology, arguably a more tempered and rational tactic, relies on a highly polished and trained consciousness, and thus is restricted to cohorts of the adept.

Denial is by far the most available and accessible resort against witchcraft and other occult forces.

***

Not everyone is susceptible to witchcraft. Those who fortify their minds and bodies, in particular, can escape the characteristic debilitating fear and the panicked search for healing. In a widely influential book, the anthropologist Adam Ashforth grappled with the distinction between those who are susceptible and those who are not. His discussion in *Madumo: A Man Bewitched* (2000) takes up a dichotomous perspective between the irrational and the scientific, the believer and the sceptic. Madumo, a young man living in Soweto, South Africa, believes in witchcraft and has a miserable experience in his search for relief from curses. Meanwhile, Ashforth, as Madumo's friend, lends all the support he can, but himself remains above the fray, because, very simply, he does not believe. In a credo for rationalists at the dawn of the twenty-first century, Ashforth forthrightly declares, "I am not predisposed to find meaning or purpose, neither higher nor hidden, in the workings of the world. Divine Providence and witchcraft are, to me, equally abstract and empty hypotheses." Ashforth tempers his profound rejection of humanity's search for higher meaning with a casual doubt that "it all boils down to physics." Nonetheless, he expressly denied any impulse "to make sense of the world, the cosmos, by reference to any sort of Supreme Being, nor to find evidence of the supernatural powers of jealous neighbors in the ebb and flow of my worldly fortunes." His credo continues apace: "I do not talk to dead relatives and I do not fear the secret malice of the living." He ends his declaration of allegiance to Western rationalism, "As far as I am concerned, there are no invisible forces or beings that shape the lives and the destinies of the living." Then, in a nostalgic gesture he admits, "I sometimes feel a sort of envy, a feeling of tone deafness, when witnessing others communicate with beings beyond my ken" (Ashforth 2000, p. 249). Ashforth's perspective is perhaps usual, even expected, among educated Westerners, especially among university-based scholars. Indeed, he describes Madumo himself as trying to "Westernize" his thinking to fortify himself against witchcraft. Witches gain power through fear, explains Madumo, the more he thinks like a Westerner, the less he will fear witches, and therefore, the less power they would wield against him (Ashforth 2000, p. 247). To this, Ashforth remarks, "This understanding of power contains ontological presuppositions regarding the natures of thought, mind, and action radically different than those commonplace in the West, at least insofar as these presuppositions surface in the 'official' discourses of modern life" (2000, p. 247).

This present chapter proposes that this easy and familiar distinction described by Ashforth is itself built upon denial of the species-wide physiological mechanisms and inescapable unreason. If Ashforth's own personal unreason falls inside the modernist credo, nonetheless it certainly exists. Perhaps this personal magical thinking manifests in obsessive following of a sports team, or in an inordinate attachment to a particular pen, or item of clothing. There is, indeed, some force with which Madumo wrestled and there is a Western language that expresses this reality. Dr. Aubin in the mid-twentieth century called it *la crypte*, magic, and *mana*, and insisted that it was universally shared among all of humanity. In contemporary neuropsychiatry we find a related explanation via the physiological polyvagal theory (Porges 2011, 2017). Ashforth's denial of humanity's search for meaning in life, like his denial of speaking with his own dead relatives, proposes a self-contained rationality that cannot convince anyone who has suffered bereavement, nor any attuned to affective neural physiology. His claim to never have a thought for the power of jealous neighbors perhaps points to his own good luck at never experiencing such powerful jealousy, as well, perhaps, to his own sense of invincibility in his highly successful career. Certainly, however, Aubin's insights, like those of polyvagal theory, run contrary to the dominant rationalist traditions of Western modernity. Ashforth is indeed correct that modern rationalism frequently excludes this type of knowledge. We, however, only lose insight into inevitable dynamics when we repress and deny the human attribution of meaning, continuity, and relationships with those who have lived before us and who brought us into existence. Knowledge of such processes, which are inevitable because they arise from our physiology, calls for recognition and integration, not denial and repression.

***

Dr. Henri Aubin's work, largely in the 1930s–50s in French and colonial psychoanalysis, focused extensively on the processes of denial, magic, *mana*, and what he called *la crypte*. His work relied on the nineteenth-century theorist of dissociation, Pierre Janet (1894), and foreshadows twenty-first century therapy for dissociation (*e.g.* Steele *et al.* 2017; Fisher 2017). Aubin described how denial, magic, *mana*, and *la crypte* expressed affective projections and the transformations of consciousness and human relationships that arose via such projections. Aubin understood how denial could shape the human world and change realities, in a magical manner. He tapped into a way of thinking and perceiving from which he – as a medical doctor trained in Western scientific thinking – would normally be excluded. Recuperating an understanding of magic via psychoanalysis broadened the reach of Western psychiatry. Aubin's techniques allowed him to open his own scientific reason to processes scientists had fought hard to overcome and repress. However, his exploration of magic and denial was necessarily limited by his commitment to psychoanalysis. Aubin protected himself in like manner to Ashforth, as described above. Western rationality and objective empiricism defused the power of malicious spirits. Thus, Aubin felt himself somewhat immune to the power of terror. This exposes an apparent contradiction in his theory. On the one hand, he postulated that the crypt formed a part of each human mind. On the other hand, the power of the crypt seemed curiously tempered for himself and others schooled in rationalism. Re-examined through the lens of polyvagal theory, we can appreciate more clearly how affective projections never cease to arise regardless of an individual's refined consciousness. Rationalist collective representations might remove metaphysical dimensions from affective projections, but the affective power nonetheless endures – even if unnamed and underestimated – and skilled individuals can use it.

***

Contemporary psychotherapy still struggles to address the mysterious forces of dissociation and the consequent magical thinking, especially the more extreme forms of dissociative identity disorder. Kathy Steele, Suzette Boone, and Onna van der Haart's masterful instruction for working with trauma and dissociation relies, as did Aubin, on Pierre Janet, the original trauma clinician with a theory of non-realization (Steele *et al.* 2017, p. 4; see also van der Haart and Horst 1989). Despite the deep nineteenth-century roots of psychiatric treatment for trauma and dissociation, such treatment in the twenty-first century is still controversial and in its "infancy" (Steele *et al.* 2017, p. x). Indeed, they remark that current clinical training does not usually include work with dissociative disorders and that some clinicians refuse to accept that such disorders exist (Steele *et al.* 2017, pp. 22–23). The fact that treatment for dissociation is still in its infancy is remarkable given that dissociation has featured in clinical practice since at least the 1880s. As recounted by Ian Hacking, the first dissociative patient with so-called doubled personality, Louis Vivet, featured in the practice of Dr. Charcot in Paris in 1885 (Hacking 1997, p. 171). Moreover, as we know from the work of Aubin, denial and dissociation has been a prominent feature in psychiatry for West Africans since at least the 1950s, with detailed observations of dissociative events, albeit from a non-medical perspective, dating back to the mid-nineteenth century (Boilat 1853).

Steele, Boone, and van der Haart explain that the traumatized individual struggles to accept and to adapt to life as it is. That is, such survivors are caught in non-realization (Steele *et al.* 2017, p. 4). Part of non-realization is denial, such as described by Aubin, and part is dissociation. Betrayal, as when a young child is abused by caretakers, inhibits the acceptance of life as it is, and promotes denial and dissociation (Steele *et al.* 2017, p. 4). Humans normally inhabit a shared social reality, as described via the Durkheimian concept of collective representations, but it is important to acknowledge that such shared reality also contains shared denials. Instances of such shared denial are evident, for example, when a family, church, or school colludes to cover up abuse. Shared denial is also exhibited in numerous collective irrationalities such as climate change denial, or indeed, the denial of the full humanity of other persons because of gender, race, or caste. Personal truths that conflict with shared representations present the individual with especially intractable difficulties. Non-realization, denial, and dissociation are expedient solutions to ease overwhelming anxiety and pain.

Non-realization – the inability to accept the past or present features of life – can be a minor widely shared foible, or an extreme rejection of large sequences of memory and dimensions of personality. In the extreme, parts of the self separate out. Such segmentation can entail alternate ego-structures that allow a person to exhibit different personalities at different moments in time. Steele, Boon, and van der Haart follow the physiological precept that the mind lives only in and through the body, and that the body's disposition reflects and conditions consciousness. Each segmented part of the person expresses distinctive somatic dimensions. The therapist's task is to establish a therapeutic rapport that supports the integration of all the distinctive, segmented, somatisms into a unified consciousness. To maintain therapeutic rapport with the patient susceptible to dissociation, Steele, Boone, and van der Haart rewrite an old adage from "don't just stand there, do something" into a new adage, "don't just do something, *be* there." They intentionally emphasize the self-assured and well-regulated therapeutic presence, which can be a real anchor for trauma survivors. The inner turmoil of survivors can be so intense that words fail to carry meaning and "language is not possible" (Steele *et al.* 2017, p. x). Through reassuring and physiological regulated presence in the midst of the expressed turmoil, the therapist can facilitate the client's psychological integration. If the therapist reacts with physiological arousal to sudden changes in the patient's demeanor, to aggression, or to alarming narratives of events, that physiological arousal will communicate to the patient via neuroception, so that a negative spiral of co-dysregulation can ensue. A dissociative individual frequently has no conscious perception of the somatic expression of a disowned, unconscious part. The therapist needs to overcome the bias toward narrative and the brain, and to consciously promote physiological co-regulation. To promote the integration of the client's personality, the therapist needs to draw the client's conscious attention to unconscious somatic expressions. The affect carried in posture, gestures, or other physical attitudes holds keys to denied memories and disowned parts of the self. A therapist who overlooks or avoids engagement with somatic expression can act in collusion with the patient in persistent non-recognition of dissociated parts (Steele *et al.* 2017, p. 6). Even if the client can provide a narrative of past trauma, unless the somatic expressions are integrated, the patient risks remaining conscious only on an intellectual level, with on-going refusal of integration of difficult emotions.

In the late nineteenth century Dr. Pierre Janet theorized that dissociation was a syndrome of the inability to accept the facts of one's life, that is, of non-realization (Steele *et al.* 2017, p. 7). In fully developed dissociative identity disorder (DID, formerly known as multiple personality disorder (MPD)), each part of the dissociative person has its own sense of self and its own first person perspective with particular perceptions, beliefs, memories, sensations, perceptions, and predictions. These multiple first person perspectives within a single individual can be wildly divergent, with the inconsistencies either not noticed by the individual, or simply tolerated (Steele *et al.* 2017, p. 7). This type of "division of the self is a solution to unbearable and irreconcilable realities" (Steele *et al.* 2017, p. 7). The dissociative individual can experience internal emotions and memories as though they are real and powerful external events in the world. In post-traumatic stress disorder psychic equivalence is experienced as a flashback to battlefield violence. Or, a victim of domestic violence might relive a quotidian terror provoked by the sound of a garage door opening or the scrape of a key in the lock. In mild psychic equivalence, the impact might be only on the modality (or mood) of the patient accompanied perhaps by a physiological fear reaction. In more extreme cases, auditory, visual, or even olfactory sensations might intrude, accompanied by a full switch of consciousness. The trained therapist is alert to this process of psychic equivalence, and acts to aid the client's process of accepting the facts, current and past, pleasant or violently upsetting. The therapist's goal is to help the client escape the trance logic of dissociation, which suspends critical thinking and linear logic, by modeling presence in the moment, mindful acceptance, and active, conscious engagement with the psychic equivalence (Steele *et al.* 2017, p. 8).

This process of dissociation is both psychological and physiological. Steele, Boon, and van der Haart describe evolutionary action systems that organize our neural networks, primary affects, and physiological needs. The fundamental action systems include: exploration, attachment, caregiving, sociability, ranking (competition), play, energy management, and sex (Steele *et al.* 2017, p. 12). This is a considerably more comprehensive schematization than the fundamental drive for attachment. Nonetheless, Steele, Boon and van der Haart still follow the theorization by Porges of neuroception and the drive for safety and social engagement (Porges 2017, p. 43, citing Porges 2003). They recognize the disruption of social engagement via ancient autonomic fight, flight, or play dead autonomic neural reactions. The trauma victim is an individual stuck in a repetitive dorsal vagal reaction of feigned death (fainting or flagging physiology). Trauma also entails, in alliance with psychic equivalence episodes, the faulty function of neuroception.

Survivors of trauma can suffer habitual chronic physiological dysregulation, so that they cannot accurately perceive safety and danger. Stuck in a dorsal vagal fear reaction, the individual cannot engage social cues nor accurately read and respond to the social expressions of others. Social behavior reads as untrustworthy, whereas signs of danger are read as normal or even desirable. This neuroceptive confusion can lead survivors into danger again and again (Steele *et al.* 2017, p. 12). Thus, trauma victims are frequently re-victimized. They can also compulsively seek experiences that recall past trauma, perhaps motivated by a deep desire to change the course of the traumatic events. Such courting of danger inevitably entails injuries, which, once an individual persists even if conscious of the pattern, is a type of self-victimization. The task of the therapist, explored in great detail by Steele, Boon, and van der Haart, is to calmly, gently, assist the client in reintegrating painful segmented parts, so that they can accept the reality of their life and live, fully integrated, in the present. For the therapeutic process to succeed, the fear, shame, and loathing of the client toward disowned memories and parts must be overcome.

The psychotherapist Janina Fisher describes the adaptation of young children to chronic insecurity,

> Their bodies have had to be on high alert, ready for action, or to be disconnected, numb, passive, and able to endure whatever comes. When they are triggered later in childhood or as adults, their nervous systems are already conditioned to activate the same autonomic response and animal defenses that served them best as children. . . . An activity that previously has been adaptive is likely to recur because the brain functions automatically . . . to produce the [same] behavior in similar circumstances.
>
> (Fisher 2017, p. 36, internal citations omitted)

The continual activation of the autonomic nervous system represses the hippocampus, "which is the part of the brain that puts experience into chronological order and perspective preparatory to being transferred to verbal memory areas" (Fisher 2017, p. 36, citing van der Kolk 2014). The hippocampus suppression inhibits as well the prefrontal cortex and leaves experience to reside as sensory elements, unintegrated and unattached to linear time or verbal memories. "Survivors are left with a confusing array of unfinished neurobiological responses and 'raw data,' i.e., the overwhelming feelings, physical reactions, intrusive images, sound, and smells associated with the event encoded as implicit memories and therefore unrecognizable as 'memory'" (Fisher 2017, p. 36). The physiological dimensions of trauma are remembered in the autonomic nervous system, which is reactivated when the body encounters stress that sets off the neuroception and subsequent physiological mobilization. Such physiological response in turn fuels re-enactment behavior (Fisher 2017, p. 36, citing van der Kolk 2014, 1994).

***

Henri Aubin on Denial and Magic

From this twenty-first-century perspective on dissociative disorders, we return to Aubin on magic, denial, and *la crypte*. In an earlier essay, Aubin's theory of denial, *la crypte*, and magic is portrayed within the history of colonialism and post-colonialism (Bullard 2011). That essay showed Aubin's work as a departure from the Algiers School of psychiatry, to which he had some early professional ties, and portrayed Aubin as an influential precursor to the transcultural psychiatry as practiced at Fann Hospital (Bullard 2011). In the context of the problematic relationship of the French psychiatrist to colonial subjects, the doctor-patient relationship was fraught with fear, tension, and denial. An analogous force operates in the history of psychiatry, so that colonial psychiatry habitually disappeared from narratives that focused preferentially on metropolitan practices. Denial emerged again and again to shape and direct the psychiatrists' interests and relationships and even the history of psychiatry (Bullard 2011).

In general, the colonial contributions to French psychiatry have not been integrated into the broader history of French psychiatry. This is a type of denial of the vitality of work done in the colonies. Dr. Franck Cazanove's integration of ethnographic knowledge into medicine contrasts with the widespread resistance among other colonial doctors to such knowledge (Cazanove 1933). Ethnography interested and served government officials more frequently than doctors. For example, Charles Monteil's 1931 study of divination in French West Africa explored the role of magic, but Monteil sought to apply this to strategies for governing West Africa, rather than to the practice of medicine (Monteil 1931, pp. 134–136). The posthumous publication of Dr. Émile Mauchamp's *La sorcellerie au Maróc* (1911) documented various magical medical practices, but Monteil's work aimed to expose superstition and ignorance rather than to build a bridge between medical practices. In 1907, Mauchamp was murdered by a mob in Marrekesh, reportedly after a German spy spread rumors that Mauchamp's medical skills included the ability to administer poison that took two or three years to be fatal (Mauchamp 1911, p. 23). The French then took this murder as a pretext for expanding colonial rule. The imperial logic was expressed by Mauchamp's father, who reasoned that France should clean up the moral miasma that caused Moroccans to rot and become ferocious (Mauchamp 1911, p. 3). In contrast to this aggressive attack on folk beliefs and credulity, Aubin followed Dr. Cazanove's exploration of local culture as connected with healing.

Aubin created an oeuvre centered on denial, *la crypte*, and magic as universal biopsychological forces. *La crypte* expressed Aubin's conviction that a biopsychological dimension underlay all human psyches. Hidden, difficult to access, archaic, and mysterious, *la crypte* contained the sacred and the corpse, *mana* and the magical. It buried, contained, and preserved the strongest common dimensions to human psyches (Aubin 1952, p. 21). Aubin strove against Carl Jung's focus on myths and archetypes as expressions of the collective unconscious and focused instead on primal energy flow, which he thought of as magic and *mana*. Most directly, however, Aubin's evocation of species-wide processes rooted in biopsychology resonates with the physiological tradition of French psychiatry and the recent revival of physiological neuropsychiatry by Stephen Porges (2011, 2017). Thus, Aubin's work has roots in Janet's explanations of trauma, hysteria, and dissociative disorders (Janet 1894).

Although Aubin worked explicitly with psychoanalytic concepts, he did not psychoanalyze African patients.[1] He sought, rather, to bring cultural analysis into the psychiatric arena. In that project, he relied on a broad array of cultural anthropologists but most notably on the *L'Année sociologique* scholars (Emile Durkheim, Marcel Mauss, and Henri Hubert), along with their collaborator, Lucien Lévy-Bruhl. Aubin blended his focus on culture with his biopsychological perspective. Working closely with African patients, Aubin drew on cultural analysis to formulate psychiatric and psychoanalytic insights, which he also found operative in the European context. Denial, conversion, and projection drew his sustained attention.

Doctors Gaëtan Gatian de Clérambault, Frank Cazanove, and Emmanuel Régis were the doctors to whom Aubin felt personally indebted as a young psychiatrist. Dr. Angelo Hesnard, who served the dual role of bringing Freudian analysis into French psychiatric practices and of carrying it with him on his tours of duty in the colonies, must be recognized as well. Hesnard's seminal book of 1914, co-written with Dr. Emmanuel Régis, presented Freudian analysis to the French public with a critical air. Hesnard – who, in 1914, was just embarking on his career – continued on to become a major advocate of psychoanalysis in France. Hesnard's influence in the French colonial administration, where he served as a medical doctor, extended to providing training analysis for certain psychiatrists or psychologists. Henri Collomb, the founding director of the Fann Hospital, was one of Hesnard's analysands. Hesnard directed the *Revue Française de psychanalyse*, which enjoyed the explicit blessings of Sigmund Freud, from its founding in 1927. Freud, Marie Bonaparte, Hesnard, and René Laforgue figure prominently among the early contributors. The *Revue* featured explicit cross-cultural and comparative dimensions, with early contributions on the Hindu castration complex, hunting trophies and the atavistic pleasure of killing, and Chinese dreams. The famous pioneer of ethnopsychiatry, Géza Róheim, presented to the Société psychanalytique in 1928 on racial psychology and the origins of capitalism.

Aubin's success as a colonial psychiatrist carried him around the French empire, and his writings, published from the 1920s through 1970, ranged from neurology to ethnography, from organic diseases to theories of magic, denial, and repression. In 1938, Aubin reported on psychiatric services in the colonies at the Congrès des Aliénistes et Neurologistes de Langue Française in Algiers. This report parallels and updates the comparatively well-known 1912 report by Henry Reboul and Emmanuel Régis. Aubin noted the role of divine and occult forces in popular accounts of mental illness. Malaria, amoebic infections, sleeping sickness, leprosy, pneumonia: each of these, Aubin explained, could cause psychopathology. Psychiatrists, he argued, played a vital role in discovering organic infections via psychiatric diagnosis. Unfortunately, he contended, "It is still common to view psychosis as a mysterious effect of destructive Occult Forces against which no real defense is possible." Evil spirits or heavenly curses, he remarked, are as present in the minds of the civilized as among those they seek to civilize (Aubin 1939b, p. 150).

Denial in the Colonized and in the Colonizers

Reniement (denial) became one of Aubin's fundamental themes, and served as a major explanatory device for African as well as European psyches.[2] Denial developed as a point of focus for Aubin as he reflected on the psychiatric aliments of Black African soldiers who served in the French army in the First World War. Inside French psychiatric hospitals, Black African spirit crises appeared to doctors other than Aubin as unfathomable psychotic rage. Colonial doctors usually postulated the driving cause as some type of biological inferiority or weakness. Aubin, however, understood the psychotic rages and subsequent denial of them as intimately linked to the fear of demons. This link was later confirmed by Fann Hospital clinicians who worked with Wolof, Serer, and Lebou peoples suffering what they understood within their own culture as spirit crises. The Black African beliefs about spirit crises, as well as Black African therapeutic practices related to them, were not studied by French doctors in a systematic manner prior to the founding of the Fann Psychiatric Hospital at the University of Dakar in the postcolonial era (Bullard 2007). In trying to understand the causes of Black African fear and denial, Aubin broke new ground, and yet even in the identification of his patients as "Senegalese," he entertains a false sense of uniformity by overlooking the multiple geographic locales and ethnicities represented among the *tiralleurs sénégalais*.

Aubin's work at the Michel-Lévy Hospital involved him intimately with Black Africans suffering spiritual/psychological collapse in the wake of military service. Informed by these soldiers' suffering, Aubin created a portrait of Black African psychotic regression and developed a theory of the curative dimensions to the habitual denial of psychotic episodes. This study of psychotic regression can be contextualized in later medical literature that depicted a relative ease of regression and quick recovery among Black Africans, as contrasted to Europeans, who are more resistant to psychosis but in whom psychosis proves more intractable. Marie-Cécile and Edmund Ortigues later theorized that early infantile object substitutions and fixations could account for these differences (Ortigues and Ortigues

1966 [1984], pp. 105–106; Bullard 2005a, pp. 180–183). "The furious paroxysms of the Senegalese soldiers," reflected Aubin,

> are the cause of unfortunately frequent dramas. . . . These are delirious, blind explosions which quickly reach their height; the patient, beside himself, gesticulates and mutters, or, turned in on himself, sorrowful, mute, . . . he seems animated by an implacable hatred of everyone . . . insensible to all exhortations, he ferociously strikes everyone who tries to approach and destroys everything within reach.
>
> (Aubin 1939a, p. 13)

Once the paroxysm takes hold, according to Aubin, it spends itself quickly, especially if the individual has been isolated (Aubin 1939a, p. 18).

Aubin was struck by the prominence of denial and the ease and frequency with which it was used by these soldiers. Even when confronted with physical evidence of psychotic fits, they would nevertheless repeatedly deny that any such fits had taken place. Aubin reflected the common reaction among the doctors to this denial, commenting, "We are stupefied *to see them tranquilly and categorically deny all their previous claims*" (Aubin 1939a, p. 3, emphasis in the original). He singled out for discussion one case in which a man in full delirium started to describe the Lilliputian devils which were tormenting him; but terrorized, he refused to recount what they said to him, saying "that would make him die" (Aubin 1939a, p. 12). Aubin respected this man's terror, explaining that in Senegal, someone who has seen the devil must not speak of it for a period of three months, else they risk the pain of further haunting and suffering. Here, Aubin allows a difference between himself and the West Africans to remain unbridged. However, in passing over this difference in silence – that is, by not reflecting on the difference between really feeling fear of demons and merely recognizing that someone else feels threatened by demons (that Aubin does not believe exist) – Aubin is able to assimilate the version of West African denial into European denial more easily. Taking the demons seriously would have required that Aubin leave the confines of psychology to grapple with metaphysics. Raoul Allier (discussed later in this chapter) engaged in such attempts and arrived at a much stronger respect for difference and yet also with a strongly hierarchical conviction of European moral superiority. From the perspective of PVT, however, the physiological reaction to fear is a human universal as is the inexorable ideation and narrativizing of perceived experience. Thus, from the twenty-first-century perspective of PVT the power of fear can be fully acknowledged from within a scientific perspective in which metaphysics appears as a perennial option among narratives.

Aubin explained how denial functioned as a form of mental hygiene by preventing suffering. Aubin theorized that the *reniement* of the "primitives" was a tool of mental hygiene that they discovered via instinct (Aubin 1939a, p. 28). *Reniement*, he contended, liquidizes individual episodes that otherwise take up an inordinate amount of psychic energy and are liable to create automatic activities in the mind, almost completely dissociated from reflective activity, which creates a nervous exhaustion that is itself generative of neurosis. Following the insights of the nineteenth-century psychiatrist Pierre Janet, Aubin claimed, "These patients would be immediately cured if they forgot the event" (1939a, p. 28).

This case, for Aubin, exemplified the sentiment that animated systematic denial. Aubin chose the word "sentiment" deliberately, because it refers to the Durkheimian theory of collective representations (Aubin 1939a, p. 12). For Aubin, denial served as a central, collective sentiment; it was a motivating affective force in mental processes. Affect, Durkheim had theorized, occupied a visceral substratum to thinking, opinions, and even to conscious will or desires. Collective sentiments, such as denial, expressed pervasive, culturally specific underpinnings to cognition and other conscious mental processes. Aubin deployed the Durkheimian theory to express the power and pervasiveness of denial among Black Africans. He then extended his argument, pointing out that denial was highly apparent among Europeans as well. For Aubin, denial was a normal feature of the mind.

Janet's intentional cultivation of forgetting is emphasized by Ian Hacking,

> No one, I think, so systematically cultivated deceptive memory as Pierre Janet. He did so from the highest motives. His patients were in torment. Their symptoms were caused by ill-remembered trauma. His cures often relied on eliciting the trauma by discussion and by hypnosis. Once the cause of the distress had been brought to light, he hypnotized the patient into thinking that the events never happened.
>
> (Hacking 1995, pp. 260–261)

Hacking characterized Janet's emphasis on forgetting as the practice of "an honorable man" who preferred to preserve and facilitate relationships rather than to pursue a hypostatized version of truth. As Hacking wrote, "Janet had no . . . Will to Truth. He was an honorable man, and (we might say *hence*) he had no inflated sense of the Truth" (Hacking 1995, p. 195). Rather, Janet helped his patients to forget and to deny unpleasant memories. He accomplished this via hypnosis and suggestion, a process through which he substituted positive images for negative memories. In contrast, Janet's great competitor of his time, Sigmund Freud, pursued Truth with such fervor that he was willing to overlook and cover up the specific personal truths told by his patients (Hacking 1995, pp. 194–195).

In 1950, *L'Evolution psychiatrique* hosted a discussion of Aubin's general theory of denial, a discussion that ranged broadly over various psychological mechanisms of defense (Aubin 1951). By this time, Aubin had formulated a general theory of the "systematic denial of transgression," which he found to be very active. The purest form of this psychic defense, he claimed, was among unassimilated Africans for whom "denial achieves the level of 'willed forgetting' which for Janet figured as an ideal means liquidating affective traumas" (Aubin 1951, p. 31). As previously, Aubin asserted here that the half-assimilated lost this facility for denial and were given to endless pondering of perceived grievances and paranoid reactions. For Aubin, the Freudian discussion of pathological repression generative of neuroses was merely a failed form of denial. Through the denial of inopportune pregnancies, of illness, or of setbacks or defeats in one's career, Europeans routinely deployed the device Aubin found revealed so clearly among Africans.

From Metaphysical Terror to Collective Western Phobia

Spiritual beliefs carry forces that can pervade cultural systems. The protestant missionary Raoul Allier explored in great depth the implications of living under the rule of demonic forces. This preoccupation led Allier to recognize that the chief characteristic of such lives is the omnipresence of terror. Allier was a historian of religion, of conversion, and of psychology (Allier 1925). His point of view occupies a cusp position, straddling an objective, secular outlook and an outlook rooted in Christian religiosity. As such, Allier took the prospect of magic, sorcery, and witchcraft rather more seriously than did Aubin. While both men saw in such practices evidence of universal human inclinations toward magical thinking, Allier felt compelled to address the reign of terror provoked among people who lived in fear of witches. Both Allier and Aubin recognized that the conviction one had been bewitched could provoke a deep terror and ensuing death. Allier looked closely at such beliefs, arguing that the search for magical causes disrupted or prevented reasoning based in empirical causality and that it encouraged people to accept things as real when they were not real at all. This indifference to factual reality, for Allier, was at the heart of a predisposition to lying: "This indifference toward the truth that seems to characterize the non-civilized, . . . should we be surprised that it takes on its gravest feature in an inveterate predisposition for lying?" (Allier 1925, p. 87).

Allier provided long documentation of such carelessness with the truth, culled from the records of the missionary Hermann Dieterlen, who commented repeatedly on the seemingly instinctual impulse to lie. Allier recounts instances of lying that seem to be self-protective (i.e., refusing to admit a pregnancy or a venereal infection) but also uses as an example a woman's denial that she had heard the noise of a certain waterfall. In local lore, it was reputed that those who heard this waterfall would certainly die. The woman's lie, and lying in general, acknowledged Allier, "became a sort of paradoxical defense. Used without the slightest regard for the truth" (Allier 1925, pp. 90–91). In Allier's view, this psychic defense mechanism, much celebrated by Aubin, led to mental impairment, stunted intelligence, and moral decrepitude. "In the atmosphere of magic," commented Allier, "the natural candor of the mind diminishes and disappears." The belief in magic and witchcraft discouraged the development of the intellect. Allier reasoned that "a creature who finds it fatiguing to habitually use reason easily becomes the plaything of his passions" (Allier 1925, p. 91).

In the life-world of those for whom witchcraft is real, life is full of the unknown, of uncertainties, of mutual suspicions, and hence of fear. The desire for magical powers – powers to protect oneself and one's family against witchcraft and also the power to gain riches, a desirable mate, or healthy children – can push people to commit crimes (Allier 1925, p. 91). Among the wealth of examples Allier offered, the most extreme was the search for powerful medicine fabricated from human body parts seized from living victims (Allier 1925, pp. 113–115). In Allier's analysis, the penchant for dishonest and unclear thinking combined with rule of fear and avarice were the root causes of such vicious behavior.

If Allier saw lying as an understandable yet ultimately corrupting defense mechanism, Aubin focused on the positive dimensions to prevarication. Aubin's emphasis on the positive role of denial distinguished his psychiatric outlook from some of his peers, who were more likely to invoke sweeping negative generalizations of the *tirailleurs*. The widely held belief that natives were inveterate liars and not to be trusted was, from Aubin's point of view, based in a fundamental misunderstanding. Aubin was intrigued by Raoul Allier's 1927 book, *Le non-civilisé et nous*, which discussed lying by "primitives," but he commented with disappointment that Allier viewed "systematic negation" only as a "negative feature leading to moral dissolution rather than perceive its potentially positive impact on mental health" (Aubin 1939a, p. 213).

At least one other psychiatric opinion on the role of lying among the colonized should be considered here, and it is that of Frantz Fanon. In 1955, Fanon and René Lacaton delivered a paper at the Francophone psychiatric Congrès titled "The Algerian and Avowal in Medico-Legal Practice." They argued that Algerians are not prone to confession in colonial courts precisely because of their resistance to the colonial order. "The colonized does not let on," Fanon later commented, "He does not confess himself in the presence of the colonizer" (Fanon 1967b, p. 127, n.2). Fanon's view of the resistance to colonization was sharpened as the Algerian Revolution continued. In *A Dying Colonialism* (published originally in 1959), Fanon wrote unstintingly of the alienation of Algerians from every aspect of the colonial order:

> The colonial situation is precisely such that it drives the colonized to appraise all the colonizer's contributions in a pejorative and absolute way. The colonized perceives the doctor, the engineer, the schoolteacher, the policeman, the rural constable, through the haze of an almost organic confusion.
>
> (Fanon 1967b, p. 121)

Fanon's emphasis on the anger of the colonized returns a political dimension to Aubin's concept of *reniement*. Indeed, the French public were introduced to colonial anger in 1921 by René Maran's widely read novel, *Batoula, veritable roman nègre* (1921). Like Fanon, Maran was an assimilated (or *évolué*) colonial; he served as a colonial official in French Equatorial Africa. In *Batoula*, the hostility of the colonized for the colonizer enters into every aspect of their relationship: "Behind the grimacing smile of welcome is rancour, and covered by apparent good will is the hope for a liberating massacre – 'We will kill them all, one day, long from now'" (Maran 1921, p. 91).

The furious outbursts of psychotic and homicidal rage described by Dr. Hesnard, for example, take on new meaning when set side by side with Fanon and Maran. Aubin and other psychiatrists did not entirely overlook this anger, yet neither did they assign colonial politics primary significance (compare to André Ombredane on the Asalampusa as discussed in Bullard 2005b). Aubin, like many psychiatrists, asserted that it was

> *precisely the individuals relatively évolués* who have the most accentuated paranoid tendencies; this evolution, it is true, has *ordinarily been defective* and too rapid; it provoked the premature abandonment of certain ancestral beliefs and institutions (which are capable of reigning in the dangerous drives of each ethnic group), before a new civilization could be assimilated.
> (Aubin 1939a, pp. 25–26 emphasis in the original)

Aubin at least acknowledged a political grievance that often animated the heart of such rancor:

> The cult of justice, so strong among them and exalted by the predication of egalitarianism, is often stymied by the discovery of actual inequalities between whites and himself; from this a latent sentiment of *distrust, injustice and hostility* grows – all of it encouraged by the *vanity of the natives.*
> (Aubin 1939a, pp. 25–26, emphasis in the original)

Distrust, hostility, and a sense of injustice, according to Aubin's reasoning, arise among the colonized because of their resentment of racial inequality. Aubin seemed to naturalize this racial inequality so that the "native's injured vanity" that provokes their resentment, and in turn causes paranoid psychosis, appears ridiculous and unjustified. Nowhere in Aubin's medical psychiatry was there a serious appraisal of the impact of unjust legal regimes.

Aubin's leap to racialized rationalizations of colonial anger betrays his own anxiety experienced as denial seizes his consciousness. As we have seen, Aubin normally rejected racialized explanations in favor of careful case studies. This exception proves the strength of the compulsion to deny colonial injustice and reveals the anxiety that such denial will prove inadequate. At length, however, he shook himself free from the compulsive denial of the political. Without retracting his compulsive racializing, he recalled himself and his readers to his commitment to specific case studies and resolved to cut short his discussion of the paranoid psychoses of the half assimilated: "We will not pursue this psychogenetic reasoning any further, since it can only be approximate given the considerable psychological differences between the diverse primitive ethnic groups" (Aubin 1939a, pp. 25–26).

Aubin's ability to assimilate Black African denial into a global unconscious – his ability to equate African with European denial – relied on twin pillars of obfuscation. He denied the power of the occult that pervaded his patients' lives, and he denied the power of French imperialism that similarly pervaded their lives. As a man of scientific medicine, Aubin was proud of his opposition to "superstition." As a product of the colonial era, he was apparently blind to his own denial of the relevance of political oppression. In both instances, his thinking offers backhanded proof of his claim that denial itself is a universal mechanism, prominent among Europeans just as among Africans. Allier, who took metaphysics more seriously than did Aubin, cannot assimilate all humans into a universal without first extirpating evil and its pervasive effects. Fanon, the anti-imperialist psychiatrist, chooses sides with the colonized, defending difference against imperialism. Aubin's balancing act – defending the secular, the scientific, and the universal unconscious – incorporates what appears to be difference as a dimension of the universal.

Aubin's discovery of denial and magic (*la crypte*) in African colonial subjects and his integration of these into a universal psychoanalytic theory relied heavily on disempowering magic, rendering the crypt relatively harmless and thereby finding it tolerable. Religiously minded men such as Allier had comparatively little tolerance for occult forces, sensing in them a metaphysical danger. Fanon similarly viewed the repressed as deeply threatening, as containing the principle of evil. Aubin's ability to assimilate the crypt into a universal psyche relied heavily on this denial of power and danger. His access to the forces of magic and participation was occluded; the African patients he treated had a much greater access to this domain and more fearful reactions to its forces.

Magic and Mana

Secure in his denial of the terrorizing power of the occult, Aubin continued his studies, focusing increasingly on magic. In 1952, he published his major work *L'Homme et la magie*, which centered on excavating the contents of *la crypte.*[3] Professor Henri Baruk, the chief doctor at the Maison Nationale of Charenton, aptly cast Aubin's *L'Homme et la magie* as a seminal interdisciplinary investigation in ethnography and psychiatry. The magical mentality, according to Aubin, is part of the depth psychology of all humans. Civilization, he explained, caused the on-going and cumulative repression of the magical mentality so that it is more and more contained under the sediments of logic and rationality. Nonetheless, Aubin contended, human intelligence remains governed by very powerful sentiments and affects and remains, in its foundations, ridden by magic (Baruk in Preface to Aubin 1852). Notably, Aubin believed that the magical governing forces bereft of the power to do real harm to him. Aubin seemed to gain access to *la crypte* precisely because the world of the occult held little power over him. This freedom – discussed previously as established via denial or alternately understood as a reason's liberation from superstition – demonstrates the circumscription of Aubin's own point of view. He can perceive the power of magic but is protected from its realm.

At its heart, *L'Homme et la magie* is a history of human moral sensibilities – tracing the historical emergence of causality, rationality, individualized identity, and responsibility – and as such, it creates a type of universal history. The driving force of this history, the gradual distinction between self and the surrounding world, entailed the separation of mind and emotion from all the diverse elements of the environment, including from other people, animals, plants, and objects.

Through this history, Aubin placed magical thinking at the foundation of a long series of human transformations that included the emergence of concepts of justice, responsibility, rights, culpability, emphasis on individual responsibility rather than group redemption, and punishment for the one proven guilty rather than for the group arbitrarily or magically held at fault. Aubin cites Bastide's *Sociologie et psychanalyse* which argued that childhood traits are consolidated in adult "primitives." Aubin clarified, "The alienated will never turn back into a primitive, no more than the primitive could be considered a madman." He dissociated himself from any claim that there was an absolute or strong distinction between "civilized" and "primitive" peoples or that "primitive mentality" was somehow "prelogical" (Aubin 1952, pp. 16, 19, 30; Bastide 1950, p. 185). Aubin emphasized rather that the "non-civilized thinks endlessly about the occult forces that surround him" (Aubin 1952, p. 19). He believed as well that the civilized repress open belief in such magic only to have it re-emerge in countless dimensions of their lives.

La crypte, magic, and *mana*, in Aubin's estimation, all expressed the same force. In psychoanalytic terms, he rendered these as projection, sympathy, and contagion. Emotional energy can transfer from one person to another and can transfer as well to any animal or inanimate object. Aubin understood magic as the diffuse and omnipresent work of *mana* in linking the visible and invisible worlds. He described *mana*, following Robert Henry Codrington's *Melanesians* (1915), as

> the most exalted of powers; the true efficacy of things that re-inforces mechanical action without obliterating it. It is *mana* that makes the net hold, that makes the house solid, that makes the canoe seaworthy. In the field, it is fertility, in medicine it is the force for health or mortality.
>
> (Aubin 1952, pp. 21–22)

Mana, in other words, is the intentionality of the fetish-object; it is the power of something to act with will. Aubin assimilated affective projection to taboo and *mana*, explaining them as communicable (contagious), powerful charges, and supplemented these with the concept of "participation," which "implies magical connections between the individual and his or her setting, between things that for us are heterogeneous, between things, that to our eyes, have no relation to each other" (Aubin 1952, p. 23). In his most lucid formulation, he explained, "We [moderns] localize sentiments in the self and in ourselves, whereas the primitive localizes his sentiments outside of himself in the world he experiences." Aubin demonstrated affective projection by explaining that while a modern individual might claim he feels terror when confronted with a king or a priest, a primitive would say that the priest or king is taboo (possesses *mana*). A modern person would say, "I am afraid of dead bodies," whereas a primitive would say, "Cadavers are taboo" (or possess *mana*) (Aubin 1952, p. 31).

If the Durkheimians wished to see *mana* as a collective force of the social group – a force perceived by individuals that gives rise to intense collective representations – Aubin did not disagree, yet he was driven to investigate the more individualized experiences of *mana*, most particularly, of course, the highly idiosyncratic experiences of the mentally ill. His examples include one troubled young woman who believed she could fly and who broke her legs jumping out a window (Aubin 1952, p. 23). In another example of individualized magical thinking, Aubin presented the case of a young man, with an Arab father and a European mother who had converted to Islam, who developed phobic delusions after he had suffered a head injury (Aubin 1952, p. 27). He developed a conviction that he could feel the finger of God on his head and that he was destined to become a saint. Then, he became obsessed with a delusion that people were trying to prevent his saintliness by tricking him into eating pork. This phobic delusion eventually led him to murder his sister. Aubin discussed this case in psychoanalytic terms of the contagion of a repugnant impurity, the sense of revulsion at being forced to participate in this impurity, and then the attempt to free himself via transgressing an interdiction (i.e., murdering his sister), which itself brought automatic retaliation. Notably, he made no reference to racial etiologies or the special challenges of assimilating to European civilization. Aubin refused a race-based explanation, and emphasized rather the biological trauma, the blow to the head, as the origin of the illness.

Aubin's conclusion to *L'Homme et la magie* enumerated 20 or more clinical, therapeutic, political, and sociological uses of the knowledge of the magic and *la crypte*. From the point of view of psychiatry for the colonized, he pointed out that the ability to heal is culturally and geographically specific. This is an insight that the Fann group developed in its careful collaboration with traditional healers in Senegal in the 1960s. He also remarked that individuals transplanted from the colonies are likely to suffer access of spleen because of the absence of emotional participation between the individual, the group, and the country. Frantz Fanon's celebrated article "North African Syndrome" covered similar terrain in 1952, two years after Aubin's *L'Homme et la magie* was published (Fanon 1952). Aubin emphasized again that pejorative opinions regarding natives should be revised, especially with respect to the positive role of lying in maintaining mental equilibrium. The concepts of taboo and *mana*, according to Aubin, explained the phobia toward hospitals and careers as nurses and also the apparent ingratitude of some patients for the treatment they received. Indeed, the experiences of Africans trained in mental health professions demonstrate that approaching the spirit world without magical protection can incur costly sacrifices. The history of the directors at Fann Hospital – one prematurely dead, the next incapacitated for many years, both reportedly because of a spirit possession – demonstrate the power of taboo and the courage required to confront such taboos directly (Bullard 2005a, pp. 210–211).

Focused as he was on the individual, Aubin neglected to consider magical thinking widely shared among Europeans. This is a blind spot in his thinking, which is nonetheless heavily characterized by the division of populations into broad categories of moderns and primitives. For him, Africans exhibited magic; modern Europeans hid it. Black Africans played the role in Aubin's theories of illuminating the crypte that was common to all humanity. For him, Black Africans symbolized the primitive, which in turn symbolized magic. This chain of symbols contrasts to those documented and critiqued by Fanon in *Black Skin, White Masks*. First published in the same year as Aubin's *L'Homme et la magie*, Fanon's book theorized that European thinking was characterized by its own type of magical thinking, "Negrophobia" (Fanon 1967a, p. 154). Following a psychoanalytic and Durkheimian analysis closely similar to Aubin's and expressly attributed to Aubin's colleague Angelo Hesnard, Fanon pointed out that phobias arise out of prelogical thinking in which symbols come to stand for powerful affective projections. Negrophobia, as Fanon theorized, embodied the Europeans' fear and anxiety that well from within and then was projected upon Blacks so that they carried the negative affective charge. Fanon was unstinting in his confrontation with negative racializing:

> In the remotest depth of the European unconscious an inordinately black hollow has been made in which the most immoral impulses, the most shameful desires lie dormant. And as every man climbs up toward whiteness and light, the European has tried to repudiate this uncivilized self, which has attempted to defend itself. When European civilization came into contact with the black world, with those savage peoples, everyone agreed: Those Negroes were the principle of evil.
>
> (Fanon 1967a, p. 190).

Aubin's project was to focus the primal associations away from rigid pejoratives to the infinitely malleable dimensions of *mana*, magic, or fetish. Fanon's concept, Negrophobia, recalls the threatening force of the occult can work powerfully as a collective projection, even when metaphysics is denied and only a secular occult is operative.

***

Aubin on Dance, Trance, and Spirit Possession

Aubin recognized the psychotherapeutic value of other diverse African practices, in addition to denial, to liquidate the disturbing event. He remarked, in particular, on magic ceremonies, diverse forms of exorcism, the removal of an evil presence by a sorcerer or a relative, sacrifices, pilgrimages, and other techniques. In this way, Aubin marked the route for future transcultural and ethnopsychiatric studies. The inauguration of this new transcultural science was demarcated in 1957 in a World Health Organization-sponsored symposium. At that event, Roger Bastide argued explicitly for the psychotherapeutic value of the Brasilian ritual of *candomblé*; in so doing, he broke explicitly with prior medical opinion (Bastide 1960). Bastide also defended African cults as part of healthy social and mental life, arguing that better medical understanding necessitated familiarity with ethnographic knowledge and local practices of African immigrant populations (Bastide 1960, p. 227).

The fascination with possession in French anthropology itself has a pedigree, with more or less casual documentation of possession crises giving way, eventually, to ethnographic precision. Michel Leiris' 1931 account of the theatrical dimensions to *zar* rituals of Ethiopia along with his attention to the gendered dynamic at play has endured as a classic of French anthropology. Jean Rouch's earliest films, from the Upper Niger, included *Au pays des mages noirs* (1947) and *Initiation à la danse des possedés* (1949). His more famous work filmed in Ghana, *Les maïtres fous*, began showing in 1956, and brought possession rituals to Parisian cinemas.

Rouch's earliest films attracted the attention of the Parisian psychoanalytic community, which arranged a 1948 film viewing followed by a lecture by Henri Aubin. Staged at the Musée de l'Homme, this event was for Aubin a rare moment in the lime-light (Aubin 1948). Aubin relished what seemed to him a breakthrough moment in the collaboration between ethnography, psychiatry, and psychology (Aubin 1948, p. 191). Conscious of the scholarly context for Rouch's film, Aubin cites Tremearne's work on the Hausa (*The Ban of the Bori*), Dubois' work on the Betsileo, Leiris on the Abyssinian *zar* cult, and, drew from his own work too, regarding the dance of the devil in Pondicherry, India, and the Aissaouas in Morocco (Aubin 1948, p. 192). Aubin described five phases of ecstatic rites – the preliminary rites, the dance itself, the stages of reaching hysterical transport (étapes hystéro-ébrieux), possession or the capturing of a magic force (or *mana*), and, finally, the rupture of this contact via post-trance amnesia. This last stage, the instant forgetting of the possession, points toward the mechanism of automatic denial. True to the French physiological tradition in psychiatry, Aubin claimed that the physicality of possession rites cannot be separated from the psychological or spiritual. He turns to the symbolist poet, Stéphane Mallarmé, to express this insight, "the dancer is not a woman who dances, for these juxtaposed reasons: she is not a woman, and she does not dance" (Aubin 1948, p. 195). This formulation expressed the physiological truth of the intertwined mind and body, each ceaselessly dependent and echoing of the state of the other.

The cumulative effect of group rhythmic dancing, usually starting with a slow circling shuffle and then accelerating over the course of hours to incredibly rapid, collective, spinning and shaking, prompted Aubin to comment, "this is a violent excitation of the labyrinth" which produces "a special type of drunkenness" (Aubin 1948, p. 195).[4] The one word – labyrinth – signal's Aubin's casual evocation of the symbolic order, the human search for the divine, and the elaboration of meaning in life. Shaking the labyrinth, that violent excitation, allows the possession trance to inaugurate a revamped symbolic order. When the possession rite is a social event, and not a circumscribed cult of adepts, the new symbolic order is widely accepted by the community.

The music of the dance expresses a certain "*état d'âme*," giving it a temporal dimension marked out in rhythm; the dance makes this representation concrete and spatialized, creating a physical figuration of a psychological state. Ritual accessories complete the scene, which is charged with a certain potential, the same potential (power) as resides in symbols. Aubin elaborated on how symbols carry condensed magic power that can be amplified as they travel through time, passing through generation upon generation (Aubin 1948, p. 197). Indigenous mystical dancing, Aubin suggested, translates emotion into movement, with the intent not just of making a desire known, but of realizing the desire (Aubin 1948, p. 198). Dance is to mimicking as poetry is to prose, explains Aubin, intimating that just as poetry expresses with certainty that which it does not say, dance communicates with certainty that which it does not express (Aubin 1948, p. 198). Honing in on the psycho-biological processes of the dance, Aubin turns to Paul Valéry's insights in his 1936 book, *Degas, Danse, Dessin*, on bodies in motion, "limbs can execute a series of figures that enchain them one to the other; this repeated intertwining producing a sort of *drunkenness* which changes from languor to a sort of fury. The state of Dance is created" (Aubin 1948, pp. 206–207). Valéry himself intimated that the neuro-muscular transformation in dance was ripe for analysis, though he himself did not venture into this terrain. Aubin, however, took up this challenge, opining that dance is a form of *sorcellerie*, a magical expression and means of obtaining unstated desires (Aubin 1948, p. 198).

Like the triangle, the square, the pentagon, or the six-pointed star, circles represent special occult powers. Circle dancing accesses this power, bringing it to life in the rhythmic incarnation of dancing bodies. When we add to these symbols the ancient swastika and weigh its use in Nazi Germany, the potentially dangerous dimensions of this type of spirit possession are readily apparent. Citing Carl Jung as well as relatively obscure ethnographers (such as Loefler-Delachaux), Aubin describes how the one who creates the circle encloses and takes possession, mastering the power inside the circle. That which is enclosed is subjected, reduced to impotence (Aubin 1948, p. 199).

The frequent hysterical scenes at the Salpétrière in Paris' rather recent past, according to Aubin, are not dead nor in the past. They are still found in North Africa and in military hospitals that serve indigenous peoples (Aubin 1948, p. 199). The famous Morzine possessions, however, Aubin attributed to carbon monoxide poisoning. Frustrated by the lack of medical insight into these conditions – hysteria had fallen out of favor as a diagnosis, and yet neither delirium nor neurosis were adequate to such events – Aubin pursued a psychoanalytic interpretation, linking the drunken excess of possession/hysteria with a frequently camouflaged erotic charge (Aubin 1948, p. 211). The sublimation of this eroticism into religious supplication – in the imitative magic of fertility rites, for example – was identified in Kretschmer's *Psychologie médicale* (1956). In European Christianity, this sublimation is notable already in Medieval lyric poetry dedicated to the Virgin Mary, which is indistinguishable otherwise from love poetry. St. John of the Cross explained the Christian love of God as so encompassing that it involved the entire body so that "sensual movements often arise during their spiritual exercises." While the soul is contemplating the most sublime oration, the body responds as well:

> that which the Christian entirely gives to his God he gives with his inferior tendencies as well as with his superior inclinations; he loves all at once with

> his body, his Heart and his mind; and, because each operates according to its own way of being, the superior part tastes God and draws spiritual pleasure, but the sensuality of the lower parts finds a satisfaction and a sensual delectation, incapable as it is to appreciate or to withstand the other [i.e. the other, spiritual, satisfaction].
>
> (Aubin 1948, p. 201; Bastide 1931, p. 173)[5]

This erotic beatitude, which channels the religious impulse and the mystery of reproduction and sexual attraction, is akin to hysteria. Sharp emotional loss, a betrayal of the heart or of the body, which cuts libidinal energy loose from its object, is the most frequent trigger for hysteria. Such a loss is now a component of trauma: the traumatic event deprives the person of physiological safety, whether that trauma is physical (a blow to the head) or emotional (a betrayal of nurturer). The libidinal energy escapes its normal channel of expression, and can take the form of painful or self-castigating symptoms. The condition, like mystical transports, is contagious. Aubin's analysis recognizes the power of curative rites such as dancing (Aubin 1948, pp. 212–213). He is not explicit, however, regarding how dances and other ecstatic rites of possession attempt to capture this energy, and to fix it within new, socially sanctioned practices, locations, or "vessels." Such possession rites, indeed, would be a manner of creating a *mana*-bearing object, a fetish of some sort. In Senegal the Serer *lup* and the Lebou *ndöep* and *samp* are powerful examples of such curative processes. Less than two decades after Aubin's publications, *Psychopathologie Africaine* published studies on the Senegalese rites (*e.g.* Gravrand 1966; Zempleni 1966). The person in need of healing participates in song, dance, and ritual rebirth. As well, a *mana*-infused altar is created in these processes, an altar which must be tended regularly for the afflicted to heal.

Aubin's views translate easily into the point of view of Porges' polyvagal theory (PVT). Progress from Aubin's theories into the contemporary, nonetheless, has not been robust. The contemporary therapeutic approach, we should remember, does not always even train clinicians to work with dissociative individuals. Some clinicians do not believe in dissociation and do not work with it. The integrative process described earlier in this chapter is presented by its leading advocates, Steele, Boon, and van dar Haart, we recall, as a science "in its infancy." Despite that characterization, the science has progressed beyond clinically induced forgetting, preferred in the nineteenth century by Dr. Janet. At the same time, rituals and curative rites continue to attract numerous adherents, whether those rites are Senegalese or derive from other traditions. Adepts who blend the science of dissociation, from Aubin through PVT, with ritualized traditions, no doubt exert considerable influence. Unreason continually impacts and embroils our consciousness. Denying that physiological dimension to our species only undermines our science.

Notes

1 Some might contend that Wulf Sachs was the first to publish, in 1937, a psychoanalysis of an African. See Sachs, W., 1996. *Black Hamlet*, with a new introduction by

S. Dubow and J. Rose. Baltimore: Johns Hopkins University Press. However, Ortigues and Ortigues, in *Oedipe Africain*, argue convincingly that true psychoanalysis must be driven by the questions and demands of the analysand, and by that standard, their own work takes precedence over that of Sachs. For an extensive discussion, see Bullard 2005b.

2 Of course, few now would agree that denial is an appropriate route toward mental health. It might be considered more appropriate in honor-based cultures (*e.g.*, see R.A. Nye, *Masculinity and Male Codes of Honor in Modern France* (Berkeley: University of California Press, 1998)). See also Hacking's discussion of Pierre Janet's therapeutic encouragement of forgetting as a dimension of his adherence to honor and then his later argument against this induced false consciousness (Hacking 1997, pp. 195–197, 260–265).

3 Aubin dedicated this comprehensive study to Dr. Henri Ey, Professor Henri Baruk, Dr. Angelo Hesnard, Daniel Lagache, Antoine Porot, and Léon Pales. These men represent a cross-section of the most prominent psychiatric and ethnographic practitioners of that era. Hesnard and Porot, we have encountered previously; Ey was the chief editor of *L'Evolution psychiatrique*, Lagache was a leading French psycho-analyst, and Pales was the associate director of the Musée de l'Homme.

4 Daedalus built the labyrinth on Crete to house the Minotaur. Imprisoned so that he could not reveal its secret, he and his son, Icarus, built wings to fly away. The psychophysiological effects of the rhythm of such dances fascinated others as well as Aubin. Aubin cites K. Brucher, *Les Rythmes et la Vie* (Paris: Plon, 1947), 253; R. Suaudeau, *Les méthodes nouvelles de l'Education physique* (Paris: P.U.F., 1951), 110 and forward; and H. Derville, *L'Ame noir* (Paris: Livres Nouveaux, 1941).

5 This view of the sexual functions as inferior and almost negligible contrasts with the modern outlook that places sexuality at the center of one's identity. The history of such imagery also highlights the sexualization of physical love. For example, the warm love of God, rendered tangible and maternal in breast imagery was prominent into the nineteenth century. The demise of the divine maternal breast marks as well the dawn of the sexualized breast (breast as fetishized sex object). The negligible importance of sexual misconduct in the eyes of the Catholic hierarchy, even in the early twenty-first century, could also be linked to such a view of the common, though differentiated, roots of spirituality and sensuality.

Works Cited

Allier, R., 1925. *La psychologie de la conversion chez les peuples non-civilisés*. Paris: Payot.

Ashforth, A., 2000. *Madumo: A Man Bewitched*. Chicago: University of Chicago Press.

Au pays des mages noirs, 1947. Film. Directed by Jean Rouch. France: Ministere de la culture.

Aubin, H., 1939a. Introduction à l'étude de la psychiatrie chez les noirs. *Annales Médico-Psychologiques*, 97 (1), 1–29, 181–213.

Aubin, H., 1939b. L'Assistance psychiatrique indigène aux colonies. *In*: P. Combemale, ed., *Congrès Médecins Aliénistes et neurologistes de France et des pays de langue françiase XLIIe session, Alger, 6–11 avril 1938*. Paris: Coueslant Masson, 147–176, 196–197.

Aubin, H., 1948. Danse mystique, possession, psychopathologie. *L'évolution psychiatrique*, 4 (numero exceptionnel), 191–215.

Aubin, H., 1951. Réfus, Réniement, Répression. *L'Évolution psychiatrique*, I, 31–40.

Aubin, H., 1952. *L'Homme et la magie*. Paris: Desclée De Brouwer et Cie.

Ba, M., 2015. Sénégal: Abdoulaye Wade, égaré entre "esclaves" et "anthropophages." *Jeune Afrique*. Available from: www.jeuneafrique.com/225676/politique/s-n-gal-abdoulaye-wade-gar-entre-esclaves-et-anthropophages/ [Accessed April 2021].

Bastide, R., 1931. *Les problèmes de la vie mystique*. Paris: Colin.

Bastide, R., 1950. *Sociologie et psychanalyse*. Paris: Presses Universitaires de France.

Bastide, R., 1960. Psychiatrie, ethnographie et sociologie: Les maladies mentales et Le Noir brésilien. *In*: *Désordres mentaux et santé mentale en Afrique au sud du Sahara*. London: Commission for Technical Cooperation in Africa South of the Sahara (CCTA), 223–230.

Bloom, M. and Moskalenko, S., 2021. *Pastels and Pedophiles: Inside the Mind of QAnon*. Palo Alto, CA: Stanford University Press.

Boilat, P.D., 1853. *Esquisses sénégalaises*. Paris: P. Bertrand.

Bullard, A., 2005a. Oedipe Africain, a Retrospective. *Transcultural Psychiatry*, 42 (2), 171–203.

Bullard, A., 2005b. The Critical Impact of Frantz Fanon and Henri Collomb; Race, Gender and Personality Testing of North and West Africans. *Journal for the History of Behavioral Sciences*, 41 (3), 225–248.

Bullard, A., 2007. Imperial Networks and Postcolonial Independence: The Transition from Colonial to Transcultural Psychiatry. *In*: S. Mahone and M. Vaughan, eds., *Psychiatry and Empire, Cambridge Series in Imperial and Post-Colonial Studies*. London: Palgrave Macmillan, 197–219.

Bullard, A., 2011. La Crypte and Other Pseudo-Analytic Concepts in French West African Psychiatry. In: W. Anderson, D. Jenson and R. Keller, eds., Unconscious Dominions: Psychoanalysis, Colonial Trauma, and Global Sovereignties. Chapel Hill, NC: Duke University Press, 43–74.

Cazanove, F., 1933. Les conceptions magico-religieuses de indigènes de lAfrique occidentale française. *Les Grandes Endémies Tropicales*, 5, 38–48.

Clark, J., 2018. *The Catch-22 in Our Medical/Legal System That Criminalizes Mental Illness*. Arlington, VA: Treatment Advocacy Center. Available from: www.treatmentadvocacycenter.org/fixing-the-system/features-and-news/4012-personally-speaking-my-son-is-mentally-ill-so-listen-up [Accessed 17 April 2021].

Fanon, F., 1952. Le Syndrôme nord-Africain. *L'Ésprit*, 20 (2), 237–251.

Fanon, F., 1967a. *Black Skin, White Masks*. New York: Grove Press (1952. *Peau noire, masques blancs*. Paris: Éditions du Seuil).

Fanon, F., 1967b. *A Dying Colonialism*. H. Chevalier, trans. New York: Grove Press.

Fanon, F. and Lacaton, R., 1955. Conduites d'aveu en Afrique du Nord. *Congrès des médecins aliénistes et neurologistes de France et des pays de langue française*, 53, 657–660.

Fisher, J., 2017. *Healing the Fragmented Selves of Trauma Survivors: Overcoming Internal Self-Alienation*. London and New York: Routledge.

Foucault, M., 1961. *Histoire de la folie à l'âge classique*. Paris: Gallimard.

Gagné, A., 2020. The 'Spiritual Warfare' Worldview of Trump's Conspiracy Doctor Is Part of a Transnational Movement. *Religion Dispatches*. Available from: https://religiondispatches.org/the-spiritual-warfare-worldview-of-trumps-conspiracy-doctor-is-part-of-a-transnational-movement/ [Accessed August 2021].

Gravrand, H., 1966. Le 'Lup' Serer: Phénoménologie de l'emprise des Pangol et psychothérapie des 'possédés'. *Psychopathologie Africaine*, II (2), 195–225.

Hacking, I., 1997. *Rewriting the Soul: Multiple Personality and the Sciences of Memory*. Princeton, NJ: Princeton University Press.

Initiation a la danse des possedes. 1949. Film. Directed by Jean Rouch. France: Le Centre National de la Cinematographie Francaise.
Janet, P., 1894. *État mental des hystériques: Les accidents mentaux*. Paris: Rueff et Cie.
Kretschmer, E., 1956. *Psychologie médicale*. Paris: Payot.
Leiris, M., 1931. *L'Afrique fantôme*. Paris: Gallimard.
Les maitres fous. 1955. Film. Directed by Jean Rouch. France: Films de la Pleiade.
Maran, R., 1921 [1938]. *Batoula, roman*. Paris: Albin Michel.
Mauchamp, É., 1911. *La sorcellerie au Maroc*. Paris: Dorbon-Ainé.
Monteil, C., 1931. La Divination chez les noirs de l'Afrique occidentale française. *Bulletin du comite des études historiques et scientifiques*, 14 (1), 27–136.
Nagle, L.E. and Owasanoye, B., 2016. Fearing the Dark: The Use of Witchcraft to Control Human Trafficking Victims and Sustain Vulnerability. *Southwestern Law Review*, 45, 561–600. Available from: www.stetson.edu/law/studyabroad/netherlands/media/Trk2.Wk3.Day3.Nagle.Fearing-the-Dark.pdf [Accessed August 2021].
Ohanyon, A., 1999. *L'impossible rencontre: Psychologie et psychanalyse en France, 1919–1969*. Paris: La Découverte.
Ortigues, M.C., Martino, P. and Collomb, H., 1966. Intégration des données culturelles Africaines à la psychiatrie de l'enfant. *Psychopathologie Africaine*, II (3), 441–450.
Ortigues, M.C. and Ortigues, E., 1966 [1984]. *Oedipe Africain*. Paris: Plon (3rd ed., Paris: Harmattan).
Porges, S.W., 2011. *The Polyvagal Theory: Neurophysiological Foundations of Emotions, Attachment, Communication, Self-Regulation*. New York: W.W. Norton.
Porges, S.W., 2017. *The Pocket Guide to the Polyvagal Theory: The Transformative Power of Feeling Safe*. New York: W.W. Norton.
Reboul, H. and Régis, E., eds., 1912. *L'assistance des aliénés aux colonies*. Rapport au Congrès des médecins aliénistes et neurologistes de France et des pays de langue française, XXII session, Tunis. Paris: l'Académie de Médecine, 1–7 avril.
Róheim, G., 1928. La psychologie raciale et les origines du capitalisme chez les primitifs. *Revue française de psychanalyse*, 2 (1), 173–174.
Steele, K., Boone, S. and van der Haart, O., 2017. *Treating Trauma-Related Dissociation: A Practical, Integrative Approach (Norton Series on Interpersonal Neurobiology)*. New York: W.W. Norton.
Stuart Hughes, H., 1958. *Consciousness and Society: The Reorientation of European Social Thought, 1890–1930*. New York: Vintage Books.
van der Haart, O. and Horst, J., 1989. The Dissociation Theory of Pierre Janet. *Journal of Traumatic Stress*, 2 (4), 1–11.
Zempléni, A., 1966. La dimension thérapeutique du culte des rab (Ndöp, Tuuru et Samp: Rites des possessions chez les Wolof et les Lebu). *Psychopathologie Africaine*, II (3), 295–439.

8 Ancestors

***

Among patients at the Fann Hospital, reckoning with the ancestors often featured in their treatment. The clinicians at Fann took an interest in the role of ancestors in creating and curing illnesses, and followed at least some of their patients in their quest for cures. Ancestry can appear as a powerful, conditioning force, bringing good fortune or misery, or sometimes both, into one's life. Discussed via multiple registers – whether in the language of genetics, psychology, or history – ancestry can be viewed as determining illness or health, happiness or chronic depression, proud traditions and brave reckoning with subjection and humiliation. As often as not, it seems that in the Western outlook one's ancestry is something to reckon with, to overcome if need be, and, more or less frequently, to celebrate. Mental illness, whether caused by genetic traits or milieu, threads through family ties in diverse manners. Who one is, one's place in the family and in the community, one's role in life, this is wrapped up in the gifts and sometimes heavy legacies bestowed from one generation on the next.

This chapter takes stock of the roles of ancestors in the lives and illnesses of the Fann Hospital's Senegalese patients. The spirits of the ancestors, by the accounts of patient case studies, could cause many types of illnesses, the cure of which involved various forms of appeasement of the spirits.[1] We cannot anticipate any overall uniformity of practice historically or between ethnic groups in this discussion. The Fann accounts of ancestry grapple with diverse changes in ancestor worship as these rites confronted migration, urbanization, and stronger ties to Islam (and much more rarely, to Christianity).

Viewed in retrospect, it appears that Fann researchers often sought to describe fixed, viable traditions to which they could attribute expertise and effective curative techniques. These researchers less frequently focused on change and historical flux, and even in those instances, the researchers seem largely secure in a classical vision of modernity – rooted in the autonomous individual and inclusive of market economies, urbanization, and Western education. In their version of modernity, progress is clearly identifiable and mostly good. The praise for individuation, for the assumption of individual responsibility and choice in the face of one's mental illness, are norms in almost all Fann case histories. From our

DOI: 10.4324/9781003112143-9

contemporary perspective, progress is less certain, and the good is often open to debate. Individuation is frequently questioned or subject to criticism as a by-product of modern, disciplining forces rather than heralded as an unalloyed historical achievement.

Disrupted relationships with the ancestors could provoke a wide array of illnesses or misfortunes. For example, in writing about the privations endured by West African migrants – whether to urban centers within Africa or abroad – Henri Collomb and Henri Ayat observed that the absence of relationships with the living as well as the dead was a chief source of mental illness. Young men frequently moved across territories and borders in order to find work to raise enough funds to achieve a desirable marriage. Delusions of marriage, of pregnancy, and of childbirth among men and women figured prominently, Collomb and Ayat observed, precisely because of this failed goal of getting married and assuming one's place as within the ancestral lineage (Collomb and Ayat 1962, p. 596).

The prominence of ancestors in the Senegalese sense of place, order, and myth suffered because of colonialism and migration. Islam, for some a bulwark against French imperialism, also discouraged ancestor worship. However, despite the widespread embrace of Islam in Senegal, the veneration of ancestors continued in various forms. The stereo-typical French colonial school lesson, in which colonial subjects were taught to revere *nos ancêtres gauloises*, takes on a powerful charge given the role of ancestor worship and ancestral spirit possessions in Senegalese cultures. Though only a small proportion of West Africans experienced such schooling, the impact on those who did could be powerful (*e.g.* Kane 1961). The development of the psychiatric profession through the nineteenth and twentieth centuries also increasingly designated spirit possession as a form of mental illness. In France, the popularity of spirit seances, in which mediums contacted and communicated with the dead, prompted the psychiatrist Joseph Lévy-Valensi to characterize spirit mediums in the popular spiritualism movement in France as voluntarily mentally ill. Spiritism drew adherents across the U.S.A., where it originated, and throughout Europe. W.B. Yeats, the Irish nationalist poet, communicated within his marriage via spiritualism. Night after night his young wife channeled counsel and oracles via automatic writing that the couple used to direct their lives (Maddox 1999). The spirit medium, according to the psychology Lévy-Valensi, voluntarily enters a hypnotic state that accesses psychologist automatism, which he compared directly to dissociation (Lévy-Valensi 1910, p. 697). This practice of inducing "mental illness" Lévy-Valensi felt was highly dangerous, even though any effort to ban it would invariably force the growth of a substitute practice.

Sometimes referred to as the "women's cult," ancestor worship in Senegal continued despite religious pressure to abandon such habits.[2] The Lebou *ndöep* rite and the Serer Lup are often discussed as a singularly robust and popular pre-Islamic practices. Because of the broad array of afflictions the ancestors could inflict, *ndöep* and the Serer counterpart, *lup*, became a major interest among Fann Hospital clinicians.

A Colonial Possession Crisis

On 19 May 1848, Boilat witnessed a possession first hand. As he describes the event, he and his companions had gone to bed for the night and just fallen asleep when "infernal cries that made our hair stand on end and made us shiver despite ourselves" awoke them (Boilat 1853, pp. 449–450). M. Vidal, the préfet apostolique, stricken with uncontrollable trembling, instructed Boilat to find out what was going on. Father Boilat went with another priest, Father Carmarans, to investigate the source of the cries in a neighboring house. There they found a young woman, about 22 years old, lying on a straw mattress, a pillow under her head. A crowd of people filled the house. The young woman's head was like a pendulum racing at an incalculable pace.

> In a tone that one could feel in an inexpressible way, she chanted all sorts of prophesies. All the Blacks were beside themselves, deeply inhibited, and could not aid her. What ails her? I asked. They responded, "a spirit has seized her body; you who are educated, you might be able to find a way to drive it out."

Responding to this challenge, Father Boilat began by asking the woman's name and he was told it was Sophie. But when he addressed the woman directly, "Sophie, Sophie, in the name of Jesus-Christ answer me, Sophie," the response came, "I am not Sophie, I am not a girl to have such a name, I am Samba-Diob, the great demon worshiped by the Serers in the village XX in Baoul. I am a spirit, I go where I like on the wings of the winds" (Boilat 1853, pp. 451–452). Samba-Diob, or Sophie, continued to chant. Suddenly he/she began a different song in a language unknown to Father Boilat. Father Carmarans, who was there as well, claimed in an astonished voice that it was a shepherd's song from his home in the Aveyron. Overcome with emotion, Father Camarans asked Boilat to stay with the young woman while he went to the chapel to pray for her. Boilat stayed watchfully by her side, but sent someone to his room for his Virgin Mary medal. When Camarans returned and the medal arrived, Boilat proceeded to perform an exorcism. Only with great difficulty could he get the Virgin's medal to stay on the woman's contorting body. Six men helped to hold her steady, while Father Boilat placed the medal on her head, only to have it thrown to the other end of the room by her violent jerkings. They found it, brought it back, and fixed it again in the same place. This time the convulsions stopped immediately. "We could not help admiring the power of Mary," reflected Father Boilat (1853, p. 452).

Next, Samba-Diob began chanting that he would leave soon if the medal were removed and flour was put on Sophie's feet. Father Camarans cautioned that this was a ruse of the demon, and that he should not be given anything at all. "The Negresses were already arriving with their flour, but we prevented them from throwing it. The evil spirit, forced by the name of Mary to depart, sounded a song of leave in a voice loud enough to be heard down the whole street, and continued, gradually in softer tones, as though he were further and further away." The Wolof words to the song were, "I am a spirit, I came here on the wings of the winds, I fly where I like, and in the blink of an eye I disappear, I return to my realm where the homages of divinity are given me" (Boilat 1853, p. 452). After this song, Sophie lay on the bed as if she were dead, then fell into a deep sleep. The next morning, Sophie was exhausted, looking as though she had not slept in a long time.

> She was very surprised to find a Virgin's medal attached to her hair, and she threw it off, saying that already in Dakar someone had given her one, and that her mother had made her get rid of it. She had no memory of what had happened the previous night.
>
> (Boilat 1853, p. 453)

"Was this a possession, an obsession, or a simple epilepsy?" asked Boilat, yet he self-consciously refused to resolve this puzzle, writing, "It is not for me to decide" (Boilat 1853, p. 453). Boilat's primary desire seems to be to reveal the different possible understandings of the experience of Sophie – Samba-Diob – that is, whether that this one experience can alternately be understood as a possession crisis, an obsessive disorder, or as epilepsy. But he later recounted what he portrayed as a less ambiguous case of a young Wolof girl, about 12 years old, who was subject to such seizures during which she made frequent prophesies in many different languages. In this instance Boilat did not credit the European view of such possessions as medical crises, but relied instead on a belief in speaking in tongues. The "demonic" origin of these possessions was not doubted by Boilat, who pointedly remarked that the most prominent languages of prophesy were either Serer or Nones, that is, languages "spoken by people who are fetishists." The term fetishist, which has held derogatory implications, refers to the use of sacred objects in ancestor worship (Mann 2003). This girl's spirits, however, also seemed related to the Islamic world, since while prophesizing she demonstrated superb knowledge of the Qu'ran and of Arabic, although she was in fact illiterate (Boilat 1853, pp. 453–454).

The possession of Sophie by the spirit Samba-Diob presents a female-male pairing that at times is characterized as a marriage. Channeling the male spirit confers on Sophie prestige and power, just as demonstrating polyglot skills and in-depth knowledge of the Qu'ran and Arabic would have conferred status on the unnamed young Wolof girl. These dimensions to the possession escape Boilat's discussion, focused as he was on categorizing the nature of the possession; an obsession that he shared – as it turns out – with transcultural psychiatry. Translation surfaces again and again as a persistent difficulty in cross-cultural psychiatry; but translation of words is only the tip of the iceberg, as deeply different life-worlds allowed experiences and meanings that sharply diverged. Boilat's account moves us from the search for language equivalents, to a search for adequate expressions for Senegalese experiences, and to the search for a clear understanding of what is potentially lost in translation and how it is lost.

Boilat describes how for many years as he had traveled around Senegal he had heard of demon possessions. The crises were viewed very differently by

Europeans and Africans; as he writes, "the Negroes remove the possessed person to a quiet house, while the Europeans comment simply that it was an epileptic attack." Epilepsy? Possession by a "subtle spirit"? Such a possession, he reports, "was like a wind which seizes the body, shakes it violently, and makes them able to foretell the future" (Boilat 1853, p. 449). Boilat's Catholic faith led him to consider these events as demon possessions, but his knowledge of local cultures and languages forced him to consider the discrepancy between a "demon possession" and the more apt translation "to be seized by a spirit." If Boilat's Catholicism provided him a certain degree of access into the spiritual view of the Senegalese, it also limited this access. In the Catholic point of view, demons are unequivocally bad or evil. Spirits in the animist worldview, on the other hand, can be good or bad, playful or mischievous, troublesome, helpful, or perhaps even neutral. Boilat's hesitancy in his translation – between demon possession and "to be seized by a spirit" – reveals his own tensions between his Senegalese ancestry and his allegiance as a Catholic priest to a metaphysical world clearly divided between the good (including God, Jesus, Mary, and other recognized saints) and evil (including Satan and other demons). The animist religions underlying Islam in Senegal, meanwhile, sustained a spirit world in which spirits did not align so neatly into Good and Evil.

The earliest French medical observations of such West African possessions date from the first half of the twentieth century (Cazanove 1933; Aubin 1939a, 1939b). Colonial psychiatric interpretations of such crises tended to try to look past the cultural beliefs in spirit possessions in order to identify a more fundamental (usually biological) cause of the crises. French doctors frequently pointed to organic diseases as the source of mental afflictions, and dismissed local understandings of spirit crises. Dr. Huot, for example, opined "that this is nothing other . . . than the doctrine of demonic possession, as old as the world" (Huot quoted in Reboul and Régis 1912, p. 101). The competing understandings of these crises exemplify tensions in colonial Senegal that go far beyond simple problems of translation. The tensions between life-worlds entailed deep discrepancies between the nature of experience, meaning, spirituality, and health. The effort to supplant the local understandings of such spiritual crises and to use in its place a Western biomedical perspective was an integral, if not highly successful, part of the colonizing process, which gradually gave way to the accommodation and co-existence of the two systems of healing.

Boilat's frank confusion and open speculation about the metaphysical nature of the possessions he witnessed express aspects of transcultural understanding that have not entirely receded over the years.

Serer Pangol and the Lup Ritual

The priest Henri Gravrand described Serer convictions that most of the spiritual crises, or mental difficulties, are related to activities of Pangol (plural, singular: Fangol) (Gravrand 1966, p. 195). Gravrand notes that his is the first systematic study of Serer possession rituals. Within French scholarship, Gravrand followed in the wake of Roger Bastide's study of *candomblé* and Michel Leiris of Ethiopian possession rituals (Bastide 1931, 1960; Leiris 1958). A cure for such spirit troubles is normally achieved by creating a new relation between the person afflicted and the Pangol. Translated literally, Fangol means serpent or snake, but understood as a metaphysical presence, the Pangol (plural) are intermediate spirits between the supreme diety, Rôg Sène, and human beings. The Serer recognized two basic types of Pangol, either unknown spirits that personified a force of nature, or known spirits of renowned ancestors who had been transformed upon death and were capable of astounding feats (Gravrand 1966, p. 199). Pangol of renowned ancestors had established rites and locations for worship; individuals possessed by such Pangol often received the spirits via inheritance and knew the necessary forms of worship to keep the spirits satisfied. The Lup ritual for identifying Pangol, fixing their place of worship at a domestic altar or shrine, and prescribing the rites for worship, composed the healing technique in instances of unexpected possession.

The dimensions of Lup that Gravrand points to as therapeutic and spiritually elevating are, to some extent, counterbalanced by the detailed stories he recounts of how Pangol succeeded in creating relationships with individuals; the disease, deprivation, and desperation he reveals display an immense variety of suffering, all of it attributed to Pangol. Possession could arise via heredity (seemingly the least traumatic possibility), punishment, contract, or the free choice of the spirits who decide for reasons of their own to demand a relationship with an individual. Most hereditary *Pangol* were *Pangol yayay*, which followed the maternal lineage, possessing an individual in each successive generation. The less prevalent *Pangol mbafap* followed the paternal lineage. Hereditary possession resulted in dysfunctional symptoms only when the possession was resisted, for example because of conversion to Islam or (more rarely) to Christianity.

Gravrand tells the stories of two men, both converts to Islam, who resisted this hereditary possession because serving as a *Yàl Pangol* – tending the altar and praying to the ancestral spirits – would offend their new religion. After much sickness and suffering the first man relented, and assumed his role as an officiant in the ancestral religion even while maintaining a professed allegiance to Islam. The second, however, resisted more strenuously and finally died rather than accept the spirits. His death was relatively quick, which the neighbors attributed to the fact that the *Pangol* loved him and did not want him to suffer more than necessary (Gravrand 1966, pp. 196–198).

Transgression of the *Pangol*s' orders could produce possession. For example, Latsuk Faye violated the orders of the *Pangol* at the village of Languème. Once he had transgressed, the one-eyed, one-breasted female *Pangol* of the village appeared before him, never to leave him again prior to his death a few short days later (Gravrand 1966, p. 205). Those who stole from the *Pangol* might become rich, but the vengeance of the *Pangol* was certain to arrive sooner or later. *Madag* (*voyants* or deviners) were especially likely to try to steal from the *Pangol* because their special sight could offer them some protection. However, even a *Pangol* deceived for a short while could obtain vengeance, if not directly on the thief, then perhaps by killing off his or her children (Gravrand 1966, pp. 205–206). If an individual sought out the *Pangol* for a special favor, the rules of engagement stipulated that the *Pangol* never give, but rather they sell at a dear price. To obtain a bountiful harvest, a man might sell his son. Once the harvest was brought in, the son might drown, or be killed by lightening. The child killed by a *Pangol*, so it was said, would be born again and invariably enjoy a rich new life (Gravrand 1966, pp. 207–208).

Pangol could choose specific individuals who for some particular reason incited their love. Resistance to possession by enamored *Pangol* produced various debilitating and/or painful symptoms. This could be mental illness manifested by laughing and crying nonsensically, running about the woods at night, disappearing from home for several days, or confused or foreign speech. Physical illnesses attributed to the *Pangol* included local or total paralysis, the loss of one or both eyes, the atrophy of a hand or foot, genital swelling, sterility in men and women, repeated miscarriages, stomach ache, gastro-intestinal infections, and more (Gravrand 1966, p. 209). This suffering—produced by resistance to *Pangol*'s impassioned possession, as distinct from suffering brought on when *Pangol* were punishing an individual—could be alleviated by a *lup*.

The *lup* aimed to discover the name and the abode of the *Pangol*, thereby providing a means of integrating them into the human community. Knowing the spirits' names allowed humans to propitiate the spirit and thereby to gain influence with it. Gravrand, who was a Catholic priest, recalls that when God told Moses his name this created a pact between God and Moses' people. All religions, he remarks, are based in the intervention of a spirit into the world of humans, but so long as the spirit has not revealed its name, this relationship is one-sided. The ancient question, "Who are you?" must be answered so that the relationship between the spirits and the person can be reciprocal (Gravrand 1966, pp. 217–218). Knowing the spirits' names creates the ability to interact with them, to pray to them, to supplicate and placate them.

The Serer *lup* ceremony identified those possessed by ancestral spirits known as *Pangol*. *Pangol* is the plural form of *Fangol*, which translates literally as snake (Gravrand 1966, p. 198). During *lup*, the officiant (known as a Lulup) first detected and discovered the name of the *Pangol* and then discovered the residence of the *Pangol* so that they could be properly worshipped. The possessed individual undergoes a simulated death during which his faults and sickness are transferred onto a sacrificial animal. The person is then reborn with a new personality, he becomes a *Yàl Pangol* and can henceforth control his illness with the aid of his *Kamb*. He is no longer a sick person to be pitied, but an officiant of a vital religious rite that is valued by the community and commands monetary recompense. Nonetheless, the burdens of the *Yàl Pangol*'s life as a mystic could be resented. Such was the case with one *Yàl Pangol*, who cautioned his sons against certain games that could incite the *Pangol* to possess them (Gravrand 1966, pp. 203, 225).

After the successful ritual everyone present feasted together on the cooked sacrificial animal. The *lup* celebrated and enshrined the status of the possessed individual as an abode of the ancestors, and of this individual's family as one that hosts the ancestral spirits in their home and worshipped them at their altar. Those present witnessed the divination and feasted with the family. This was a communal event which made all part of the same sacred community. *Lup* acted to confer a specific, recognizable status on the possessed (who, prior to the ritual, had likely been acting in a manner that ill-conformed with their status). Once installed securely in their new status, this individual and his or her family could resume untrammeled social bonds.

Father Gravrand was far from alone among Fann investigators in emphasizing that social existence among the various Senegalese ethnic groups is conferred by having a specific, demarcated status. Conforming to that status formed an essential dimension and aspiration to everyone's life. This is frequently contrasted to a broadly evoked "European" style of achieving identity via individual striving and merit. The Western emphasis on individual achievement seems to overlook the vital role of class, education, occupation, sex, and race (to name just the most obvious) as constraints on status. The ability of *Lup* to effectively rework social symbolics so as to affirm the special status of the possessed demonstrates how status validated individuals even when they were outliers and more in touch with spirits than with their fellow human beings. This power diminished during colonization, with Islam offering alternative status categories and urbanization contributing to the loosening of status and the rise of (more or less) self-fashioned identities. Andràs Zempléni took up these same themes, as discussed below, with respect to the Lebou rites.

These Serer *lup* beliefs and rites, Gravrand remarks, are found in variant forms across Africa and in Central and South America, and he suggests were present on other continents during earlier times. The age-old Serer practices, for Gravrand, pointed to a common human striving to know a higher power, and the belief in the possibility of a Higher Spirit to intercede in the affairs of man (Gravrand 1966, pp. 225–226). Louis Mars, the Haitian psychiatrist, placed such rituals firmly within the context of therapeutic psycho-drama as sketched by Michel Leiris in his book on *zar* possessions in Ethiopia (Mars 1966, p. 241, citing Leiris 1958). The ritual of possession by the healer and curative dialogue with the possessed, created a mixed scene of lived-drama and played-drama. Playing and replaying a dramatic event, as Mars believed, could dissipate trauma, disperse threatening spirits, lift up human spirits, and solidify community. Emphasizing the strength of interpersonal bonds on the African continent as well as in Haiti, Mars foresaw a prominent role for psycho-drama within African psychiatry. The work at Fann Hospital signaled how traditional healers, families, and doctors, might together orchestrate such healings.

Lebou *Rab* and *Ndöep*

It is within this already crowded field that Zempléni offered his ethnography of the various rituals of the *ndöepkat*. Driven by a desire to demonstrate the therapeutic dimensions of *samp*, *ndöep*, and *tuur*, Zempléni made palpable the therapeutic body-work of the *ndöepkat* (Zempléni 1966, 1968, 1977). Working with Jacqueline Rabain, Zempléni had previously studied the peculiar relationship that could form between an ancestral spirit and an infant or child (Zempleni and Rabain 1965). The goal of this present discussion cannot be to reproduce Zempleni's legendary documentary detail, but aims rather to reflect on the historical nature of Zempleni's research, and to consider its role in creating transcultural psychiatric practices. Leiris' *L'Afrique Fantôme* (1934) reads like a later-day voyage of discovery by an accidental ethnographer. Aubin's "Danse Mystique" (1948) chronicles the psychoanalytic universality of trance rituals. Zempleni's work provides careful consideration of the micro-processes of Lebou possession rituals in order to reveal their therapeutic value and potential role in biomedical psychiatric and therapeutic work.

Zempleni resisted the temptation to separate the therapeutic dimensions of *ndöep* rituals from the religious. The intertwining of Lebou religion and therapeutic ritual, however, reveals a barrier to the transcultural value of Zempleni's labors. That is, if his exhaustive ethnographic endeavors were truly to be fully usable by clinicians at the Fann Hospital or elsewhere, a separation of the therapeutic from the religious would need to occur. Or, at least that is the case if we can assume (apparently safely) that not all clinicians at Fann or other medical establishments were prepared to become true believers in Lebou-style ancestor worship. As a secular sociologist-ethnographer, Zempleni avoids entanglement in metaphysical discussions of ancestral spirits and their worship. He focuses on the bodies, on the physicality of the rites: the cloth is wrapped in such a way, the gourd is buried here, not there, the herbs are chewed and spit, the drums are played, the *ndöepkat* (priestesses) dance. As his detailed descriptions accumulate, there is a certain emptiness that takes the place of religious mystery at the center of his study. In Aubin's psychoanalytic work the fetish was explored as a powerful object that carries socially symbolic value and is imbued with intentionality. This type of animation of the inanimate is at the heart of the possession rituals.

The therapeutic work, Zempleni points out, begins even prior to consulting with a *ndöepkat* (priestess), because significant family tension and disagreements need to be reconciled in order to undertake a consultation. The individual's crisis is a family affair, and the diverse points of view within the family must be brought to agreement in order to embark on the path of ritualized healing. The afflictions suffered by an individual can be attributed to Islamic or animist magic or *sorcellerie*, to simple illness, or even to Western-style biomedical causes. Overcoming the resistance of Islamic family members who object to the animist rites often formed the most daunting barrier to accessing *ndöepkat* services. While the clinicians at Fann often dealt with fractious families who advanced conflicting interpretations of an illness and pursued various paths toward healing, those who chose the rituals of the *ndöep* needed the explicit consent of their extended family (Zempléni 1966, pp. 318–319, 345–347). This consensus, sometimes arrived at only with great difficulty, was essential not only because the rites worked through collective mechanisms calling upon the maternal and paternal ancestors, but also because the costs of the ceremonies imposed a heavy burden, normally shouldered by an extensive network of relatives.

In these matters, Islam was an obstacle but not an insurmountable barrier, as demonstrated by the case of Moussa (Zempléni 1966, p. 349). This young man worked hard to persuade his father, who was an Islamic marabout with his own healing practice, to allow a *ndöep*. A pared down ritual provided Moussa with some relief from his symptoms, but his father objected to the installation of a spirit shrine at their home, fearing that it would offend his Islamic clients, and insisted that the shrine be left at the *ndöepkat*'s home. Moussa's father also encouraged him to neglect the prescribed offerings to the shrine. Finally after Moussa's symptoms reappeared and grew more severe, the father assented to a full *ndöep*, saying that he would not stand in the way of necessary prayers and that the cow could be sacrificed. This family consensus underlay the successful ritual, the installing of the shrine at their home, and Moussa's eventual cure (Zempléni 1966, p. 349). In another case, however, an Islamic father proved intractably opposed to bringing a divided family together (he and the animist mother were divorced) in the *ndöep* ceremonies. The son, torn in his affiliations by the family's bitterness and dissension, fell into lasting psychosis (Zempléni 1966, p. 349).

The rapidly changing social structure in Senegal, including urbanization and the spread of a commercial market, produced in the *ndöepkat* an emergent commercialization of the ceremonies. The elevated cost of treatment, in Zempleni's analysis, was an adaptation that allowed the reconstitution of families within and through the very forces (urbanization and commercialization) that tore families apart and created strife. The goods and money that proved fodder for family quarrels, provided, through the unifying and conciliatory spirit necessary for undertaking and funding a *ndöep*, the route to reunification and renewed family cohesion (Zempléni 1966, p. 348).

Zempleni's emphasis on the gender dynamics at work during the eclipse of ancestor worship by Islam (or, more rarely, Christianity) is particularly notable for the 1960s. Zempleni compares the Serer possession rite, the *lup*, as a deeply similar practice in which Islam did not play a significant role. The chief differences between *lup* and *ndöep* revolve around gender. Matrilinear ancestors are overtly recognized among the Serer in Gravrand's study, and men and women participate equally in the possession rites. The end-result of these rites among the Serer is reintegration of the sick individual into a family milieu. The importance of the illness is entirely collective, involving the entire family or even the community, and its resolution marks the acceptance into the family of a reborn, perhaps deeply altered, individual. In contrast, the Lebou and Wolof populations, who had largely converted to Islam by the late nineteenth-century, no longer recognized matrilineal ancestors and the possession rites provoked a sense of conflict with Islam. The rites were often characterized as "a woman's affair," and yet nonetheless a majority of Muslims judged them powerful ceremonies, or at least accepted them as vital to preserving peace within their families (Zempléni 1966, p. 429).

In Islamic milieux, the prominent therapies were performed by maraboutic men, schooled in the written word of the Qu'ran. Hence, from the Muslim point of view, the cult of the *rab* was essentially feminine. Men who wanted to be an officiant had to dress as women (Zempléni 1966, pp. 428–429). Muslims preferred the *samp*, because it was a private, discrete ceremony that allowed for a partial recognition of the animist worship inclusive of matrilineal ancestors (Zempléni 1966, p. 429). The *samp* did not infringe Muslim sensibilities of dignity, cleanliness and order, as did the public drumming, singing, tumultuous jostling, dancing, agitation, crises, and falls of the *ndöep*.

Zempleni pointed out that Senegalese men, bound to Islam in the interest of obtaining social status and attracted by the freedom it offered from maternal lineages, generally turned away from the ancestor cults. Women, in contrast, tended to maintain the ancestor shrines and rituals. The women officiants, the *ndöepkat*, reworked the symbolic and social order. From the psychoanalytic point of view, in Lacanian language, they wield the power of the phallus (Bullard 2015). During the early years of Fann, this role suffered circumscriptions by marabouts, themselves extending their dominion and under-cutting the authority of women in the realm of ancestral healing and social symbolics. The *ndöepkat*, however, persists as a powerful force in contemporary Senegal, continuing to provide women with the ability to rework social status.

The spread of Islam did not suffice by itself to explain why the ancestor rites were feminized. Zempleni explained, "the strong position of the uterine lineage in the past seemed to be the second condition for the continuation and the essentially feminine character of the current Wolof-Lebou rites" (Zempléni 1966, p. 432). The possession rites acted as an equalizing force because they reasserted matrilineal ancestry within the context of the overtly patrilineal Islamic system. However, the contemporary practice of these cults, Zempleni noted, was somewhat compromised by the breakdown of the ability to reintegrate individuals into family systems and the rise, in contrast, of congregations of the possessed.

Khady Fall, A Wolof Priestess

Zempleni's study of the role of the spirits in the life of Khady Fall, a possessed Wolof priestess, describes the intersection of gender, animism, Islam, and French colonization. The dynamics revealed are unusual. As presented by Zempleni, Khady Fall's personal journey through illness, years of peregrinations, and, finally, into a successful practice as a *ndöepkat* in Dakar, expressed a struggle for recognition and empowerment. Normally *rab* are transmitted via maternal lineages. In Khady Fall's family, her father's lineage transmitted *rab* and as well produced male guardians and officiants of the *rab*. If inheriting *rab* via the paternal lineage was somewhat unusual, tracing out Fall's lineage reveals even more surprises. Contrary to the dominant trend, possibly because Fall's heritage was largely Muslim on her maternal (Toucoleur) side and largely pagan on her paternal (Wolof) side, in her family the ancestor cults were more associated with men than women. In Fall's family the paternal transmission of the *rab* produced, in turn, male heritors of the spirits. Fall's prolonged illness and difficulty in assuming the roles of guardian of the *rab* and healer hinged on the struggle to assert her destiny over and against the paternal lineage and presumed male inheritance of healing powers. As an example of the interactions between gender, Islam and the *rab*, then, Fall's story is unusual. The paternal lineage of Fall's *rab* contrast with the more common maternal *rab* lineage. Nonetheless, Khady Fall's life demonstrates how women could forge empowering alliances with the *rab*.

Fall encountered at least one male *ndöepkat* who insisted that women should not have *xam-xam* (knowledge from the spirit world). Moreover, she struggled with her maternal cousin to regain ownership of Ardo, a powerful healing fetish that was her rightful inheritance from her father (Zempleni 1977, pp. 114–115). These struggles call into question the extent to which the ancestor cults were considered "women's affairs." Certainly some of the men Fall encountered – a misogynist male *ndöepkat* and her male cousin – participated as spirit world officiates and guarded their status jealously against her encroachments.

Among Fall's many shrines, three were dedicated to inherited *tuur*; all of whom were male. The other *rab* whom Fall acquired were also male; these included eight spirits, one of whom was a European who had appeared to Fall as a ship's captain. Fall's relationship with this European *rab*, named Alamdu, was in Zempleni's view so overtly sexual as to present a challenge to Fall's brothers, in effect forcing them to view her as a mature, sexual woman. This European *rab* is free of entanglements between Islam and paganism, between maternal and paternal lineages; indeed, Zempleni goes as far as to suggest that Alamdu represents Fall's autonomy (Zempleni 1977, p. 118).

Khady Fall lived entirely outside of the psychologized sphere of the Fann Hospital and its personnel. In this her life differed from the case studies more normally presented in *Psychopathologie Africaine*. Those who sought treatment at the hospital in some sense invited (or at least acquiesced to) the psychological interpretation of their spiritual struggles and crises. Many patients implicitly transferred interpretive authority to their doctors. They sought the doctors' aid in sorting out the pathogenic effects of witchcraft, *rab*, and magic, and chose to adopt some (perhaps limited) version of the biomedical outlook on mental illness. Khady Fall participated in none of that. She lived fully within the world of *rab* and the *ndöep*, and for a long time refused to reveal her world to Zempleni. That Zempleni finally did gain Khady Fall's confidence – at least to the degree necessary for her to explain her ancestral shrines, their origins, and types of power – is a testimony to his perseverance. Zempleni also demonstrated formidable ability to overlook Fall's intentional insults, such as broken appointments. At length, Zempleni gained Fall's confidence. Through leisurely conversations, Zempleni collected as much information as he could about her *rab*, how they were identified, what characteristics they had, and how she had become a *ndöepkat*. He explained to Fall that his goal was to understand healing better, so as to improve European methods for treating illness (Zempleni 1977, p. 91). Fall's concern, above all, that Zempleni respect the power of the *rab*, is challenged by Zempleni's translation of the idiom of the *rab* into the language of psychoanalysis. Zempleni characterized the *rab*'s idiom as the traditional language of persecution, which allowed Fall to "say whatever she wished . . . aside from what would have forced her to recognize her own desires in the will of the *rab*, and would have obliged her to assume her individual fate" (Zempleni 1977, p. 89).

Zempleni's presentation of Fall's story within the context of the projection and inversion of aggression is at odds with the strict respect for the *rab*, but nonetheless provides us with a clear understanding of what, from Zempleni's perspective, is at stake in participating in the "idiom of the *rab*" versus participating in the psychologizing language of the hospital. For all the attention to detail about Fall's *rab*, Zempleni believes that individualizing experience, accepting responsibility and agency, and making oneself to the extent possible, master of one's own fate, is in some sense a more "true" explanation for the crises, power struggles, and eventual ascendance of Fall's life. This preference for individual psychology over the meddling roles of the ancestors is revealed not just in Zempleni's deployment of the psychologizing language of his scholarly and hospital milieu, but also in his final estimation of Khady Fall's life story. He portrays her repeated crises of possession as dimensions of her personal life progress and focuses on the status she gained as a respected priestess and practitioner of possession rites. It is possible, however, to alter the emphasis in the story as recounted by Zempleni to reassert the power of the *rab*, of fate, and of family. In that story, Khady Fall's life is truly not about her individual striving, or her intimate desires, or her veiled search for autonomy, but is actually about fate, family, ancestral ties, and healing. That, it appears, is the story Khady Fall told to Zempleni. To emphasize the role of the ancestors, after all, is not necessarily to occult the desires of the individual, but rather it recognizes the texture of Fall's lived life, and the meaning of the struggles through which she eventually emerged as a healer. To cut the agency of the ancestors out of Fall's story removes depth, history, and meaning from her life. It seems that even if worship is not offered, living and achieving within a framework that meaningfully incorporates one's ancestors remains an ideal. Life as an isolated, self-seeking, self-promoting individual incarnates an emptied-out existence. Perhaps this is characteristic of some globalized individuals. Yet by no means is it universal, mandatory, or necessarily desirable. Why not, then, leave Fall's story of struggle, growth, and mature empowerment within the idiom of the *rab*? Why not accept her power struggle as one that reconciled her own life with the divergent forces of her ancestry?

***

Further Perspectives on Ancestors

At the Fann Hospital, the temptation to look for enlightenment and inspiration from traditional understanding of spiritual crises stumbled against the historical reality of the demise of ancestor cults. The remnants of ancestor cults sometimes appeared relatively robust in individual case histories, but the overall decline of these practices was inescapably evident, even when ancestral spirits and ancestor worship were evoked by individuals. Recuperating various traditions related to ancestor worship embroiled the personnel at Fann in an odd dynamic that involved appealing to traditions that were falling into disuse. In retrospect, it is provocative to see these European researchers assiduously documenting animist traditions, while at least some Senegalese appeared to be walking away from them. During colonialism and even after independence, Islam has offered a refuge from the hegemony of French (and, more generally Western) civilization (Diouf and Leichtman 2009). In this sense, the Fann fascination with healing rites rooted in non-Islamic beliefs is a faint echo of the 1950s colonial policy of supporting animist religious movements over and against Islam (Mann 2003, pp. 278–279).

Danielle Storper-Perez, a sociologist at Fann Hospital who published *La folie colonisé* in 1974, stands out because of her concern to uncover historical dynamics at work at Fann and personal strategies of the patients it served. Incorporating the work of other Fann personnel, Storper-Perez's perspective is distinctive because she attributes Senegalese (primarily Wolof in her book) actions to self-interested calculation. Most Fann scholarship did not identify individual motivation within the cultural structures or lexicons they were so careful to catalogue, but Storper-Perez analyzes Wolof strategies in relation to seeking treatment (or, sending family members for treatment) at Fann and how such strategies responded to the historically evolving social realities in Senegal. Benchmarks in Fann case studies tended to hold out individuation as a primary accomplishment of the therapeutic encounter. Distinct from most Fann case studies, Storper-Perez's sustained discussion of treatment strategies chosen by Wolofs, along with the individual needs and desires satisfied in pursuing particular treatment paths, reveals astute maneuvering within a field of possibilities.

Storper-Perez perceived a historical shift, from social bonding to myth to individual maneuvering within ideology, in Wolof milieux. This shift, she argued, arose from the combined forces of Islam and French colonialism that disrupted pre-existing Wolof social forms (Storper-Perez 1974, pp. 135–136). From a society based in solidarity and established status, the Wolof were developing a more individualized, competitive social order. To this standard sociological analysis, Storper-Perez added depth and texture by the competition she identified between the adaptive strategies of Wolof men and women. Echoing and adding detail to Zempleni's remarks on gender and the *ndöepkat*, Storper-Perez (1974) depicted that Wolof men during colonialism shore up their identities and prestige by turning to Islam. Tightening their relations with Islam insulated them from the French colonial hierarchy and also freed them from their maternal lineage and their wife's (or, wives') lineage(s). Islamic denial of matrilineal ancestors, however, produced an incentive for Wolof women to resist Islam. Instead, Wolof women tended to celebrate ancestor cults. Whether we call these animist or pagan, the worshipping of ancestors rooted women in pre-Islamic practices that provided distinctive healing rituals for those suffering spiritual crises. If Islam barred the worship of ancestors and the practice of these healing rituals, it proposed instead the healing powers of *marabouts* and their magical invocations of the Qu'ran and of *djinns*.

Seeking treatment at Fann, according to Storper-Perez, arose from the intra-family conflict over the origins of spiritual crises. Men typically expressed their understanding of the crises in the terms of *djinns* and magic. Women more frequently expressed their understanding of the crises as various types of possession by ancestors. This conflict was resolved, in effect, by not resolving it. Instead they put their family in the hands of the hospital personnel.

This family conflict over how to understand spiritual crises was intensified by the historical dislocation of economic power from the older to the younger generation. Status-based Wolof society lodged familial authority firmly in the patriarchal head of the family. However, the market-oriented, competitive economy promoted through French colonialism produced a young generation with an earning capacity that far outstripped their elders. The African healers – whether Islamic marabouts or animist – were expensive whereas treatment at Fann was free. Pursuing an Islamic or animist healing, then, would involve not only reconciling the differences between the men and women in the family, but also enlisting the cooperation of younger family members to pay for the treatment. Choosing Fann cut short these confrontations and removed a substantial burden from the family. Confiding their family member to Fann, Storper-Perez argues, was akin to confiding a child for adoption: henceforth that person more or less belonged to the medical team at Fann. Too much family involvement in their treatment would signal disrespect.

If Storper-Perez's analysis fails to account for the often discussed parallel treatment – Fann biomedical coterminous with Islamic or animist healing – nonetheless her gendered analysis of adaptive strategies in relation to Islam and French colonialism is provocative. Storper-Perez's analysis builds upon Zempleni's observations a decade earlier, but she emphasizes how women suffered as men tightened their relation to Islam, because they lost their personal rights and the support of their brothers, both of which had been inscribed in the pre-Islamic religions. The gendered conversion to Islam produced a corresponding gendering of allegiance to ancestor worship and pre-Islamic rituals. Women tended to cultivate their ancestral beliefs as a means of preserving their rights. This created a female-dominated practice ranged in competition with the Islamic *marabouts* (Collomb 1979, p. 353; see also Collomb 1974, 1975; Picard 1985, p. 30). If the ascendancy of Islam impeded *samp* and *ndöep* rituals, what Collomb called "traditional healing" certainly transformed in response (Collomb 1974, 1975). Nonetheless, traditional healers offered by far the majority of mental health care in Senegal in the 1970s.

In refusing recognition of ancestral spirits (that could possess individuals and cause madness) and classifying them as demons, Islam operated in a manner similar to Christianity, if with much broader impact. Women aligning with the pre-Abrahamic religion presents us with the situation of women aligning with demons, that is, with "evil" demons rather than the beneficent, patriarchal, deity. In casting their allegiance with the pre-existing ancestor worship, women also align themselves with the "archaic," that which is situated previously in historical time, and is assumed to be less evolved, less modern (and, not often expressed in the twenty-first century but nonetheless still widely assumed, less respectable). Perhaps the patriarchal dimensions to monotheism motivated the assumptions of

Catherine Clément and Julia Kristeva as they embarked in their exploration of women and the sacred. At any rate, the gendering of ancestor worship and ancestral healing via rites is central to the controversy between Julia Kristeva and Catherine Clément on the one side and Molara Ogundipe on the other. The epistolary volume, an exchange of reflections by Kristeva and Clément, that is *The Feminine and the Sacred*, opens with Clément describing a Catholic mass held outdoors in a suburb of Dakar. As the mass progresses in the hot sun, increasing numbers of Serer women fall to the ground in fits of screaming and thrashing about. First aid medics, standing at thc ready, bind the flailing women to stretchers and cart them away, attempting to staunch the crisis. Clément perceives these women as porous, susceptible to invasion by the pre-Christian sacred, and performing a trance akin to *candomblé*. The upper-class African man sitting next to her at the mass, however, insisted to her that the women were having hysterical fits (Kristeva and Clément 1998, p. 6). Clément characterizes his view as "*toubab*," the Wolof expression for "white" or "European," and disparages his white-African outlook even while she acknowledges being disconcerted by it. Clément imagines, she frankly admits, "a particular porousnes in black women, . . . a fulminating access to the sacred" (Kristeva and Clément 1998, p. 7).

While Clément wants to compare these possessed Serer women to Brasilians in the throes of *candomblé*, she is stymied by the medical response to the Serer women. Rather than anticipated and welcomed possessions of *candomblé*, in Popenguine (a small town outside of Dakar), the women are strapped down and subdued. Clément sees here a strange reversal of the role of slavery, where the previously enslaved Brasilians now celebrate their possession rites freely, whereas the Serer in Senegal are bound tightly under the auspices of the Catholic clergy in alliance with biomedicine. The Serer sacred disorder ("from the past" as Clément says) is treated as a medical emergency.

This intersection of the Christian and Serer sacred, mediated by medical authority, does not contradict the historical trends of transcultural psychiatry. Aubin, for example, was called to treat Carmelite noviates in a convent in the south Indian town of Karikal who were suffering hysterical crises (Aubin 1948, p. 202). While a certain degree of syncretism is accepted by the Catholic Church, to ask or expect the Church to openly embrace Serer possession rites during mass would be naïf. The enduring rifts between spirit worlds, monotheistic rituals that cast the African spirit world as demonic, and biomedical views, are perhaps surprising. Boilat's mid-nineteenth sketch of these epistemic rifts is notably still in effect even if the advocates of various interpretations have changed location, with Clément identifying a spirit trance and her unnamed African colleague seeing biomedical hysteria.

Clément's experience in Popenguine reminds her of a Breton peasant woman she once witnessed have a full-blown hysterical fit at the St. Anne psychiatric hospital in Paris. This was in 1964, and the attending physician had remarked that such fits – common in Victorian psychiatry – were virtually unheard of anymore, except in illiterates new to the bustling city of Paris. In Clément's view, the

Breton woman, like the Serers, exhibited the archaic art of the acrobatic trance. She lamented that

> [i]n psychiatry, no one knows how to deal with a "secular" trance; and, since the sacred is not among the classifications, it is declared an opisthotonos. That's a technical term, and a bluff.[3] A lot of good it did her, that Breton woman . . . Elsewhere she might have used her gift for the trance to religious ends; perhaps she might have attained the status of a visionary. But she was a patient in the emergency ward of a psychiatric hospital in Paris. There you have it.
>
> (Kristeva and Clément 1998, p. 9)

Reading the trance as a revolt, Clément feels that the Serer at the Catholic mass are right to rebel. Openness to this form of the sacred, in Clément's view, is peculiar to lower class and illiterate women.

> I think that the capacity to accede violently to the sacred truly depends on one's minority status or on economic exploitation. "*Id*" must find an out somewhere, and, in the absence of education, that place of expulsion is the sacred. Or crime. Or both.
>
> (Kristeva and Clément 1998, p. 10)

The "both" here – the sacred and crime as the *id*'s outlet – is demonstrated by Clément by the case of the Papin sisters, maids in Paris in the 1930s, who murdered their employer and her daughter one stormy night and then cut up their bodies in a state of rapturous trance (Kristeva and Clément 1998, p. 10; this historical event informed Jean Genet's play, *The Maids* (1947)). Clément presents the displacement of desire in such transformative moments – desire let loose that seems to emanate not from the self but from someplace or someone else – as evidence of oppression and repression. Regarding incomplete repressive mechanisms, that is, what Clément called the porousness of African women, Kristeva suggests instead using the word "perfume." Oozing sensations that escape the boundaries of language, identified by Husserl as the porous boundary of being, and taken up by Merleau-Ponty as a type of limitation on the utterable, underlay Kristeva's proposal. A subject with imperfect repression, woman is herself subject to generalized vapors; Kristeva evokes the poet Charles Baudelaire's *Fleur du mal*, reflections on strong perfumes "for which all matter is porous. It is as if they penetrate glass" (Kristeva and Clément 1998, p. 16).

If questions of how to interpret "trance" or "fits" are widespread, the equations drawn here – between rebellion, trance, *id*, and class oppression – are not easily recognizable in other accounts of spirit possession. The two of them reject any sense of a world of the spirit – whether of the individual or the collective – distinct from the primal *id*. However, *id* is already an abstraction, an idea, and a belief. PVT points to physiological neuroception and a predisposition for dorsal vagal dissociative reactions as the fundamental origin of such a somatic reaction.

Kristeva's response to Clément compared the Serer women of Dakar to women of color in New York city, and, further on in their exchange, to speculate on their fixation on a "sacred" that is increasingly "black":

> [b]lack women, black religions: our journey continues to link the three enigmas – the *feminine*, the *sacred*, and the various fates of *Africanness* – in a metaphor that becomes more substantial as we write, and which further complicates, if need be, what Freud in his time called the 'dark' – that is, the black continent.
>
> (Kristeva and Clément 1998, p. 21)

Kristeva's astonishing invocation of the Victorian trope of the dark continent in twentieth-century feminist theory is just the strongest signal in this text that Kristeva, in particular, is insufficiently attuned to post-coloniality.

Molara Ogundipe deplores the "shades of *The Heart of Darkness*" in Kristeva's letter, and sets about correcting the imprecision and mistakes of Clément's and Kristeva's discussion. Ogundipe dismisses the speculations about *id*, oppression, illiteracy, porousness, and perfume, and points instead to a simple superimposition on Serer religion. She writes of the possession as Rokh consciousness within Catholic ritual (Ogundipe 2007). A Catholic practice, Ogundipe explains, such as reciting the Lord's Prayer, can be performed in the tones and rhythms of Rokh worship so that possession can result. This altered consciousness, according to Ogundipe, is not related to class, caste or oppression; despite Clément's argument that the trance allows *id* to manifest in people otherwise beaten down. Ogundipe further argues for careful distinction among activities Clément jumbles together, including candomblé, macumba, Serer worship at masses, and the healing ritual of *ndöep*. Indeed, the only clear point on which Ogundipe agrees with Clément is that *ndöep* is dominated by women, such that male healers can only partake dressed as women. The patriarchal preferences of Abrahamic religions, remarks Ogundipe, have thrust ancestor cults and possession rituals into the power of women. Striving to retain the power of maternal lineages, women cultivate the practices abandoned by their men.

Clément and Kristeva see *id* where Ogundipe sees Rokh consciousness. In the mid-nineteenth century Père Boilat could not distinguish if he had witnessed a spirit possession, obsession, or epilepsy. From the PVT perspective, we could say that each of these narratives regard physiological state change and autonomic dorsal vagal fear reactions. The narratives are contingent. However, narrative is not optional. Insofar as we are conscious of events, our consciousness creates narratives. PVT recommends co-regulation in order to regain physiological equilibrium from which the social engagement system engages optimally. PVT also connects us to our ancestors, including our most distant, evolutionary ancestors. Those ancient, long-extinct ancestors from whom we inherit our unmyelinated dorsal vagal system, live within each human being. PVT offers us the ability to narrate a relationship with ancestors that is scientific, includes all of humanity, and also accounts for the long human history of spirit possession and/or dissociative crises. There is, as well, room for more than one narrative regarding ancestors, spirits, and physiological equilibrium.

In a sense this chapter ends where it begins, with an array of possibilities for understanding possession and the role of the ancestors in health and illness. The ancestral possession rites reveal powerful techniques as well as powerful healers, including women healers. This chapter ends with multiple perspectives and interpretive possibilities. What are we to make of possession? What are the roles of the ancestors? Most especially, what are the stakes for women in possessions and ritualized healing?

Notes

1 The focus here is not on religious history. Not wanting to vest significance in the terminology, I use in this chapter a variety of terms. Ancestor worship seems the most direct expression. Animism is frequently used in the documents, and so it is used in this chapter, while fetishism appears in the documents only rarely.

2 Compare to Adam Ashforth's discussion, focused on Soweto, South Africa, of the ambivalent relation between Christian sects and ancestor worship, and his explanation of how Christians view the ancestors as demons. Broadly speaking, a newly ascendant or conquering religion habitually demotes the previous deities to demonic status. However, Jean-Paul Colleyn (1996), argues that possession cults in Mali demonstrate no tension with Islam. Likewise, the syncreticism of Senegalese society is often emphasized, but nonetheless tensions between Islam and other forms of worship are documented in Fann studies.

3 Opisthonos, meaning arced figure, refers to a fit in which the body goes stiff, arced backward, eyes vacant.

Works Cited

Aubin, H., 1939a. Introduction à l'étude de la psychiatrie chez les noirs. *Annales Médico-Psychologiques*, 97 (1), 1–29, 181–213.

Aubin, H., 1939b. L'Assistance psychiatrique indigène aux colonies. *In*: P. Combemale, ed., *Congrès Médecins Aliénistes et neurologistes de France et des pays de langue françiase XLIIe session, Alger, 6–11 avril 1938*. Paris: Coueslant Masson, 147–176, 196–197.

Aubin, H., 1948. Danse mystique, possession, psychopathologie. *L'évolution psychiatrique*, 4 (numero exceptionnel), 191–215.

Bastide, R., 1931. *Les problèmes de la vie mystique*. Paris: Colin.

Bastide, R., 1960. Psychiatrie, ethnographie et sociologie: Les maladies mentales et Le Noir brésilien. *In*: *Désordres mentaux et santé mentale en Afrique au sud du Sahara*. London: Commission for Technical Cooperation in Africa South of the Sahara (CCTA), 223–230.

Boilat, R.P., 1853. *Esquisses sénégalaises*. Paris: P. Bertrand.

Bullard, A., 2015. Neither Melancholic nor Abject: A Lebou (West African) Inspiration for Feminine Empowerment. *Studies in Gender and Sexuality*, 16 (1), 63–81.

Cazanove, F., 1933. Les conceptions magico-religieuses de indigènes de lAfrique occidentale française. *Les Grandes Endémies Tropicales*, 5, 38–48.

Colleyn, J.-P., 1996. Entre les dieux et les hommes: Quelques considérations atypiques sur la notion de culte de possession. *Cahiers d'études Africaines*, 36, 144, 723–738.

Collomb, H., 1974. Psychiatrie moderne et thérapeutiques traditionnelles. *Ethiopiques*, 2, 40–54.

Collomb, H., 1975. Rencontre de deux systèmes de soins: À propos de therapeutiques des maladies mentales en Afrique. *Social Science and Medicine*, VII, 623–633.

Collomb, H., 1979. L'avenir de la psychiatrie en Afrique. *Psychopathologie Africaine*, IX (3), 343–370.

Collomb, H. and Ayats, H., 1962. Les migrations au Sénégal: Étude psychopathologique. *Cahiers d'Études Africaines*, II (8), 4th cahier, 570–597.

Diouf, M. and Leichtman, M.A., 2009. *New Perspectives on Islam in Senegal: Conversion, Migration, Wealth, Power and Femininity*. New York: Palgrave Macmillan.

Genet, J., 1947 [1963]. *The Maids*. B. Frechtman, trans. London: Faber.

Gravrand, H., 1966. Le 'Lup' Serer: Phénoménologie de l'emprise des Pangol et psychothérapie des 'possédés'. *Psychopathologie Africaine*, II (2), 195–225.

Kane, C.H., 1961. *L'aventure ambiguë*. Paris: René Juillard.

Kristeva, J. and Clément, C., 1998 [2001]. *The Feminine and the Sacred*. J.M. Todd, trans. New York: Columbia University Press.

Leiris, M., 1934. *L'Afrique Fantôme*. Paris: Gallimard.

Leiris, M., 1958. *La possession et ses aspects théâtraux chez les Ethiopiens de Gondar*. Paris: Plon.

Lévy-Valensi, J., 1910. Spiritisme et Folie. *L'encéphale*, V (1), 696–716.

Maddox, B., 1999. *Yeats's Ghosts: The Secret Life of W.B. Yeats*. New York: HarperCollins.

Mann, G., 2003. Fetishizing Religion: Allah Koura and French 'Islamic Policy' in Late Colonial French Soudan. *The Journal of African History*, 44 (2), 263–283.

Mars, L., 1966. La psychiatrie au service du tiers monde: Novelles Considerations. *Psychopathologie Africaine*, II (2), 227–248.

Ogundipe, M., 2007. The Sacred and the Feminine: An African Response to Kristeva and Clément. *In*: G. Pollock and V.T. Sauron, eds., *The Sacred and the Feminine: Imagination and Sexual Difference*. New York: I.B. Tauris, 88–110.

Picard, P., 1985. *Réflexions su le phénomène de la double demande*. Dakar: Faculté de Médecine, 170.

Reboul, H. and Régis, E., 1912. *L'assistance des aliénés aux colonies*. Rapport au Congrès des médecins aliénistes et neurologistes de France et des pays de langue française, XXII session, Tunis. Paris: l'Académie de Médecine, 1–7 avril.

Storper-Perez, D., 1974. *La folie colnisé*. Paris: Maspero.

Zempléni, A., 1966. La dimension thérapeutique du culte des rab (Ndöp, Tuuru et Samp: Rites des possessions chez les Wolof et les Lebu). *Psychopathologie Africaine*, II (3), 295–439.

Zempleni, A., 1968. *L'interprétation et la thérapie traditionnelle du désordre mental chez les Wolof et les Lébou du Sénégal*. Thèse pour le Doctorat de troisième cycle. Paris: Sorbonne.

Zempleni, A., 1977. From Symptom to Sacrifice: The Story of Khady Fall. *In*: V. Crapanzano and V. Garrison, eds., *Case Studies in Spirit Possession*. New York: John Wiley, 87–139.

Zempleni, A. and Rabain, J., 1965. L'enfant nit ku bon; un tableau psycho-pathologique traditionnel chez les Wolof et Lebou du Sénégal. *Psychopathologie Africaine*, I (3), 329–441.

9 *Bouffée Délirante*

Living Myth and Madness

***

The experience that Dr. Henri Collomb called *bouffée délirante* involved frenetic anxiety, fears of persecution, and other disruptive behaviors. This crisis befell Africans who migrated from their home villages to urban centers, whether within Africa or overseas. Collomb subdivided *bouffée délirante* into four distinct kinetic phases: 1) loss of homeland or ethnic milieu; 2) fear of *sorcellerie*, *rab*, *djinn*, or magic; 3) intense anxiety; and 4) delusions. Loss of a safe and familiar home was always at the origins of *bouffée délirante*. That loss, perhaps even a sense of being lost in the wide world, led to fear. In the case of West Africans the fear is expressed in metaphysical terms, and leads to an anxiety reaction characterized by internal decompensation. Finally, the more severe episodes entail delusions, whether auditory, olfactory, and/or visual. *Bouffée délirante* shares dimensions of depression (object loss), general anxiety disorder (intense, usually frenzied anxiety), and schizophrenia (psychotic delusions). The supernatural dimension to *bouffée délirante* – that is, the belief that one is bewitched, possessed, or under a magical spell – is the feature that is most obviously out of step with Western European disorders. However Western populations, particularly those from more rural and/or religious communities, also narrate with metaphysics. The intense anxiety generated by such fears could be enough to kill an individual. When the physiology of fear and anxiety are considered, we are forced to admit the incredible power of ideation and narrative to infuse dysregulation and loss of social engagement with meaning that endures, propagates, and at times escalates to alarming degrees.

Soul theft or vampiric death – the chief symptom of bewitchment – typified the onset of many mental crises treated at the Fann Hospital. Soul theft is a common feature across cultures. Robert Jay Lifton, in *The Broken Connection*, cites the famous autobiography of the Austrian jurist who suffered from psychosis, Daniel Paul Schreber, who reflected that

> the idea is wide spread in the folklore and poetry of all people that it is somehow possible to take possession of another person's soul in order to prolong

DOI: 10.4324/9781003112143-10

> one's life at another person's expense, or to secure some other advantages which outlast death.
>
> (Lifton 1979, pp. 227–228; see also, Saks and Litt 1991)

Characterized as psychotic breaks, or *bouffée délirante*, these events commonly began with a sense of having one's vital organs eaten, blood drunk, or living within a dead body.

This chapter presents *bouffée délirante* as a diagnosis that captures the peculiar crises suffered by those uprooted from deeply familiar lives and locations. From its origins, which trace to the work of Valentin Magnan in 1886, *bouffée délirante* was strongly associated with degeneration (Ey *et al.* 1963, p. 245). *Bouffée délirante*, however, is always distinguished – as a diagnosis and as a mental crisis – from schizophrenia. Generally, the acute psychosis of *bouffée délirante* allowed for rapid and complete recovery, whereas schizophrenia is longer lasting and often chronic. Collomb, as we shall see, extolled the resilience of Africans who could so easily return from psychosis. This skillful resilience seemingly arises from the cultural truths expressed in Léopold Sédar Senghor's formulation, "Je con-naît l'Autre"/"I know/give birth to the Other" and provides a model for other cultures. Westerners more easily get permanently stuck, to use Stephen Porges' language, in the extreme fear dorsal vagal physiological state (Porges 2011, 2017).

The life habits and relational self to which Senghor refers when he writes, "Je con-naît l'Autre," are expressed in the psychiatric literature as "lived space," "hallucinated space," or "myth." For example, the early theorist of this diagnosis, Dr. Henri Ey, presented *bouffée délirante* as an acute disorder characterized by the disorganization of lived space (*éspace vécu*) (Ey 1955; Ey *et al.* 1963). The concept of "lived space" (*éspace vécu*) refers to how a person's habitual environment is bound up with affective perception and projection. This communal hallucinatory space of mythic meaning allowed the Senegalese to reintegrate the afflicted back into their families and societies. This mythic space, however, could deteriorate under forces of social change. Such rupture contributes to epistemic anxiety, a chief marker of modernism (Ashforth 2005, p. 127). The impact of such loss cannot be ignored or underestimated. During Collomb's era, ancestral village culture could be inaccessible to individuals living far from their natal land.

If *bouffée délirante* captured the experience of deracinated Africans in the 1960s, tracing the history of this diagnosis entails considering the changed phenomenology of these crises. Wrapped up with the colonial – post-colonial continuities and ruptures in psychiatry, forming a complicated, misshapen package that we like to call "history," are the changing manifestations of mental crises themselves. Psychiatry not only grapples with itself as a scientific clinical practice, but also with the patients and the world(s) from which they come. *Bouffée délirante* is frequently viewed as a transient psychosis, akin to and yet markedly different from schizophrenia. Other theories of *bouffée délirante* describe it as more akin to hysteria, although it does not carry the gendered dimensions to the hysteria diagnosis (Hollender and Hirsch 1964; Micale 2008). These debates continue to develop, with recent scholarly opinion reflecting a belief that *bouffée délirante*, or its cousin in the International Classification of Diseases manual, acute transient psychotic disorder (ATPD), bridges schizophrenia and affective disorders. Some studies suggest a continuity between *bouffée délirante* and depression, pointing to a culturally induced psychotic masking of depression. This so-called "Black mask of depression" expresses a cultural preference for frenetic confusion over morose apathy and prolonged anhedonia (Hanck *et al.* 1976). Another theory is that *bouffée délirante* ceded ground, from the 1950s into the 1980s and beyond, to depressive conditions. Investigating the fault lines between acute psychosis, hysteria, depression, and schizophrenia leads us to deeper insights into the nature of the experience and into the evolving historical context of the diagnosis. The *bouffée délirante* diagnosis is enmeshed in these psychiatric debates, and in historical trends that include racism, migration, and urbanization. Thus to the global visceral unity of humanity, the discussion in this chapter adds these increasingly globalized forces of social change. The visceral species-wide need for a safe home is a personal experience for every human being. The absence of a lived space redolent with sentiment, especially intimate sentiments that are shared widely with the community, so-called collective sentiments, is at the root of the disorder.

The studies and data about *bouffée délirante* reveal the curious process by which localized forms of suffering were adopted into debates that span the globe. Whether viewed as a dysfunctional symptom of modernization, a malady of migration, or as induced or exacerbated by racism, *bouffée délirante* has figured prominently in the globalization of Senegalese spiritual crises. This diagnosis links into global experience, whereas collective sentiments and narrated beliefs – along with the enormous consequences of such narration – are inflected by and nourish cultural specificities. Even local narrative, however, shares modalities and themes prominent around the globe – for example, themes of intense fear and anxiety, the mystical, and the felt need to propitiate meddling spirits. In conclusion, we emphasize the remarkable resilience to psychosis afforded by this disorder, and consider how these attributes contribute to open global civilization.

Collomb's *Bouffée délirante* and Schizophrenia

Collomb's place in the history of psychiatry is deeply tied to his theory of *bouffée délirante*. The diagnosis is a platform on which he staked his claim to innovation and from which his further, frequently collaborative, research was launched. His valorization of the adaptive advantages of *bouffée délirante*, and his respect for cultural details and social circumstances related to these mental crises, belies the origins of his theory in earlier, less forward-thinking studies. The murky ties of Collomb's theory of *bouffée délirante* to works in the 1950s and before, strengthen our sense of transcultural psychiatry as a practice rooted in the colonial past, and yet attempting to transform the errors of colonialism. The dependence of subsequent research on Collomb's formulations reveals the extent of his insights and influence.

Dr. Collomb considered *bouffée délirante* among the most common ailments of Fann Hospital patients. Accounting for 30–40% of the psychotic cases in Africa, *bouffée délirante* accounted for only 5% of French metropole psychotic reactions (Collomb 1965, p. 167). The *bouffé délirante* diagnosis continues within French psychiatry, and yet remains excluded from Anglophone psychiatry as described in the very tongue-in-cheek spoof by J. de Leon, "The French attempt to include the bouffée délirante in the DSM-V during 2006: a recollection in the year 2050" (2009). However the diagnosis has been integrated into the ICD-10 (Castagnini and Berrios 2009). This diagnosis distinguished acute psychosis from the chronic suffering experienced in schizophrenia. Collomb's defense of the *bouffée délirante* diagnosis self-consciously positioned his psychiatry as culturally sensitive, and yet it still preserved French categories within the Senegalese milieu. His post-colonial perspective is distinguished from American psychiatry of those same years, in which psychosis in Black men represented a dangerous, atavistic disease that threatened social discord and upheaval (Metzl 2009).

Collomb proposed *bouffée délirante* as a quintessential aspect of "African psychiatry," stretching his Dakar-based case studies to underpin a theory meant to cover the entire continent. If this seems an overly ambitious generalization, it is worth considering that in years since Collomb's theorization, *bouffée délirante* has become a prominent diagnosis in developing countries around the globe, and continues to be a prominent diagnosis for African and Caribbean immigrants to France. This widespread use of *bouffée délirante* owes much to the processes of globalization, that have taken local psychiatric insights and adopted them into wide-ranging theories and that have also increased the migratory flows of people, uprooting individuals and relocating them in foreign lands, with strange laws, climates, and habits. As a malady of migration, dislocation, and loss of home and of familiar settings, *bouffée délirante* is apt for the era of globalization. Its transitory nature exhibits resilience that Western psyches frequently lack.

Bouffée délirante has remained a diagnosis peculiar to French-language psychiatry, and this has contributed to on-going confusion of it with schizophrenia in international studies. For example, Collomb pointed to drastic inconsistencies in the diagnosis of schizophrenia across the continent. Whereas the frequency of schizophrenia in Europe was relatively stable, in the African context the frequency varied between 56.7% in South Africa and 6.8% in the Sudan (Collomb 1966). Too frequently, according to Collomb, Western doctors interpreted routine references to ancestral spirits, cannibalistic witches, *djinns*, and magic, as signs of paranoid delusions. He urged his co-practitioners to distinguish the cultural systems of representation – which could be established by psycho-sociologists or anthropologists – from mental illness. In many cases paranoid outbursts (*bouffée délirlantes*) were frequently confused with true schizophrenics.

If *bouffée délirante* is a diagnosis peculiar to French-language psychiatry, it nonetheless has close cousins in a number of other psychiatric traditions. However, these were often assimilated to schizophrenia. British doctors did not distinguish between acute psychotic attacks and schizophrenia, leading to exceptionally high numbers of British-ruled Africans diagnosed as schizophrenics. In the U.S.A.

hysterical psychosis was an operative category in the 1960s, if not one that was officially recognized. However, its theorists remained open to the probability that hysterical psychosis was a form of schizophrenia (Hollender and Hirsch 1964, p. 1072; Hirsch and Hollender 1969). Swiss psychiatrists described an acute psychosis similar to *bouffée délirante* in relation to rural southern Italian immigrants who migrated to Swiss cities and experienced mental illness featuring fears of witchcraft (Labhart 1963; Risso and Boeker 1964). The Nigerian psychiatrist, T.A. Lambo, described similar crises as a version of schizophrenia (1965).

Collomb's advocacy of *bouffée délirante* as a diagnosis was rooted in his conviction that it is particularly responsive to syndromes evident in Africans and entirely distinct from schizophrenia. The *bouffée délirante* is characterized by sudden onset of a transitory crisis through which the patient either emerges subject to continued psychotic episodes, which can lead to schizophrenia, or experiences a type of explosive expression of conflicts, the resolution of which permits the emergence of a new personality (Collomb 1965, pp. 167–169). *Bouffée délirante* can thus function as a transitional mechanism in cultures that tolerate or even favor it (Collomb 1965, p. 169). Disregarded or even argued against by some diagnosticians, *bouffée délirante* regained ground in France during wartime psychiatric treatment of North Africans and West Africans because of the prominence of "the brutal, delirious explosions among Africans in migratory situations, that is, among Africans in the military during colonial times"(Collomb 1965, p. 169).

In English language psychiatry, the diagnoses of acute, transitory psychosis, and schizophrenia continue to merge into each other, and sometimes – as in Jonathan Metzl's *The Protest Psychosis* – are used virtually interchangeably (2009). Metzl, throughout his book, discusses schizophrenia as though it were psychosis, or *vice versa*, even though the scholars he cites (Bromberg and Simon 1972) carefully upheld a distinction between the two. The U.S.A.-based Diagnostic and Statistical Manual has never included *bouffée délirante*. The World Health Organization-sponsored cross-cultural study of schizophrenia as well as the follow-up study viewed a single psychotic episode followed by complete remission as "schizophrenia" (Jablensky *et al.* 1992, pp. 57–58). Using that standard, and following the insights of Collomb's work on *bouffée délirante*, it is not surprising that the WHO studies revealed better prognoses for those in the developing world, who had higher rates of single psychotic episodes. From the perspective of Collomb's theory, these episodes most likely were not schizophrenic in nature, but rather instances of *bouffée délirante*. The WHO studies, moreover, viewed the diagnostic data in isolation from the surrounding culture, completely by-passing any ability to discern the deeper process of psychotic regression, ego re-constellation, and recovery, offered in Collomb's study (Jablensky *et al.* 1992).

Moreover, schizophrenia as an illness remains mysterious – neither its cause, nor its range of symptoms is entirely understood – even as the diagnosis enjoys frequent use. Indeed, David Healy remarked that schizophrenia was the default diagnosis in the U.S.A. in the 1960s (Healy 1997, p. 47). One of the root debates – that schizophrenia is somehow intrinsically linked to the rise of urban, individualistic, industrialized civilization – has endured over the decades. That debated is the motor-force for much historiography of psychiatry. These issues have been posed variously as whether "madness" rose along with civilization, whether modernism caused madness, or, as Louis Sass would phrase it, whether schizophrenia reflected the traits of high modernism. Sass defined the high modernist schizoid traits as an aesthetic slanted toward hyper-reflexivity, multi-perspectivalism, play with conceptual categories, and logorrhea (Sass 1994). Finally, a number of diverse anti-psychiatrists from Thomas Szasz (1961), through Frantz Fanon (1952, 1961), Erving Goffman (1961) and Michel Foucault (1961, 1975) focused on the restrictive institutions and professional disciplines of modernity which identified certain traits or even phenotypes as "mad." That is, the rigid, Western, white, rationalist institutions categorized madness as beyond the pale of acceptable behavior, and relegated symptomatic individuals to institutions cordoned off from mainstream society. Fann practitioners in the 1960s worked within this maelstrom of psychiatry, modernism, and anti-psychiatry, and were far from sheltered from these debates. The anti-psychiatry influence, for example, appears in Collomb's creation of psychiatric villages, the invitation of family members and healers into the hospital, and the use of the hospital courtyard for palavers and traditional houses.

Nonetheless, Collomb's outlook on the debates about the nature of mental illness and modernization were highly nuanced, deeply engaged in psychoanalysis, and not at all predisposed toward rejecting biomedicine. Far from a thoroughgoing anti-psychiatrist, Collomb sought to bring the best methods to the treatment of human suffering that to him was all too evident. Collomb's theory of *bouffée délirante* emphasized its positive, ego-transformative capacities, and thus refuted the broad, European psychiatric and psychoanalytic brush that equated so-called "primitives" with the irrational, and fundamentally akin to the insane. The displacements Collomb presented as causative of *bouffée délirante* themselves reflected some degree of increasing integration into colonial or post-colonial networks of military, schooling, and work either in urban centers in Africa, in France, or in some other French colonial region. In this way, he inadvertently contributed to a general conviction that migration and urbanism increased the rate of mental illness. While some studies conflict on whether migration or urbanism increases rates of mental illness, Beiser and Collomb (1981) indicated no increased rate of mental illness in migrants. This was confirmed in a 1996 study which found no increased incidence in schizophrenia between first and second generation immigrants to France from North Africa (Taleb *et al.* 1996). These results are sustained, as well, in the International Pilot Study of Schizophrenia (Jablensky 1992).

Combined with irrationality, the threat of uncontrolled emotional outbursts figured large in traditional portraits of schizophrenia. Anti-psychiatrists who celebrate the Dionysian, exuberant, irrational dimensions to madness reveal the flipside of the same psychiatric coinage, valorizing the so-called "primitive" whom the psychiatrist has disdained. This link of the "primitive" to schizophrenia was challenged in the 1990s by Louis Sass, who argued passionately that in fact chief markers of schizophrenia pointed to hyper-intellect and lack of emotive qualities (a so-called "flat affect"). Sass removed the comparison of the primitive to the schizophrenic, and in doing so his theory presented a conundrum for explaining the schizophrenic individuals in traditional societies. Sass himself believed that the occurrence of schizophrenia correlated with the rise of industrialization – hypothesizing that perhaps some biological predisposition to schizophrenia is activated by the type of demands on individuals in urban, industrialized, and highly individualized societies. For Sass, the schizophrenic individual exemplified aspects of the society that elicited his or her mental disease – hyper-individualized, hyper-intellectual, disaffected, alienated, bizarre, and disconcerting.

Like psychiatrists practicing in Western countries, Collomb and his research team struggled with explaining schizophrenia, presenting many alternative perspectives on the illness and yet reaching no definitive insights. Reflective of Collomb and other Fann personnel findings, John Cooper and Norman Sartorius, writing in 1972, theorized that schizophrenia existed, although was not recognized as a distinct disorder, in pre-industrial times (Cooper and Sartorius 1977). They present several reasons for this delayed recognition, arguing that these are more plausible explanations than accepting that such a ubiquitous condition as schizophrenia arose only late in the nineteenth century (Cooper and Sartorius 1977, p. 51). Unlike *bouffée délirante*, Collomb found little to no functional dimension to schizophrenia, and it is perhaps this dimension that is its most salient characteristic.

The Work of Hallucinations and Delusions

Collomb's work in Dakar confirmed in him the belief that *bouffée délirante* was a type of mental illness central to the African experience, whereas he viewed schizophrenia as peripheral. Transitory delusional states, for him as for Georges Devereux, were essential in understanding what they called the "African personality" (Collomb 1965, p. 170). Collomb's theory of *bouffée délirante* has largely withstood the test of time, prompting elaboration and fine-tuning but no fundamental re-theorization. *Bouffée délirante* continued in the first decades of the twenty-first century to be the prominent diagnosis of African and Afro-Caribbean immigrants admitted for the first time to psychiatric treatment in France. A study in 1991 in Swaziland confirmed acute transitory psychosis as a dominant reaction to stresses of acculturation (Guinness 1991). The diagnosis is also used in Latin American contexts, and has been adopted into the International Classification of Mental Disorders as "acute, transitory psychosis" (Villaseñor Bayardo 1993; Jilek 2001). The widespread use of this diagnosis, however, does not resolve the continued confusion about the nature of *bouffée délirante*. Is it a type of anxiety crisis? Does it present as psychosis conditions that, fundamentally, are akin to depression? Or, is it, after all, a version of schizophrenia? Or, might we more fruitfully recall Stephen Porges' emphasis on the physiology of fear, and remember how physiological fear states and the shut-down of the social engagement system give rise to diverse symptoms which psychiatrists have tried to separate out into discrete disease entities (Porges 2017, pp. 74–75).

Collomb sought to reach beyond the level of description of the phenomena to understand the structure of acute psychosis and the relations of it to other structures of the African personalities and social organization (Collomb 1965, p. 170). Negative and positive dimensions to *bouffée délirante*, theorized by Dr. Follin, were appropriated by Collomb (Collomb 1965, p. 170). The negative dimensions include a disorganization of the functions which organize one's relation to the world. The consciousness disengages from inter-subjectivity and falls under the sway of structures of subjectivity that constitute the private world. This is the irruption of the individual into the world, akin in Klaus Conrad's expression, to the replacement of the Ptolemaic by the Copernican cosmology (Collomb 1965, p. 170). The negative dimensions include as well an alteration of the peripheral zone around the personality, that is, of the zone in which the person expresses him or her self as a person in a role recognized by others and hence authenticated for him or her-self (Collomb 1965, p. 170). The positive dimensions to *bouffée délirante* include the formation of new types of relationships organized through the delirious crisis.

Collomb's presentation of his theory in 1965 was prefaced by an earlier work published in collaboration with a colonial psychiatrist, Dr. L. Planques, who was senior to him in the military. Published in 1957, this study of "Psychosis among Blacks" bears traces of a colonial psychiatry that Collomb later worked hard to overcome. The reliance on John Colin Carothers is overt and uncritical (Planques and Collomb 1957). Carothers published several works on psychopathology derived from his work at the Mathari Mental Hospital in Kenya, in which he infamously compared the normal psychology of "primitive" Africans with sociopathic Western Europeans (Carothers 1953, 1954; for Carothers' political context see Mahone 2007; Elkins 2005, esp'y pp. 106–108). The "primitive" African, he argued at length, resembled in many crucial respects, a leucotomized European (Carothers 1951). Planques and Collomb echo this view directly, writing that among rural Blacks, cerebral activity is limited to sensory and motor functions in the cortical structure and to the cerebral stem (Planques and Collomb 1957, p. 199). In "Les psychoses des noirs," Planques and Collomb adopt as well a view of African thinking, rooted especially in rural milieux, in which psychological processes rely on collective representations of a magical and emotional nature. The dominance of emotional or affective over individual and logical thinking allow condensed and symbolized content to simplify psychic processes. The division of images of the self and of the exterior world is made imperfectly, so that strong emotions can confuse this distinction entirely, facilitating hallucinations and illusions (Planques and Collomb 1957, p. 198). Thus, to the infamous Carothers thesis, we must add Planques and Collomb's adherence, as well, to Lucien Lévy-Bruhl's "primitive mentality" as translated into psychiatry by Dr. Aubin. Dr. Rainaut's contribution on acute psychotic reactions, in 1958, relied heavily on Collomb's work (Rainaut 1958). And yet, predating Collomb's major publication on *bouffée délirante* in *Psychopathologie Africaine* by nearly a decade, Rainaut's presentation reflects a coarse and at times unpalatable vision.

It is tempting to relegate Collomb's authorship of "Les psychoses des noirs" to an act of youthful indiscretion. His co-author, Dr. Planques, was his senior in the hierarchy of military doctors, and could well have exercised a heavy influence on this paper, which at any rate contains little original material. With respect to colonial relations, Planques forthrightly advocated for overt collaboration between psychiatrists and colonial government. Psychiatry, in Planques estimation, could and should aid colonial governments by providing expert and reliable insights into the personalities and habits of the subject populations: "the role of the psychiatrist in the colonies should not be confined to the hospitals and should not be envisaged in the narrow perspective of curative medicine, the psychiatrist should be a councillor to and a collaborator with the Administration" (Gallais and Planques 1951, p. 6).

Comparing the early "Les psychoses des noirs" with Collomb's 1965 article on *bouffée délirante* reveals numerous aspects that changed, developed, and contradicted or corrected his early article. While we cannot speak of an absolute break from the earlier scholarship of Carothers and Aubin, we can nonetheless point to specific developments in psychiatric knowledge that changed Collomb's outlook. For example, mythic consciousness replaced the discredited idea of primitive mentality. Further, Collomb jettisoned the comparison with Carothers' work. He cited instead to Jacqueline Rabain's research on mothering, published as a book *L'enfant du lignage* in 1979. Rabain focused on nursing and weaning as a means of understanding the development of subjectivity, and time-space orientation among the Senegalese (Rabain 1979). Added to Rabain's research were studies of migration and mental crises suffered in migration, that aimed to refine the understanding of both the causes of the crises and their nature (Benyoussef *et al.* 1974; Beiser and Collomb 1981; Beiser *et al.* 1976). Collomb's 1965 article on *bouffée délirante*, hence, represents a critical departure from Carothers, and to a lesser extent from Aubin, as well as a research platform for further investigation.

The explosive, frequently violent, and frightening *bouffée délirante* forced the attention of psychiatrists who treated Black Africans. Collomb's efforts to treat psychotic patients at Fann Hospital relied upon his sympathetic appreciation for their narratives of the crises, as well as upon his biomedical knowledge of psychopharmaceuticals. The symptoms recorded in the case histories amassed by Collomb are rich and varied. The expressed beliefs by patients and relatives invariably entailed *rab* (ancestors), *djinn* (spirits), *sorcellerie* (witchcraft), or *maraboutage* (magic) as the cause of the illness. The treatment tended almost invariably toward anti-psychotics and, in 50% of the cases, electro-shock. This biomedical and pharmacological treatment was almost always combined with maraboutic sessions or rituals such as a *samp*, *khamb*, or *khalva* (Collomb 1965, pp. 202, 211, 213). Collomb admitted that the frequent use of (ECT) might surprise some, but argued that daily experience revealed its (to him as yet unexplained) efficacy. A robust 90% rate of cure emerges from Collomb's statistics (Collomb 1965, p. 211).

The 16-year-old girl, Bintou, was a third wife who lived with her family rather than with her husband and was four months into an ambivalent pregnancy. When her mother left home for a trip Bintou suffered a *bouffée délirante*. She first complained that her soul had been stolen. After she named those responsible, she lost her sight due to a veil "they" had dropped in front of her eyes. Bintou's mother, who returned immediately upon learning of her daughter's illness, alleged that Bintou's co-wives had bewitched her. Suspicion fell on the wife who had already been forced to leave by their joint husband because, he said, she had bewitched him. This wife had returned when Bintou joined the marriage, and yet Bintou's arrival caused the returning wife to lose her status. Bintou claimed status as second wife, leaving the returning wife status as third wife. This situation of contested status, soul theft, and mutual hostility formed the background for Bintou's hospitalization of 40 days. The doctors treated her with neuroleptics and electro-shock. Reportedly she was discharged in excellent condition (Collomb 1965, pp. 180–181).

Fatou was 32 years old and divorced when she was hospitalized because of a sudden onset of *bouffée délirante*. Her symptoms included intense agitation, logorrhea, covering herself with sand, and dancing semi-nude while singing the *ndöep* possession-ritual songs. She complained of soul theft, stating that that her body felt dead. She and her aunt complained that she was tormented by *djinn* who visited her disguised as various animals. This was all caused, they explained, by her ex-husband who had bewitched her because he was still in love with her. Fatou, like Collomb's other patients suffering *bouffées délirante*, responded well to neuroleptics and electro-shock (Collomb 1965, pp. 181–182).

Symptoms and beliefs vie uneasily in the case reports with the habitual resort to anti-psychotic drugs and electro-shock. Indeed, anti-psychotic drugs and electro-shock composed the standard Fann treatment for Senegalese patients. Those suffering *bouffée délirante* might complain of *rab*, of *djinns*, of magic, or of witchcraft, and a rich compendium of symptoms were carefully relayed for posterity, but most cases recounted in Collomb's searching essay are accompanied by a brief note on how the patient responded (mostly positively) to neuroleptics and electro-shock (1965). From this incongruence it is evident that the priority at Fann was to master the physical symptoms so that the mind might achieve equilibrium. The liberal use of ECT and anti-psychotics reflects as well that clinical practice at Fann Hospital marched in step, to some significant degree, with standard Western psychiatric practice. However there is no evidence that clinicians at Fann abused ECT as, for example, the historian Richard Keller describes in colonial Algeria (Keller 2007, pp. 104–108). In the 1980s neuroleptics were still used in France to treat immigrants suffering *bouffée délirante*, but ECT was no longer used (Leroy *et al.* 1982, p. 286). Indeed, by the 1980s anti-depressives were increasingly used to treat this condition, as symptoms in at least some individuals more closely resembled depression (Leroy *et al.* 1982, p. 288).

One of Collomb's singular achievements at Fann appears to be his successful cultivation of a safe and welcoming atmosphere, so that the individuals who arrived for treatment actually divulged details of their inner experiences. This contrasts to the experience of Henri Aubin in the 1930s and to metropole psychiatric practitioners well into the 1980s. Aubin described the numerous similar cases he had treated of *tirailleurs sénégalais*[1] who had arrived for treatment after episodes of rage, depression, attempted suicide, and self-mutilation (Aubin 1950, pp. 566–567, 1939a, 1939b). These individuals refused to discuss their experiences, even during months of hospital treatment. Rather than offering details of the metaphysical forces that assailed them, Aubin met with resolute denial of untoward events. Nothing had happened, his patients would say, I am not sick, I bear no wounds, I did not destroy any furniture. This denial was so prominent that Aubin seized upon it as a cornerstone of his theory of universal magical thinking (Aubin 1952; Bullard 2011). The blocked communication between Aubin and his patients is notable, and likely reflected not only impulsive denial, but also the distrust of his patients, the inhibiting impact of colonial racial hierarchies, and the chasm between cultures reflected (for example) in the outlawing of many healing and occult practices. This type of denial persisted in metropole French psychiatric services at least into the 1980s. Immigrants to France from Guadeloupe, Martinique, Senegal, and Mali refused to discuss their delusional experiences at metropolitan psychiatric services. Apparently fearful of a negative medical record that might impede their obtaining legal immigration status, these individuals remained largely silent about their interior mental states and simply attributed their troubles to physical illnesses (Leroy *et al.* 1982, p. 285; Lalive and Zivojinovic 1987, pp. 229–230). Already in 1956, Collomb had proven adept at overcoming his patients' hesitancy to speak (Bullard 2005, p. 241 and for a comparison with the technique of Frantz Fanon, pp. 234–237). The details of delusional experiences he was able to access in his study of *bouffée délirante* testifies to his success at cultivating a non-threatening therapeutic environment at Fann. The location in Senegal (as opposed to France) must have helped, but added to this was the welcoming of healers, of family members, and of traditional architecture into the hospital. Collomb himself attributed this openness, at least in part, to his clients' evolving understanding of mental illness, and of their readiness to use a medical doctor to help them in their own understanding of *sorcellerie*, *rab*, and *maraboutage* (Ortigues *et al.* 1967, pp. 144–145).

Spatial Psychosis and Timely Neurosis

Collomb theorized that *bouffée délirante* constituted the most common mental illness among migratory or uprooted Africans, including those enrolled in the military, students and workers living abroad, or those living in the urban and industrial landscape of Dakar (Champion 1958 is the seminal post-war French scholarship on migration and mental illness). In contrast to the strict order and limits on personal identity in village life, uprooted individuals faced pressures and demands that challenged their public persona (Collomb 1965, p. 215; see also Collomb and Ayats 1962). These events can be characterized as a type of existential challenge. The changed social relations and changed physical and human environments reconfigured the experience of time and of space, deeply challenging the fundamental dimensions to expressed personhood (compare to Constant 1972; Leroy *et al.* 1982; Sizaret 1987; Jilek 2001). Such reconfigured time and space can be understood in a literal manner as well as much more abstractly. As, for example, a life lived by the rhythm of the sun and moon, compared to a life lived by a railway timetable, a factory clock, or a school and office schedule. A location deeply different from home and not only ruled by different laws and authorities, but animated by very different concerns, ideas, and values. This is a profound shock to a person who had not previously known such a shock might exist or even be possible. In comparison, denizens of globalized capitalism are inundated by change; they are used to such shocks, and many seek them avidly. In such difficult situations of lost milieu, "being for the other" – that is, the persona that one presents to society – is fundamentally questioned, and *bouffée délirante* can take hold. The transition in the individual moves from loss, to fear, to full-blown anxiety reaction that in its most serious forms becomes psychosis. Carothers explained the frequent outbreaks of "frenzied anxiety" (compared by him to the Indonesian crisis of "amok") in the following:

> Behind the carefree façade and constantly restricting behavior there lies the ever-present fear of bewitchment. So long as all goes well it lies dormant, but when things go wrong this fear inevitably develops side by side with the more obvious misfortune, and the subject frequently reaches a pitch of helpless terror which cannot be mitigated by a larger understanding to the total situation. In these circumstances an explosive reaction must result and the frequent occurrence of frenzied anxiety is the result.
>
> (Carothers 1951, p. 43)

Collomb compares the crisis of acculturation experienced by Africans with identity crises that Europeans experienced as they made a transition to adulthood, or from a dependent to independent situation. Emotional maturity in traditional societies, recounted Collomb, is characterized by strong bonds that fused the individual into the communal fabric. Choice is restrained to a small number of possibilities for the person; social roles or status are fixed "once and for all" and the individual invests the whole of his or her existence in this role. Once removed from such a highly structured community, the demands of renewing or creating a person in a fluid situation, and of bridging the distance between the old, lived personage and the emerging personage are significant (Collomb 1965, pp. 216–217). In the late nineteenth and early twentieth centuries, Collomb remarked, Europeans who languished and flagged under such demands received the diagnosis of neurasthenia (Collomb 1965, p. 217).

Within the context of Dakar, the meaning, course, and outcome of *bouffée délirante* was so deeply contingent on social forces that Collomb remained uncertain whether it could be correctly characterized as an illness. *Bouffée délirante* was explained invariably in ways that did not implicate the patient. If the patient demonstrated symptoms, this was only because some outside force manifested itself through the patient. The patient – him or herself – was in no way implicated. If a person is not sick, Collomb asked, can he or she suffer an illness? *Sorcellerie*, ancestral spirits, *djinn*, or *maraboutage* explained the irregular actions of the individual. These external causes could appear independently or simultaneously. When simultaneous, the various forces might work in collusion or in conflict. Or, in other cases, a person complaining of *sorcellerie* might improve, and then begin to allege *rab* as the causal force. Further improvement would lead to comparatively mild allegations of *maraboutage*. Such successive interpretations, often facilitated or formulated by one or more healers, achieved quick acceptance. Socially accepted reality was reconfigured to resolve the crisis, to dissolve social tensions surrounding the crisis, to avoid guilt, to reduce anxiety, and to reintegrate the symptomatic individual into society. From the perspective of Collomb and other medical personnel, the succession of allegations – from *sorcellerie*, to *rab* or *djinn*, and finally to *maraboutage* – indicated a progressive lightening of the psychotic episode. Notably the most severe stage, attack by an anthropophagic witch, involved soul theft or inner death. This experience of soul theft is most akin to Western schizophrenia. Nonetheless, Collomb emphasized that such experiences do not meet the European standard of delirium, which in its very conception is a "type of existence radically separated from the social order" (Collomb 1965, pp. 204, 218). In Africa, Collomb reflected, "deliriums are not emancipated from the social; they do not become a form of individual existence, but are taken up in a representational system which bestows social reality, and thereby reintegrates the sick into society" (Collomb 1965, p. 210).

Searching for an adequate expression of the experience of *bouffée délirante*, Collomb turns to artistic and philosophical evocations of primal existence and mystical oneness. He departs from the Bantu term "*ntu*," which conveys the confluence of beings in things expressed, and then turns to André Breton's *Second Surrealist Manifesto*, which declared

> everything leads us to believe that there is a state of mind where life and death, the real and the imaginary, the past and the future, the communicable and the incommunicable, the high and the low, all cease to be perceived as contradictory.

Collomb also found inspiration in Paul Klee's search for a single expression for man, animal, plant, fire, water, air, and all the forces that surround us, and in Léopold Sédar Senghor's "rediscovered unity." "Here return very ancient times, rediscovered unity," wrote Senghor, "the reconciliation of the Lion, the Bull, and the Tree./The idea bound to the act, the ear to the heart, the sign to meaning." Aimé Césaire's poem, "À perte de corps," expressed this unified plane of existence as well, "each drop of water makes a sun/in which the name is the same for all things/will discover all" (Collomb 1965, p. 219, internal citations omitted). One word, Collomb reflects, can signify everything. The verbal fluidness of the psychosis, in Collomb's view, allowed utterance to proceed meaning, so that sounds dominated and any sound could carry any meaning.

Souleymane Bachir Diagne brings out the philosophical, Bergsonian, dimension to time – space psychology. Diagne's discussion of Senghor's deep affinity for time as duration places the philosophical insights of Bergson at its core. The perspective of polyvagal theory is also present in the lines quoted from Senghor: "The idea bound to the act, the ear to the heart, the sign to meaning." The vagal neural connection of ear to heart is extremely direct (Porges 2017, pp. 114–118). As physiological state is narrativized, the body is connected intimately to thought and belief that directs action, and there is no division nor duplicity of sign and meaning. Bergson's philosophy of time hones in on consciousness as determinative of the time – space in which we live (Deleuze 1966, pp. 29–44; Diagne 2017, pp. 22–26). Thus Diagne knits the connection between Senghor and Bergson, who wrote of, "the flow of meaning which runs through words" in which "two minds which, without intermediary, seem to vibrate directly in unison with one another" (Diagne 2019, p. 16). In like manner, Porges emphasizes that prosody in speech carries the meaning (Porges 2017, p. 109), Diagne writes that comprehension is literally a "rhythmic attitude." As Senghor expressed, we dance meaning (Diagne 2019, p. 16). Prosody and dance implicate time because such an experience of life, informed by philosophy and encouraged by poetry, is only possible via duration. That is, only because of our living bodies do we experience, and only through our bodies do we participate in life and consciousness. Life is a "force that cannot be decomposed" (Diagne 2017, p. 24). The character of this life is that of duration of inter-penetrating moments. Life endures. Every moment includes the infinite. Each drop of rain opens onto the cosmos. Live intelligence comprehends this duration. Intelligence can also apprehend time quite distinctly, as a type of expanse or field, in which analytic segmentation operates (Diagne 2017, p. 23). Time as an expansive field is, indeed, the dominant Western apprehension, and it is this that Bergson aimed to shift. Diagne emphasizes how Senghor viewed analytic reason (*ratio*) as drying up the "humid" and "vibratory" *logos* (Diagne 2017, p. 25). The *bouffée délirante* accesses this humid and vibratory duration at a point that is almost pre-verbal. Joined to the simultaneous dilution and concentration of words during *bouffée délirante* is extreme proficiency at identification and metamorphosis: "the all powerful word gives rise to the image, the symbol becomes reality, the signifier becomes the signified" (Collomb 1965, p. 221). For example, Abdoulaye, a 34-year-old Wolof, married with five children and a practicing Muslim, presented transforming, megalomaniacal personas including the traffic chief of Dakar, the president France, the president of Senegal, the president of the world, and director of the hospital (Collomb 1965, p. 220).

Myth is a conceptualization used in this context, which is admittedly difficult to put into words for the very reason that it is a state of consciousness that is nearly pre-verbal (compare to Campbell 1996, p. 132 on monosyllabic twilight language). Myth expresses space textured by meaning, a world in which the word is not yet separated from the thing to which it refers (Gusdorf 1953; Wyrsch 1958). The sensorial word, indeed, is itself close to hallucination, as Collomb found expressed by Carl Jung and Hans Driesch in their theory of an early human capacity for collective hallucination. This collective hallucination is a power of those living within a myth-saturated world (Collomb 1965, p. 221). Maurice Leenhardt evoked the myth-laden world in *Do Kamo* by writing,

> the gods do not go places that are untouched by Kanak hands, they do not go beyond the space where Kanak reside. The dead are still there, dead mixed with the living, the space of the one and the other, side by side.
>
> (Leenhardt 1947 cited by Collomb 1965, p. 221)

The powerful intertwining of the individual and the social and mythic environment is a great reassurance for the Kanak, but one that is unavailable for those transplanted from their natal lands. Mythic, collective hallucinatory space recedes, remarks Collomb, as rational thinking gains ascendance (Collomb 1965, p. 222). Collomb writes this as though the Western order is not another mythic structure within which individuals live and think (Barthes 1957). If exceptional individuals can escape myth via enlightenment, nonetheless mythic dimensions to life continually re-form, support, and ensnare.

Overlooking or denying the power of myth in Western thinking remains a perennial topic. If overlooked by Collomb, the mythic dimensions to European lives and how that was implicated in European therapeutic interactions with West Africans received pride of place in a 1972 study by an interdisciplinary team of three psychiatrists (J. Broustra, Paul Martino, and M. Simon) and one ethnologist (J. Monfouga-Nicolas) (Broustra *et al.* 1972). These authors described life in all cultures organized between the poles of rational thought and mythic knowledge and belief (also described as affective knowledge), emphasizing that both types of time can be lived simultaneously. In some cultures the mythic pole is highly organized, widely known, and recounted with formal precision. In other cultures, myth resides in informal domains, and can be highly individualized rather than encompassing of all of society. This type of myth, indeed, tends to be denied by a rationalizing veneer (Broustra *et al.* 1972, p. 76). Magical thinking in Western cultures is bound up with this rationalizing veneer, remark the authors. This is a style of thinking that attempts to obliterate myth and in the process perpetuates diverse myths of rationality.

Time and space are lived within the realities encompassed and defined by myth and consciousness.[2] The *bouffée délirante* functions as a dynamic and salutary process because Senegalese cultures grant it status as a significant event, with status-bringing consequences. In contrast, Europeans suffer more frequently from neuroses – whether obsessional, phobic, or hysteric – in which the present seeks ceaselessly to create a future which itself dissimulates a dangerous and ignored menace from the past that forces repetition via obscure mechanisms (Broustra *et al.* 1972, pp. 80–81). The rare European who suffers a *bouffée délirante* (only 5% of all recorded psychotic episodes) is marked with a completely different psychic structure, characterized by tight emotional bonds with others, lack of independence, and inability to rely upon his or her own judgment. This type of "immature" personality is incapable of real creativity, lives a life of disharmony, and fluctuates in poorly defined time and space. Akin to the old neurasthenic, this type of taciturn or morose personality can be relatively stable so long as their environment is not disrupted, but once thrust into a tumultuous situation, psychological breakdown can occur. Among Europeans, such a breakdown is experienced as ineffable and inaccessible to all cultural understanding.

In light of the African success in navigating *bouffée délirante*, Collomb extolled African resilience and highly adaptive strategies in the face of mental illness. Among Senegalese, the osmosis between time and space constitutes a barrier to neurosis and chronic psychosis, and a means of accessing and employing collective myth in the remaking of one's personality. Broustra, Martino Monfouga-Nicolas and Simon, however, feel that this interpretation does not sufficiently reveal Collomb's ethnocentricity. Europeans prioritize time over space, arriving at their diagnosis through a lens that focuses on an organism in crisis, confronting degeneration, rather than flourishing in the pursuit of life. This prioritization of time is the reason Europeans suffer from neuroses rather than *bouffée délirante*. In times of crisis or difficulty, a European chooses to respect the problematic of time, whereas Africans use space to compensate for their deprivations. Africans seek refuge from anxiety in highly subjective and hallucinatory space which, however, can be adopted into the social mythic order, "dis-alienated," and rendered meaningful. The European who experiences an acute psychotic episode finds her future completely blocked off (impossible), and is invaded by a menacing space populated by various phantasms. Illusions without end fill up this space that is uncoordinated in time, oriented neither toward the future nor the past, but ceaselessly bound to a terrifying present (Broustra *et al.* 1972, p. 82). The European who experiences psychosis is not able to exploit collective beliefs to reintegrate his ego, nor able to exploit collective beliefs to reintegrate into society. He or she bears the suffering as an individual, with the added burden of knowing they appear to wider society as defective or diseased.

Broustra, Martino, Monfouga-Nicolas, and Simon argued that the ethnocentric emphasis on time had invaded even Collomb's view of *bouffée délirante*. These researchers present a self-reflexive and phenomenological consideration of the introjection of time and space via European-style education. They argue that the resistance among Western psychiatrists to the *bouffée délirante* diagnosis is rooted in a resistance to the recognition that a pathology can exit the temporal domain and reside within a cathartic, hallucinatory space (Broustra *et al.* 1972, p. 84). Referencing Merleau-Ponty's discussion of pre-predicative thought, and more generally the phenomenological and psychoanalytic traditions, the authors insist that there is a Western suspicion or distrust of space, which originates in our educational systems (Broustra *et al.* 1972, p. 84; Merleau Ponty 1945, see also Kullman and Taylor 1958). This resistance to space and its possibilities causes Western medicine to overlook and under-diagnose *bouffée délirante*, even while, as the authors admit, the valorization of space in Africa perhaps leads to an over estimation of the diagnosis.

The Case of I.G.

The reinterpretation of the case of I.G. illustrates for this research team that, in the Senegalese context of a *bouffée délirante*, not only the content of the psychotic episode but, more importantly, the spatio-temporal dimensions to the *bouffée délirante* are impregnated with meaning. While those who originally treated I.G. at Fann had discussed his case as possibly one of a *nit ku bon* or as one marked by trouble with his father, for Broustra, Martino, Monfouga-Nicolas, and Simon, the most remarkable aspect of I.G.'s troubles and recovery was the auspicious return to health. That return was facilitated by a marabout. The whole community participated by accepting an understanding of I.G.'s troubling events as part of a mystical experience. I.G. was 30 years old when in 1967 he came to the Fann Hospital for treatment. Prior to his recent troubles, he had made a successful life for himself as a small business man who supported three wives as well as contributing to his parents' family. Poor harvests and an economic downturn, however, led to a reversal of I.G.'s fortunes, and he risked the loss of his business and public humiliation because of unpaid debts. I.G. appealed to his *marabout* for aid, but he was unable to help. At that point I.G. began to suffer from bizarre behavior, including verbally assaulting the *marabout*, and claiming publically to be God, come to serve the happiness of everyone (Broustra *et al.* 1972, p. 85).

Brought to the hospital on the recommendation of the *marabout*, I.G. was soon calmed, treated with anti-psychotics, and after three weeks was discharged. I.G. remained troubled by his behavior, however, because in his fit he had dared to insult the *marabout* by looking him in the eyes. This social tension was resolved when the *marabout* received I.G. back into the community with the declaration that God had really inhabited him (that is, I.G.) for a few moments. This declaration valorized I.G.'s behavior and breakdown, as it was now understood as the reaction of a mere human possessed by the divine. Following this explanation, I.G.'s fortunes soared. He became a privileged person. He moved his business close to the mosque, and obtained the means to pay off his debts. The follow-up visits with Fann personnel revealed nothing in his speech or behavior that marked him as mentally ill. On the contrary, I.G. gained social status because he had been visited by God. His *bouffée délirante*, then, attained meaning in and through the collective understanding of I.G.'s privileged moment; this moment of being "touched by God" – understood from the Western perspective as a psychotic break – became incontrovertible fact for the community (Broustra *et al.* 1972, pp. 86–87).

Depaysement, Depression, and Nostalgia

Depression links to *bouffée délirante* through object loss. In Collomb's early article on black psychosis, co-written with Planques, they acknowledged the common connection between reactional psychosis and depression due to *depaysement*, isolation from one's ethnic group, and disappointments or emotional traumas (Planques and Collomb 1957, p. 204). In contrast to this depression brought on by loss of home or homey conditions (such as living among a lively expatriate community), classical melancholy, conceived as a despairing fount of self-accusation, was quite rare among Africans. This link of *bouffée délirante* to depression due to a lost object receded from Collomb's 1965 theorization of the crisis, but re-emerged in a 1976 study he co-authored with Charles Hanck and M. Boussat. These authors theorize a "black mask of depression" adopted because the direct expression of classic symptoms of depression – specifically, isolating tendencies that signal a retreat from the community – would be interpreted in Senegal as acts of aggression. Recent scholarship on depression in the Maghreb sustains this theory that *bouffée délirante* can be a mask for depression (Zouari *et al.* 2010). The frenzied anxiety of *bouffée délirante* is tolerated and viewed with sympathetic interest, and hence is adopted as a mask for depression. In this study all the subjects exhibited delirium and hallucinations, and only half demonstrated sadness, a sense of guilt, or psycho-motor inhibition (Hanck *et al.* 1976, p. 38). The psychotic regression is achieved, they theorize, because of the weak anal fixations, and the ease of accessing the oral level (Hanck *et al.* 1976, p. 41). If anti-psychotics are administered to a masked depression, the psychosis will recede and reveal an individual possessed of sadness. Imipramine led to rapid recovery of these individuals, and the authors indicate that many, if not all, suffering *bouffée délirante* might respond equally as well (Hanck *et al.* 1976, pp. 41–42). Whereas anti-depressants had previously appeared to be counter-indicated for *bouffées délirantes*, these authors recommend that doctors be alert to signs of depression, and unfearful of administering anti-depressants.

Hanck, Collomb, and Boussat overtly linked their (re)discovery of the depressive dimension of *bouffée délirante* to psycho-pharmaceutical treatment. Indeed, discovering the power of imipramine to alleviate the symptoms of *bouffée délirante* is the driving force behind their study. Diagnosis and psycho-pharmacology in this instance are deeply, mutually implicated. Another possible perspective on the relation of *bouffée délirante* to depression entails a change in the subjective experiences of individuals seeking treatment. As Hanck, Collomb, and Boussat remark, the direct expression of depression demands individualistic action on the part of the sufferer; it is these individualistic demands that force the masking of depression as *bouffée délirante*. If this is true, then a culture or society in evolution toward more individualistic forms could increasingly tolerate the expression of depression. At least one study has pointed to this conclusion, noting that in France anti-depressants are increasingly used with *bouffée délirante*, and that some patients' symptoms are evolving toward classic symptoms of depression (LeRoy *et al.* 1982, p. 286). However, at least one study, by Sizaret, Degiovanni, and Faure, theorizes that the syndrome will evolve – as societies become more urban and traditional healing falls into disuse – to more closely resemble schizophrenia (1987). Meanwhile, David Healy has shown that anti-depressants might more accurately be characterized as anti-anxiety medication, which returns us to anxiety as a root dimension of both *bouffée délirante* and of (masked) depression (Healy 1997, pp. 211–213).

Whereas the African *bouffée délirante* was compared by Collomb to Europeans with the same diagnosis, the longer term history of the diagnosis – flourishing only in the mid-twentieth century and then fading, according to Leroy, Alby, and Ferreri, into depressive conditions in the 1980s – encourages a broader perspective on mental anguish and uprootedness (Leroy *et al.* 1982, p. 288). Seeking to situate *bouffée délirante* within the history of psychiatry, Collomb suggested a comparison to neurasthenia, which was characterized by an overwhelming nervous exhaustion suffered in conditions of modern urbanism. Jilek, writing in 2001, suggested comparing *bouffée délirante* to *folie hysterique* (a French diagnosis) or *amentia transitonia* (a Viennese diagnosis), which he characterizes as transient psychotic episodes that occurred in early phases of industrialization (Jilek 2001 citing Fraser 1899). Looking deeper into the history of psychiatry, into the seventeenth century, uprooted Europeans, most notably those serving in foreign military campaigns, suffered greatly from nostalgia so severe that it could be fatal (Bachet 1950; Bullard 2000, pp. 182–209; Rosen 1975; Starobinski 1963). The symptoms of nostalgia could involve depression, psychosis, and prolonged dream-like states. Interpreted literally as "homesickness" the temptation is to equate nostalgia with depression in the face of a lost attachment. However, this loss of home entails not just a loss of place, but of a place imbued with meaning and sustaining of meaningful life, comparable to the spatio-mythic qualities discussed by Collomb and others. Psychiatrist and psychoanalyst Henri Aubin recognized this connection when he described the complicated participation between the individual, the group, and the landscape, and how such participation structures the routines of daily life. Aubin was impressed by the immense diversity of objects and phenomena the ambience of which informed the native and which gave him warnings or orders. Great meaning could be communicated from "the slightest detail in the configuration of the terrain, of the soil, of springs, wild-life or plants, atmospheric changes, or movements among neighboring settlements" (Aubin 1951, p. 45). Removal from the immersion in this communicative medium occasioned a deep shock to the individual. As Aubin reflected,

> hence the difficulty experienced in living outside of his country. Hence the anxiety, the depression, *the spleen*, that we have observed so clearly among the *tirailleur sénégalais* transplanted to our land – above all when he is isolated from comrades of his own race. . . . It is not difficult to describe, even among our own compatriots, facts of the same order.
>
> (Aubin 1951, p. 45)[3]

Aubin compared the travails of the uprooted *tiralleurs* to cases of psychosis among French recruits from isolated rural regions, especially Brittany, and refers these back to the eruption of nostalgia during the first Empire. The nostalgia diagnosis reached its height sometime in the late eighteenth or early nineteenth centuries. It faded from prominence as technologies of transportation and communication became faster and Europeans developed more capacity for moving their lives from one place to another.

Living in the Present? The Case of Abdou

Collomb worked with a team of mental health practitioners, including Marie-Cécile Ortigues, Paul Martino, Danielle Storper-Perez, and M.-T. Montagnier, to describe a family in Dakar, several members of which apparently suffered schizophrenia (Collomb *et al.* 1966). Their struggles to make sense of this family centered on the younger son, Abdou, who came to the hospital for treatment. Collomb distinguished the narrative or recitative troubles of *bouffée délirante*, involving the self told to others and to oneself, from the more profound disturbance of schizophrenia, which involved a perturbation of the origin of the person, which is situated before the narrative (*récit*), and even before the prohibited (l'interdit) (Collomb 1965, p. 171).

This study approaches the case of Abdou, age 18 when he entered the hospital, from multiple angles: psychiatric, life history, family history, analysis of the delirium, psychological testing via Rorschach, and a follow-up study after one year. For all of the intense study of this troubled youth, the insight into his case remained stymied. The constellation of studies accumulated information, but this resulted more in a communal report than in increased insight (Collomb *et al.* 1966, p. 10). As with other cases of *bouffée déliriante*, Abdou was treated with neuroleptics and also with anti-anxiety medication. This medication ameliorated his situation, but did not effect a cure. In the one-year follow-up study, Abdou was still taking the neuroleptics and still caught up in his delirious projects to change the world via a magical language he had discovered.

After the death of his father, Abdou's mother returned to her family home with her children. It was then that Abdou fell into a delirious state. The medical analysis of Abdou's family remarks that three of Abdou's four maternal uncles are mentally ill, one of them so seriously that he has been paralyzed and mute for more than 20 years. Ruled by the elder maternal uncle, who lived a solitary and idle life, Abdou's family seemed to the Fann researchers to reject the present in its entirety (Collomb *et al.* 1966, p. 64). This interpretation sits uneasily with the family's embrace of Islam and rejection of Lebou animist rituals. Generally in Fann scholarship, the use of *xamp* (sacrifice on a domestic altar) and *ndöep* (a six- or seven-day ritual of rebirth, and possession-ritual dance) to conciliate *rab* appears as a redemptive treatment, especially when combined with hospital stays. Here, curiously, the family that allegedly "rejects the present" also refuses the *xamp* and *ndöep*. When Abdou's mother began to organize a *xamp* to appease the ancestral spirits which possess him, she was opposed by both her mother and her brothers because these rituals conflicted with Islam. After this interruption, Abdou's condition worsened (Collomb *et al.* 1966, p. 22).

Abdou's grandmother revealed her own conflicted feelings about *rab* and Islam, recounting at length how all Lebou have *rab*, but because of Islam, the rites are no longer practiced. "We send the sick to the hospital," she explained, "even if that means they might die of their neglected *rab*." But she concluded this revealing story by averring that she had never practiced the "women's cult" (Collomb *et al.* 1966, p. 26). Naming the *ndöep* and *xamp* rituals as the "women's cult" hints at deeper power struggles in Dakar's early post-colonial society. If Islam displaced the ancestral cults to greater or lesser degree, this displacement entailed a power shift from maternal ancestral spirits to paternal lineage. In Abdou's case, one could observe that he was cut off from his paternal lineage by his stern father who abandoned Abdou when he died abruptly. Abdou's return to his mother's compound may have resulted in an identification with his maternal lineage, but this too was blocked by the prohibition of animist rites by Islam. His maternal uncles – taciturn, unproductive, shut up in their decaying compound – enforced the prohibition on accessing the maternal lineage without offering any viable alternative route of empowerment and identity. However, Islam also stood for opposition to French authority and a rejection of a post-colonial clientele relation between the Senegalese and the French. That is not a rejection of the present, but rather an attempt to choose an alternative path to the reigning cultural and racial hierarchy.

The Muslim interdiction of animist ancestral worship allowed, however, a substitution of magic for spirit possession. *Maraboutage* could be alleged, discussed, and treated, while remaining within the boundaries of Muslim religiosity. Abdou's mother and grandmother hence began speaking openly of Abdou's sickness as the result of a bewitching by a jealous wife of Abdou's father's younger brother (Collomb *et al.* 1966, p. 27). She had a son Abdou's age who was in competition with Abdou to succeed at school exams. Allegedly, to make Abdou fail and her own son succeed, she put a curse on him. The Fann team commented on this interpretive preference, noting that it accounted for fewer of Abdou's symptoms than *rab*, and that it emphasized dualistic competition rather than familial and social integration throughout the generations. Abdou's mother resorted reluctantly to this witchcraft accusation, turning to it only after her brothers had adamantly opposed organizing a *ndöep* and *xamp* for Abdou. Meanwhile, Dijbril, Abdou's older brother, invented a system of interpreting r*ab* within Western psychological terms. He coupled this system with theories of physiognomy and parapsychology. Dijbril, who worked as a teacher at the time Abdou fell ill, eventually fell ill himself, suffering manic crises that led to his hospitalization. The multiple and conflicting explanations for Abdou's illness resulted in a family entente grounded in hospitalization. At least while Abdou was in the hospital the family was not disturbed by his screams, or fearful of his seemingly random violent attacks.

Not finding a coherent interpretation of Abdou's illness via family history and life story, the medical team at Fann undertook a psychoanalytic interpretation of Abdou's delusions. Like most schizophrenics, Abdou was not sufficiently communicative to participate in an analytic relationship, so the analysis proceeded only via the delusions presented, not via a transferential relationship. Abdou lived in isolation, burying himself as much as possible in books and the cinema. He worked in solitude to discover a secret language that revealed potent words, a type of magical, all-powerful language in which personal names produced godlike and prophetic powers. Abdou believed himself to be a prophet, destined to have a powerful son. He believed he held the keys to the future, that he would be a miracle worker. He believed that he could be anything he would like, that he could possess any knowledge he desired (Collomb *et al.* 1966, p. 42). Resorting to the Lacanian theorization of foreclosure, the Fann team interpreted Abdou's relationship with his father as pre-conflictual or elided. This foreclosed conflict with the father accounted for Abdou's eternal search for a name, as the name serves dually as the marker of the place of the father and of the son. Without acceptance of the paternal name, Abdou lived in a world of endlessly possible, endlessly cycling names, unlimited and without direction, the names proposed and replaced themselves continuously. Along with this limitless possibility of names, Abdou perceived a sense of limitless power. The foreclosing of the castrating relationship with his father left Abdou adrift in a sea of endless potentiality. No reality principle intervened to order or limit his sense of self and place in the world (Collomb *et al.* 1966, pp. 42–43).

These characteristics of Abdou's psychosis seem relatively culture-free, no particularities of his Lebou lineage are apparent. His psychosis was distinguished, however, by a maternal complex, centered on the mother's potentially schizogenic relationship with Abdou and her role in denying him "the thing"/*la chose*. Abdou's mother set off Abdou's first psychotic crisis when, as a young boy she would not allow him to play with a long stick. "She spoke to me," Abdou explained, "she took my spirit." The Fann team explains this as a deprivation of "the thing"/la chose rather than as castration. The father's relationship with the child imposes the castration complex, but in Abdou's situation that relationship was foreclosed. Rather than castration, the clinicians described deprival of "the thing"/la chose, a primal deprivation in the symbiotic mother/child relationship. Their relationship fell short of the desirable gratification combined with an ability to distinguish himself clearly from his mother. Abdou identified deeply with his mother and at the same time expressed fear and horror of her. He told the doctors, "I feel like, if I talk with my mother, my spirit will fly away, it will go into her" (Collomb *et al.* 1966, p. 44). To cleanse himself of his crises, Abdou attacked his mother, violently hitting her.

Abdou's endless search for an unlimiting name appeared displaced into an Egyptian tale he told the doctors:

> a woman wanted to know the many names of Ra. She finally discovered his real name, and this discovery made her into a goddess. I mocked this God who allowed himself to be fooled by a woman. It seems I'm destined to be like him, but I won't go with women. Women are always mocking men.
>
> (Collomb *et al.* 1966, p. 43)

In this story, the one who searches for the empowering name is a woman who finally becomes a goddess, whereas in Abdou's life it is Abdou who searches for an empowering name and wants to become god-like. Here also, Abdou mocks the God, while in life it is women who mock Abdou. The denial and consequent denigration of his maternal lineage is echoed here in the mocking of the woman who aspires to know God. And yet, in this fantasy, Abdou identifies as that woman, aspiring to divinity. His inner conflicts are thus revealed.

Racism as Symptom and Cause of Psychosis

The addition of racial antagonism to the other difficulties of uprootedness are passed over in silence by Collomb and those who follow his theory of *bouffé délirante*. Frantz Fanon's "North African Syndrome," which offered an analysis of psycho-somatic reactions of migrant workers in France and the misinterpretation of their symptoms by French doctors, is conspicuous for its absence in Collomb's discussion (Fanon 1952). While it is true that Collomb presents a more comprehensive and in-depth medical study than did Fanon, nonetheless the contributing dimension of racial unease or antagonism which Fanon addressed directly is overlooked by Collomb. Indeed, it can be argued, that focusing on ethnic differences in psychological crises promotes relative silence on the role of racism in mental health problems.

Collomb and his Fann personnel practiced with sensitivity to psycho-somatic conditions, in effect seconding Fanon's call to arms in 1952 in "The North African Syndrome." They were also sensitive to the marginal position of white doctors in post-colonial Senegal, and highly aware that although people came to them for treatment, they placed their real confidence in traditional healers. Nonetheless, their silence when confronted with symptoms that bore overt racial dimensions is remarkable. B. Ousmane, a Diolan Muslim, was 27 years old and still single when he was admitted to Fann for treatment (Collomb 1965, p. 179). An officer in the army, B. Ousmane was to direct a shooting session along with a European sergeant on February 23, 1963. On that day Ousmane ordered all the African soldiers to get down into the trenches, and then ordered the European soldiers to shoot them. Eschewing their frequently extensive discussion of symptoms, the Fann team pass over this remarkable episode in silence. As well, the extensive presentation and discussion of Abdou and his family overlook the impact of race and post-colonial relations. Abdou's sketches of powerful, world-creating prophets carried typically Caucasian characteristics (smooth hair, small lips and noses) (Collomb *et al.* 1966, figure 2, p. 23). His uncle had studied decorative arts in France and seemed destined for a satisfying career, but he returned to Senegal, refused to work, and shut himself off from the world. The difficulties of Black Africans in France, described in 1954 in Frantz Fanon's *Black Skin, White Masks*, do not generate an echo from the Fann collective. The much less well-known study by Mr. Diarra, but published, after all, in the same issue of *Psychopathologie Africaine* as the schizophrenia study, is not referenced either (Diarra 1966). No context is provided in terms of psychopathology and the educational process (i.e., Donnadieu case or others). The three uncles who live without gainful employment are not considered in relation to the job market in Dakar, nor in terms of the socio-political exigencies of obtaining and retaining gainful employment in late colonial and early post-colonial Dakar. These omissions in this exhaustive case study reveal that what the Fann team characterized as a "refusal of the present" was in fact a present – from the perspective of the Fann team itself – curiously devoid of economic, political, and racial content. Refusing the present, a concrete and particular present is, after all, not equivalent to refusing the present on principle and in general. It seems at least a possibility that Abdou's uncles are caught in a refusal of particular dimensions to their contemporary present, rather than in a global rejection of any (im)possible present. At the very least the embrace of Islam over and against animist ancestor worship indicates some engagement with their present-day concerns.

This silence on racism is not because personnel at Fann were embarrassed to discuss race – they discuss endlessly the "African" psychosis, and other African or Senegalese mental crises, their effects, and how they were healed. The blockage arises specifically in relation to racism (by which I mean the devalorization of Africanism and the valorization of whites or Europeans) as a factor in mental illness. Racism as suffered by Africans and the impacts of racism on consciousness and mental illness do not appear in *Psychopathologie Africaine*. The impact of this silence is more clear than its origins: they missed a major opportunity to write honestly about the role of racism in mental illness. This omission is characteristic of transcultural French mental health services. In *Judging Mohamed*, Susan Terrio has documented that in the 1990s and early 2000s troubled children of immigrants were routinely sent for culturally sensitive psychological treatment. These same authorities overlooked the fact that the vast majority of the children they see are non-white, and rejected any suggestion that racism within French society might be a factor in maladjustment (Terrio 2008, pp. 27–28). Indeed, in general racism's link to mental illness has been under-researched whereas culture's link to mental illness has developed a niche market in mental health services (but on racism as pathogenic see Fernando 1984; Chakraborty and McKenzie 2002). S.P. Sashidharan raised the concern that focusing on psychological differences between Blacks and whites rather than on the power disparities inherent in a predominantly racist society serves only to reinforce the idea of racial differences (1993). The niche of culture and mental health is threatened by the global dominance of American culture and the U.S.A.-based Diagnostic and Statistical Manual (Watters 2010). Nonetheless, transcultural and ethnopsychiatry are practiced in many venues, large and small. Notable centers outside of Senegal include Harvard medical center in Cambridge Massachusetts, the Georges Devereux Center in Nanterre, France, and McGill University hospital in Montreal, Canada.

Neither the primitivist nor the modernist affinities of schizophrenia or *bouffée délirante* account for the racial themes to symptoms exhibited. Neither did the WHO cross-cultural study of schizophrenia grapple with the role of racism, racial hierarchies, and post-colonialism in generating schizophrenia or the specific symptoms of those suffering this disorder. Fanon, for all his attention to racial antagonism as a factor in mental illness, did not specifically address schizophrenia. However, the more recent book by Jonathan Metzl, *The Protest Psychosis*, argued that African Americans in the 1960s and 1970s were disproportionately diagnosed with schizophrenia. The anger of African Americans, he argues, was interpreted as pathological rather than political; their protests – and sometimes their mere existence – were interpreted as threatening of the social order, defiantly oppositional, and worthy of long-term confinement and heavy medications. Metzl describes an advertisement that he considers illustrative of this racist dimension to psychiatric treatment. "Assaultive and belligerent?" the ad asked, before answering its own, racially charged question, "Cooperation often begins with Haldol" (Metzl 2009, pp. 102–103). Metzl pointed out that the

> ad gives phatasmagoric illustration to . . . [the] contention that black anger corporeally threatened white authority. Indeed, the high-profile ad works by asking doctors to identify with their own projected fears – it asks its assumed white viewers to be scared. And the ad goes a step further by suggesting that a doctor's racial anxiety could be assuaged by chemically subduing the threats represented by unruly black men.
>
> (Metzl 2009, pp. 102–103)

My own research in French psychiatric journals reveals nothing akin to the racially charged advertisements in American journals. *Psychopathologie Africaine*, for the record, did not accept advertisements. Indeed, the closest comparison is *Medicine Tropicale*, in which a primitivist theme is used, but in an entirely non-threatening – indeed, in a rather bucolic – manner. The aesthetic echo is with Henri Rousseau's primitivism, evocative of an exuberant outlook. Most advertisements used modernist aesthetics, presumably to capitalize on the sense that modern science could conquer mental illness while also conveying a reassuring message of how appropriate psycho-pharmaceuticals are to modern living.

Rejecting the civilization in which one lives and which is a powerful, hegemonic force – as in protest psychosis that repudiated white civilization – in fact, could easily lead to mental instability. Acknowledging this etiology reveals the illness-generating power of racism in that civilization and in the particular institutions of that civilization that sustained the mental health practices (including police, social workers, prosecutors, judges, wardens, and doctors working mental hospitals and prisons). Metzl writes about protest psychosis as a racist diagnosis. However, it is also true to some degree that the diagnosis revealed the pathogenic power of racism.

If we compare Abdou and his family (who seemed to the Fann team to "reject the present") to the rejection of the present via protest psychosis, we can say that in Senegal and in the U.S.A. rejecting the present was viewed as a sign of acute psychosis (if not full-blown schizophrenia), and that on both sides of the Atlantic race seemed to play some role in this rejection. However, the difference in how the "rejectors" lived out their lives was profound. In Senegal, even in cases of homicide – for example, S.C. who murdered the man he thought bewitched his daughter – the psychotic outburst is determined to be short-lived and not socially threatening (Martino *et al.* 1965, see Chapter One for case discussion). S.C. was not confined to jail. He was treated for his psychosis, and, after he found a reputable witch hunter (*bilédo*) he was allowed to return to his family. An even stronger contrast is drawn by the case of a young Serer man named Guirane, published in 2010 by Papa Lamine Faye, Mamadou Habib Thiam, Idrissa Bâ, and Sokhna Seck (Faye *et al.* 2010). This young man's family had been denounced for generations as *sorciers-anthropophages* and had built their home outside the nearby village in order to avoid the hostility of other villagers. They also protected themselves from the disdain and ostracism by focusing on life beyond the village, and adopting a resolutely modern life-style. Guirane exhibited depersonalization and derealization. In the mirror he saw a hideous face. To him the world did not seem real. He was agitated, and tried to run away while crying out in terror, "cannibals are chasing me." This young man killed his parents in a fit of paranoid psychotic delusion. Guirane had six months hospital treatment, after which he was expected to return home. Faye, Thiam, Bâ, and Seck discuss with consternation the extended family's refusal to accept him back. This type of social rejection, they reflect, reinforces mental illness. They point out how the ill individual served the extended family as a scape-goat, so that the family could join the other villagers in the rejection of such "cannibalistic" violence. Thus, the outcast family felt drawn to reject their own member in order to draw closer to the villagers. The assumption that the family should accept a young man who had murdered his mother and his father contrasts completely with the criminalization of protest psychosis in the U.S.A. The basic belief by these Senegalese doctors that the homicidal mentally ill should be reintegrated into the family as soon as possible is part of why such psychosis can be healed and overcome. Meanwhile, in the U.S.A., the psychotic are cut off from family and community, incarcerated, and lapse into deepening illness. Indeed there is pervasive criminalization of the mentally ill across the U.S.A. (Roth 2018).

The schizophrenic uncles of Abdou lived in their compound, kept to themselves, and seemingly threatened no one (that is, no one other than Abdou, who seems to suffer from their disengagement with the society around them). Psychotic outbursts described as violent, destructive of physical objects, harming people through punches thrown, biting, or other means, do not lead these doctors, psychologists, and sociologists at Fann into denunciations or recommendations for locked-door internment. The contrast with the American "protest psychosis" is strong and points to the inference that race relations as embodied in medical practice in post-colonial Senegal were much better than in the U.S.A. in the 1960s and 1970s. Or, at the very least, the personnel at Fann did not enforce – that is, did not bear the responsibility for enforcing – a racial hierarchy within society through their practice of medicine as American psychiatrists acting as adjuncts to the legal system did. On the contrary, Fann Hospital under the direction of Henri Collomb sought to build bridges between French and Senegalese cultures, and in this process they valorized the Senegalese experiences of mental crises, and their healing beliefs and practices.

The tangential relationship of the personnel at Fann to social and racial hierarchy in Dakar is certainly relevant in this discrepancy. This French-run institution, after all, was located in an independent African nation, whereas the doctors and institutions studied by Metzl were located in the heartland of a nation locked in epoch-making racial struggles. The (predominantly white) doctors treating the African American "protestors" were personally vested in the rejected civilization, and, Metzl urges us to believe, personally threatened by the protests. Perhaps what makes the situation of Abdou's family so poignant is the rejection of the present – seemingly based on some racial contestation – within an independent African nation. With the French deposed from official power (if nevertheless occupying significant institutional positions) against whom could they protest? As we are reminded by the Ousmane Sembène's novel *Xala*, not all members of the newly independent nation enjoyed the fruits of independence, not everyone celebrated the new order. And yet, to whom could they protest?

Conclusion

In this chapter we have sought to illuminate the controversies surrounding the *bouffée délirante* diagnosis. Whether or not Africans or those of African descent are more susceptible to psychosis and what exactly characterizes this psychosis endures as a research topic in the psychiatry of immigrant receiving countries (Europe and the U.S.A.) and in understanding the legacy of racism, particularly in American psychiatry. Resolving this problematic would entail an assessment of the role of racism within psychiatric practice as well as a driver for mental illness. Research on ethnic differences in psychotic and schizophrenic illnesses can perpetuate notions of racial difference in mental health. It would be helpful, in contrast, to change the focus to the role of racism in causing mental illness and in causing psychiatrists and other mental health professionals to treat certain patients with lack of compassion. The impact of racism – both individually expressed racism and structural racism – produces hardships and suffering that require acknowledgement and amelioration.

This chapter has portrayed the specifics of the suffering and the historical politics of the *bouffée délirante* diagnosis. Uprooting from home, modern, urban mixing of populations, racism: all of these are situations in which a person's being-for-others is disrupted and their time-space mythic participation is lost. Alone and without secure status in a strange environment, fear takes over, and inner safety crumbles into anxiety. The ability to use psychosis creatively as a means to refashion identity and status is a valuable strategy to secure healing from this crisis. As a remarkable method of healing that is notably superior, this is a significant contribution to global culture. The contrast with Western-style schizophrenia, which is normally a chronic, highly debilitating condition, is stark. The methods for integrating the suffering individual and creating a socially valued meaning for the symptoms deserve continued recognition. Open global civilization requires such re-configuring of symbolics and status, to promote healing for more people. There is continued acute and chronic need for such healing.

Notes

1 This term, *tirailleurs sénégalais*, refers generally to Black African military troops. It was not used only for troops originating from Senegal.
2 This analysis of time and space contrasts to J.C. Carothers, who characterized the "primitive African" as living in a world of sound. Sounds from the natural world (the wind, water, animals) and sounds of people (talking, singing) comprise their main stimuli, and

are notably heavily charged with meaning and emotion. The Western European, Carothers argues, lives largely in a world of sight; a high degree of visual awareness leads to a highly developed sense of spatial and temporal relations. This visual world is more easily objectified than is the auditory (emotion and meaning laden) world. "An understanding of the world we live in, and the development of an objective attitude and of mature responsibility depend on a well-developed sense of spatial, temporal and causal relationships and these, in turn on a habit of visual, as opposed to auditory, synthesis. . . . It is by no accident that 'foresight' has visual connotation, and by no accident that vision unlike hearing is dependent on *cortical* integrity, and it is clear that verbal and musical ability alone must fail to develop most of those faculties that make man pre-eminent, must leave him grossly dependent on the aspects of the world which are of directly personal interest and emotional appeal, and must leave the frontal lobes in relative idleness" (Carothers 1951, p. 45).

3 On the same page he compares the Rorschach test to other forms of divination, such as by casting bones, reading the surface of a liquid, or gazing into a crystal or a mirror.

Works Cited

Ashforth, A., 2005. *Witchcraft, Violence, and Democracy in South Africa*. Chicago, IL: University of Chicago Press.

Aubin, H., 1939a. Introduction à l'étude de la psychiatrie chez les noirs, parts I and II. *Annales Médico-Psychologiques*, I (1) and I (2), 1–29, 181–213.

Aubin, H., 1939b. L'Assistance psychiatrique indigène aux colonies. *In*: P. Combemale, ed., *Congrès des Aliénistes et Neurologiques de France et des pays de langue française* XLIIème session. Paris: Coueslant Masson, 147–176, 186–197.

Aubin, H., 1948. Danse mystique: Possession, psychopathologie. *L'Évolution psychiatrique*, 4 (numero exceptionnel), 191–215.

Aubin, H., 1950. Conduites de réfus et psychothérapie. *L'Évolution Psychiatrique*, IV, 565–589.

Aubin, H., 1951. Procédés et processus divinatoires. *Médecine tropicale*, 11 (1), 39–56.

Aubin, H., 1952. *L'Homme et la magie*. Paris: Desclée De Brouwer et Cie.

Bachet, M., 1950. Étude sur les états de nostalgie. *Annales Médico-Psychologiques*, 108 (1), 559–587.

Barthes, R., 1957. *Mythologies*. Paris: Éditions du Seuil.

Beiser, M. and Collomb, H., 1981. Mastering Change: Epidemiological and Case Studies in Senegal, West Africa. *American Journal of Psychiatry*, 138 (4), 455–459.

Beiser, M. *et al.*, 1976. Measuring Psychoneurotic Behavior in Cross-Cultural Surveys. *The Journal of Nervous and Mental Disease*, 163 (1), 10–23.

Benyoussef, A. *et al.*, 1974. Health Effects of Rural-Urban Migration in Developing Countries – Senegal. *Social Science and Medicine*, 8 (5), 243–254.

Bromberg, W., Simon, F. and Pasto, T.A., 1972. Symbolism in a Protest Psychosis. *Israel Annals of Psychiatry and Related Disciplines*, 10 (2), 164–179.

Broustra, J. *et al.*, 1972. Réflexions ethnopsychiatriques sur l'organisationtemps-espace de la personne. *Psychopathologie Africaine*, VIII (1), 75–89.

Bullard, A., 2000. *Exile to Paradise: Savagery and Civilization in Paris and the South Pacific, 1790–1900*. Palo Alto, CA: Stanford University Press.

Bullard, A., 2005. The Critical Impact of Frantz Fanon and Henri Collomb; Race, Gender and Personality Testing of North and West Africans. *Journal for the History of Behavioral Sciences*, 41 (3), 225–248.

Bullard, A., 2011. La Crypte and Other Pseudo-Analytic Concepts in French West African Psychiatry. *In*: W. Anderson, D. Jenson and R. Keller, eds., *Unconscious Dominions: Psychoanalysis, Colonial Trauma, and Global Sovereignties*. Chapel Hill, NC: Duke University Press, 43–74.

Campbell, J., 1996. *Travellers in Space: In Search of Female Identity in Tibetan Buddhism*. London: Athlone Press.

Carothers, J.C., 1951. Frontal Lobe Function and the African. *Journal of Mental Science*, 97, 12–48.

Carothers, J.C., 1953. *The African Mind in Health and Disease*. Geneva: World Health Organization.

Carothers, J.C., 1954. *The Psychology of Mau-Mau*. Nairobi: The Government Printer.

Castagnini, A. and Berrios, G.E., 2009. Acute and Transient Psychotic Disorders (ICD-10 F23): A Review from a European Perspective. *European Archive of Psychiatry and Clinical Neuroscience*, 259 (8), 433–443.

Chakraborty, A. and McKenzie, K., 2002. Does Discrimination Cause Mental Illness? *The British Journal of Psychiatry*, 180, 475–477.

Champion, Y., 1958. *Migration et maladies mentales: Essai de synthèse des recherches en matière d'épidémiologie et de pathologie mentales concernant la mobilité géographique des populations*. Paris: Arnette.

Collomb, H., 1965. Bouffées délirantes en psychiatrie Africaine. *Psychopathologie Africaine*, I (2), 167–239.

Collomb, H., 1966. Psychiatrie et Cultures (Considérations générales). *Psychopathologie Africaine*, II (2), 259–273.

Collomb, H. and Ayats, H., 1962. Les migrations au Sénégal: Étude psychopathologique. *Cahiers d'Études Africaines*, II (8), 4th cahier, 570–597.

Collomb, H. *et al.*, 1966. Étude d'un cas de schizophrénie (approche multidisciplinaire). *Psychopathologie Africaine*, II (1), 9–64.

Constant, J., 1972. Les bouffées délirantes en Guadeloupe: Essai d'analyse sémiologique, psychopathologique et culturelle à propos de 112 Observations. *Psychopathologie Africaine*, VIII (2), 169–199.

Cooper, J. and Sartorius, N., 1977. Cultural and Temporal Variations in Schizophrenia: A Speculation on the Importance of Industrialization. *British Journal of Psychiatry*, 130 (1), 50–55.

Deleuze, G., 1966. *Le bergsonisme*. Paris: Presses universitaires de France.

Diagne, S.B., 2019. Postcolonial Bergson . L. Turner, trans., J.E. Drabinski, foreward. New York: Fordham University Press.

Diarra, S., 1966. Problems d'adaptation des travailleurs Africains noirs en France. *Psychopathologie Africaine*, II (1), 107–126.

Elkins, C., 2005. *Imperial Reckoning: The Untold Story of Britain's Gulag in Kenya*. New York: Holt.

Ey, H., 1955. Psychoses délirantes aiguës. *Psychiatrie*, 2 (37), 239, A10.

Ey, H., Bernard, P. and Brisset, C., 1963. *Manuel de Psychiatrie*, 2nd rev. ed. Paris: Masson.

Fanon, F., 1952. Le 'syndrome nord-Africain'. *L'Ésprit*, 20 (2), 237–251.

Fanon, F., 1961. *Les damnés de la terre*. Paris: Françoise Maspero.

Faye, L.P., Thiam, M.H., Bâ, I. and Seck, S., 2010. Problématique de la réinsertion d'un patient auteur de parricide dans un contexte de sorcellerie. *L'information psychiatrique*, 86 (9), 794–797. Available from: https://doi.org/10.3917/inpsy.8609.0794 [Accessed August 2021].

Fernando, S., 1984. Racism as a Cause of Depression. *International Journal of Social Psychiatry*, 30 (1–2), 41–49.

Foucault, M., 1961. *Folie et Deraison: Histoire de la folie à l'âge classique*. Paris: Plon.
Foucault, M., 1975. *Surveiller et Punir; Naissance de la Prison*. Paris: Éditions Gallimard.
Fraser, D., 1899. Hysteria as Psychosis. *Journal of Mental Science*, 45, 173–174. Available from: https://doi.org/10.1192/bjp.45.188.173.
Gallais, P. and Planques, L., 1951. Étude sur les déficiences mentales dans les territoire d'Outre-Mer; Perspectives ethnopsychiatriques dans l'Union Française. *Médecine Tropicale*, 11 (1), 5–30.
Goffman, E., 1961. *Asylums: Essays on the Social Situation of Mental Patients and Other Inmates*. Garden City, NY: Anchor Books.
Guinness, E.A., 1991. Acute Psychosis and Rapid Social Change in Swaziland. *In*: S.O. Okpaku, ed., *Mental Health in African and the Americas Today*. Nashville, TN: Chrisolith, 53–89.
Gusdorf, G., 1953. *Mythe et métaphysique*, vol. 1. Paris: Flammarion.
Hanck, C., Collomb, H. and Boussat, M., 1976. Dépressions masquées psychotique ou masque noir de la dépression. *Acta psychiatrica belgica*, 76 (1), 26–45.
Healy, D., 1997. *The Anti-Depressant Era*. Cambridge, MA: Harvard University Press.
Hirsch, S.J. and Hollender, M.H., 1969. Hysterical Psychosis: Clarification of the Concept. *American Journal of Psychiatry*, 125 (7), 909–915.
Hollender, M.H. and Hirsch, S.J., 1964. Hysterical Psychosis. *American Journal of Psychiatry*, 120 (11), 1066–1074.
Jablensky, A. *et al*., 1992. *Schizophrenia: Manifestations, Incidence and Course in Different Cultures. A World Health Organization Ten-Country Study. Psychological Medicine Monograph Supplement 20*. Cambridge: Cambridge University Press.
Jilek, W.G., 2001. *Cultural Factos in Psychiatric Disorders*. Paper presented at the 26th Congress of the World Federation for Mental Health. Available from: www.mentalhealth.com/mag1/wolgang.html [Accessed 26 April 2010].
Keller, R., 2007. *Colonial Madness: Psychiatry in French North Africa*. Chicago: University of Chicago Press.
Kullman, M. and Taylor, C., 1958. The Pre-Objective World. *The Review of Metaphysics*, 12 (1), 108–132.
Labhart, F., 1963. *Die schizophrenieahnlichen Emotionspsychosen*. Berlin and Heidelberg: Springer Verlag.
Lalive, J. and Zivojinovic, S., 1987. Une situation de crise ethno-psychiatrique: Le cas des requérants d'asile d'Afrique noire. *Annales Médico-psychologiques; revue psychiatrique*, 145 (3), 225–236.
Lambo, T.A., 1965. Schizophrenic and Borderline States. *In:* A. DeReuck and R. Porter, eds., *Transcultural Psychiatry, (Ciba Foundation Symposium)*. London: Churchill, 62–83.
Leon, J.D., 2009. The French Attempt to Include the *bouffée délirian*te in the DSM-V During 2006: A Recollection in the Year 2050. *L'Encephale*, 35 (1), 1–3.
Leroy, C., Alby, J.-M. and Ferreri, M., 1982. Dysthymie et Bouffées Délirantes chez des transplantés d'origine noire. *Psychopathlogie Africaine*, XVII (3), 281–291.
Lifton, R.J., 1979. *The Broken Connection: On Death and the Continuity of Life*. Washington, DC: American Psychiatric Press.
Mahone, S., 2007. East African Psychiatry and the Practical Problems of Empire. *In*: S. Mahone and M. Vaughn, eds., *Psychiatry and Empire*. New York: Palgrave Macmillan, 41–66.
Martino, P., Zempleni, A. and Collomb, H., 1965. Délire et représentations culturelles (à propos du meutre d'un sorcier). *Psychopathologie Africaine*, 1 (1), 151–157.
Merleau Ponty, M., 1945. *La phénoménologie de la perception*. Paris: PUF.

Metzl, J., 2009. *The Protest Psychosis: How Schizophrenia Became a Black Disease*. Boston: Beacon Press.

Micale, M.S., 2008. *Hysterical Men: The Hidden History of Male Nervous Illness*. Cambridge, MA: Harvard University Press.

Ortigues, M.C., Martin, P. and Collomb, H., 1967. L'Utilisation des données culturelles dans un cas de bouffée délirante. *Psychopathologie Africaine*, III (1), 121–147.

Planques, L. and Collomb, H., 1957. Les psychoses des Noirs. *Revue du Corps de Santé Militaire*, XIII (2), 194–205.

Porges, S.W., 2011. *The Polyvagal Theory: Neurophysiological Foundations of Emotions, Attachment, Communication, Self-Regulation*. New York: W.W. Norton.

Porges, S.W., 2017. *The Pocket Guide to the Polyvagal Theory: The Transformative Power of Feeling Safe*. New York: W.W. Norton.

Rabain, J., 1979 [1994]. *L'enfant du lignage: Du sevrage à la classe d'âge*. Paris: Éditions Payot & Rivages.

Rainaut, J., 1958. Un Aspect des psychoses transitoires en milieu Africain: La bouffée aiguë, confusionnelle et anxieuse. *In*: *Desordres mentaux et santé mentale en Afrique au sud du Sahara*. Bukavu: CCTA/CSA, WFMH, WHO Meeting of Specialists on Mental Health, 193–214.

Risso, M. and Boeker, W., 1964. *Verhexungswahn*. Bibliotheca psychiatrica et Neurologica 124. New York and Basel: Karger Verlag.

Rosen, G., 1975. Nostalgia: A 'Forgotten' Psychological Disorder. *Psychological Medicine*, 5 (4), 340–354.

Roth, A., 2018. *Insane: America's Criminal Treatment of Mental Illness*. New York: Basic Books.

Saks, E.R. and Litt, M., 1991. 'Soul Murder' as Destruction of Psychic Integrity: Further Development of the Theme of Possessiveness in Schreber's Memoirs of My Nervous Illness. *Psychoanalysis and Contemporary Thought*, 14 (3), 453–477.

Sashidharan, S.P., 1993. Afro-Caribbeans and Schizophrenia: The Ethnic Vulnerability Hypothesis Re-Examined. *International Review of Psychiatry*, 5 (2–3), 129–144.

Sass, L., 1994. *Madness and Modernism: Insanity in the Light of Modern Art, Literature, and Thought*. Cambridge, MA: Harvard University Press.

Sembène, O., 1976 [1974]. *Xala, a Novel*. C. Wake, trans. Chicago: Chicago Review Press.

Sizaret, P., Degiovanni, A. and Faure, M., 1987. Bouffées délirantes et culture. *Annales Medico Psychologiques*, 145, 753–762.

Starobinski, J., 1963. La Nostalgie: Théories médicales, expression littéraire. *Studies on Voltaire and the Eighteenth Century*, 27 (5), 1505–1518.

Szasz, T., 1961. *The Myth of Mental Illness: Foundations of a Theory of Personal Conduct*. New York: Hoeber-Harper.

Taleb, M. *et al.*, 1996. Cross-Cultural Study of Schizophrenia. *Psychopathology*, 29 (2), 85–94.

Terrio, S., 2008. *Judging Mohamed*. Palo Alto, CA: Stanford University Press.

Villaseñor Bayardo, S.J., 1993. El concepto de la 'bouffée délirante' dentro de la clasificaciones de las enfermedades mentales. *Revista del Residente de Pisquiatria (Mexico)*, 4, 26–30.

Watters, E., 2010. *Crazy Like Us: The Globalization of the American Psyche*. New York: Free Press.

Wyrsch, J., 1958. *La persone du schizophrène: Étude Clinique, psychologique, anthropophénomologique*, J. Verdeaux, trans. Paris: Presses Universitaires de France.

Zouari, N. *et al.*, 2010. Aspects culturels dans la dépression masquée par des symptômes psychotiques. *L'Encéphale*, 36 (6), 504–550.

Index

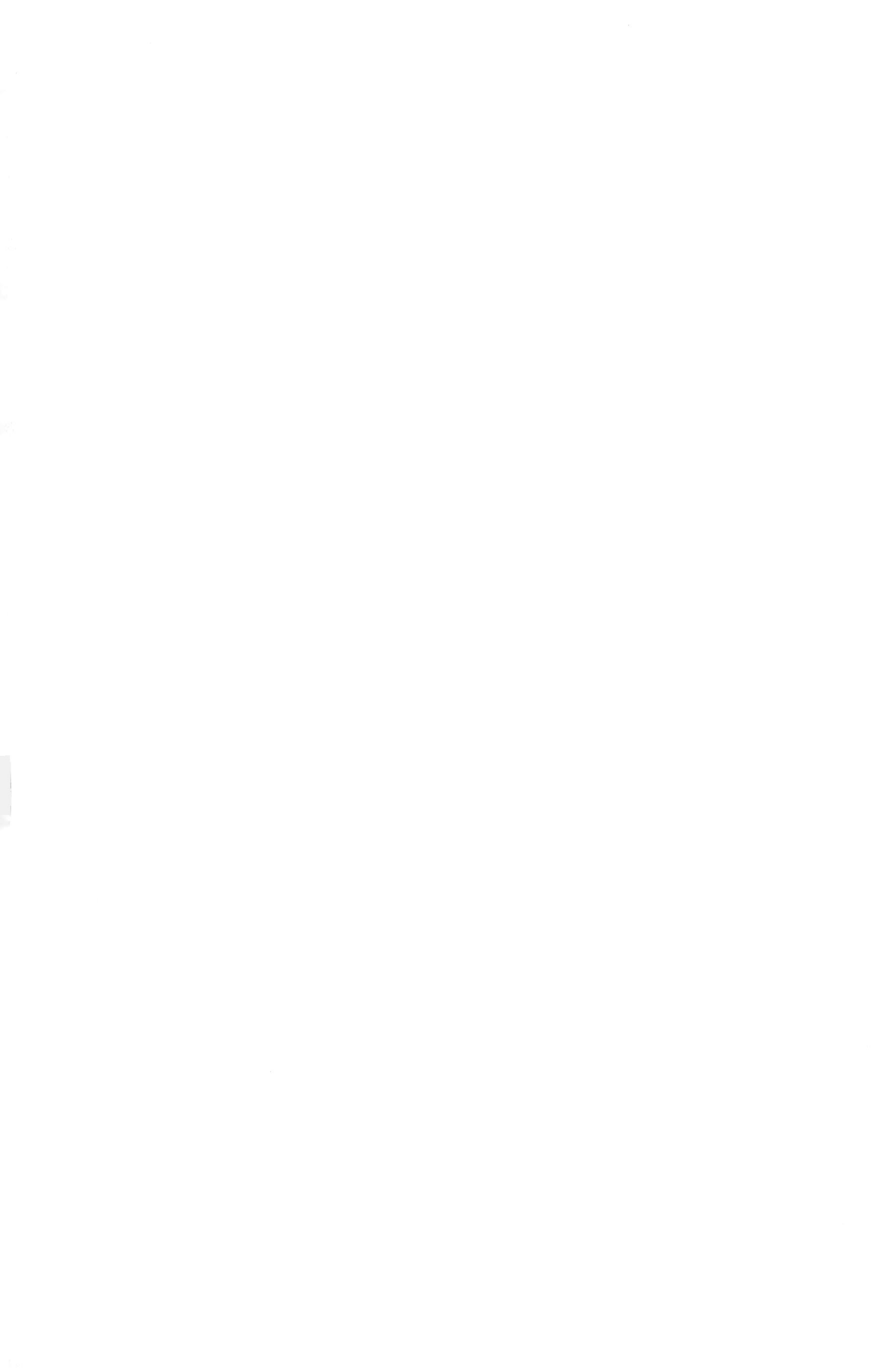